BREAST-FEEDING
a guide for the medical profession

BREAST-FEEDING
a guide for the medical profession

RUTH A. LAWRENCE, M.D.

Associate Professor of Pediatrics and Obstetrics and Gynecology,
University of Rochester,
Rochester, New York

with 110 illustrations

The C. V. Mosby Company

ST. LOUIS · TORONTO · LONDON   1980

Printed in the United States of America

The C. V. Mosby Company
11830 Westline Industrial Drive, St. Louis, Missouri 63141

Library of Congress Cataloging in Publication Data

Lawrence, Ruth A   1924-
  Breast-feeding, a guide for the medical
profession.

  Bibliography: p.
  Includes index.
  1. Breast feeding. 2. Lactation. 3. Milk,
Human. I. Title. [DNLM: 1. Breast feeding.
WS125 L422b]
RJ216.L358   612.6′64   79-17277
ISBN 0-8016-2897-0

TS/CB/CB 9 8 7 6 5 4 3   01/A/087

Affectionately dedicated to
Rob, Barbara, Timothy, Kathleen,
David, Mary Alice, Joan, John, and Stephen
for their love and patient understanding
and to **Bob**
for his boundless faith, trust, and inspiration

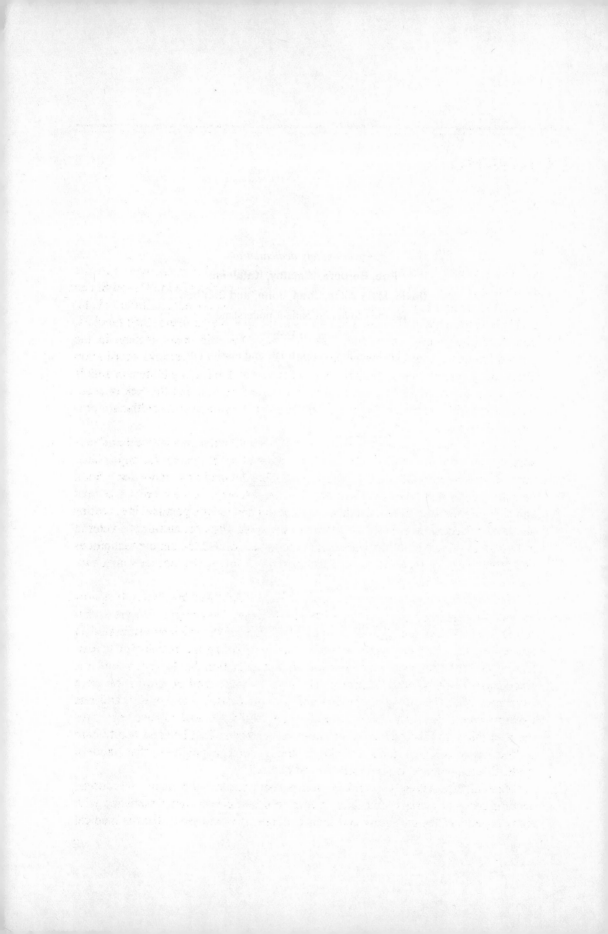

Foreword

There would have been little need for this book had it been written at the beginning of the century, when more than 50% of the mothers in the United States breast-fed infants beyond one year and a wealth of experience, cultural beliefs, and information about breast-feeding was shared by young mothers, their families, and their physicians. There has, however, been so little breast-feeding in the United States for the past four decades that the repository of cultural information about lactation has almost disappeared. Fortunately, the feeding of human milk is once again returning to its proper position of preeminence, and the lack of practical information on breast-feeding available to parents-to-be and health-care professionals is being keenly felt.

Dr. Ruth Lawrence, a physician and mother with extensive medical and personal experience in the field, designed this manual to fill the gap for physicians, nurses, and other health-care professionals. This detailed and well-written book benefits greatly not only from the author's extensive experience running a normal and sick infant nursery, but also from her special and unique personal life, rearing and breast-feeding nine healthy children of her own. Thus the author is a veteran in two areas. She beautifully documents the values of and the simple techniques and procedures for increasing, supporting, and continuing the mother's milk supply.

Health-care professionals in the United States might well ask themselves how and why we stopped the practice of breast-feeding. They might also ask themselves what factors led the educators and leaders of the medical profession to ignore (or discount) the wealth of information regarding the benefits of breast-feeding and the hazards of its discontinuation, information that has been available since early in the twentieth century. The leaders of the medical profession were extremely vocal about these benefits and hazards early in the century, and one wonders where the voices of these medical educators and leaders have been over the past thirty to forty years. Have these voices been silent because health-care professionals believed (and convinced the general population) that modern medical science could indeed improve on nature?

Medical professionals complain that parents request too many operations, demand too many drugs, and, after medicine's best efforts, are dissatisfied with many aspects of the care provided their children. It would seem that the medical profession has oversold the abilities of modern medical science and undersold the innate wisdom, resources, and responses of the healthy human mother.

Was another of the factors contributing to the trend away from breast-feeding that the "science of nutrition developed a reliance on measurement and analysis which encouraged the impression that prepared foods were superior because they could be measured and calculated to meet precise needs," as Dr. Lawrence suggests in Chapter 1? Working in a neonatal intensive care unit with young physicians, one gets the impression that they with their ever-ready calculators are frustrated because they do not know the precise caloric content or the total volume the breast-feeding mother gives her premature or sick infant. Are their attitudes fundamentally different from those of their paper- and pencil-pushing predecessors of a generation ago?

It does not seem possible that a reader can help but be overwhelmingly impressed by the information presented in this book. For example, Table 1-6 presents data on the difference in mortality and morbidity between artificially fed and breast-fed infants and the difference in survivors to age one year from the end of the nineteenth century up to 1947 with *always* a marked advantage for the breast-fed infant. Table 1-7 presents deaths and death rates in seven Punjab villages, which show that artificially fed infants had a mortality of 950/1000 in the first 11 months of life in contrast to 120/1000 of the breast-fed infants. In this decade in rural New York state the studies of Cunningham showed again the lower incidence of respiratory and gastrointestinal illnesses in breast-fed infants compared to those fed cow's milk.

We hope this book will encourage physicians and other health-care personnel to help families realize their own strengths and resources and to adapt their child rearing to the wishes and needs of the infant or child. It will still be some time before we health-care professionals can fully readjust our expectations for growth, weight gain, development, and sleeping and feeding behavior to the standard of the breast-fed infant rather than make comparisons to the bottle-fed infant. We are learning that when an anxious breast-feeding mother asks why her infant does not burp often or loudly enough (or eats too frequently or has bowel movements that are too loose), we should not respond with concern or criticism of the burping technique but should say "great!" and point out that it is wise to use the behavior of the breast-fed infant as our standard.

Several studies have suggested that the motor or mental development of breast-fed infants may be different from bottle-fed infants. There is a great opportunity for careful studies to evaluate this further at the present time. In our own research, filmed observations of mothers bottle-feeding their infants have been shocking at times and have reminded us that there can be an enormous difference between the warmth, skin-to-skin contact, and multiple sensory interactions associated with breast-feeding and the situation with some bottle-feedings, when the infant may be fed away from any human contact, fed when not hungry, and with an imposed rhythm and schedule that may conflict with the infant's own wishes and rhythms.

Ruth Lawrence points out that "one of the symbols of the emancipation of women that began in the 1920s was bottle-feeding." Our present woman's move-ment is accompanied by an increased interest in breast-feeding. However, are there other features or side effects of the changing life-styles of today that will have a comparable impact on the health and well-being of a generation from now?

We will take this opportunity to comment about the association between breast-feeding and parent-infant attachment. We believe that early mother-infant contact starts a process of mother-infant interaction that gradually builds a strong affectionate tie, first of the mother to her infant and then later on of the infant to the mother. This is most likely to proceed successfully with breast-feeding, in which close contact and interaction occur repeatedly at the times the infant wishes and at a pace that fits the needs and wishes of the mother and the infant, with gratifications for both. Thus breast-feeding provides an optimal model for the development of a strong mother-infant attachment following contact immediately after birth, which in turn has been shown to be a simple maneuver to significantly increase the success of breast-feeding.

Any nurse, physician, or health-care professional who reads this book will be more convinced than ever of the importance of breast-feeding, will have solid data to support this conviction, and will be given a wealth of information about how to help mothers succeed with breast-feeding. Ruth Lawrence points out that there are many reasons why mothers may not be willing to breast-feed, and it will be necessary for us to realize that we cannot produce a change overnight in attitudes that have developed over the last fifty years.

John H. Kennell
Marshall H. Klaus

Preface

This book was written in an effort to provide the medical profession with an easily accessible reference for the clinical management of the mother-infant nursing couple. After many decades of championing formula for the newborn and infant, the medical profession has recognized that human milk is preferable for the human infant. The world literature reflects scientists' work on breast-feeding in the fields of nutrition, biochemistry, immunology, psychology, and sociology. These researchers have demonstrated what most mothers have long believed; human milk is specifically designed for human infants.

Although reports in dozens of journals have contributed information valuable in the clinical management of lactation, it has remained difficult for the practitioner to gain access to it when an emergency arises. There are other topics, such as the pharmacokinetics of human milk, on which more knowledge and data are needed. This book is intended to provide the information that is available as well as identify areas of deficient information. The first part of this book is basic data on the anatomical, physiological, biochemical, nutritional, immunological, and psychological aspects of human lactation. The remainder centers on the problems of clinical management and, I hope, maximizes scientific data and minimizes anecdotal information. The goal is to provide practical information for managing individual mothers and their infants. It is also hoped that a balance has been struck between basic science, on which rational management should rest, and advice garnered by experience. Through use of the bibliographies interested readers may seek out the original works for details and supporting data.

I recognized some years ago that specific data were accumulating rapidly but remained in scattered, sometimes inaccessible, references. The increasing requests for consultation about breast-feeding sparked the idea for a more formal publication to replace the information sheets and brochures that I had been putting together. My interest in breast-feeding started during internship and residency at Yale–New Haven Hospital where Dr. Edith Jackson, Dr. Grover Powers, and Dr. Milton Senn expressed genuine concern for the declining rate of breast-feeding. Dr. Jackson provided excellent training in the art of breast-feeding for families and professionals in the rooming-in project in New Haven.

This book does not speak to world issues or the political issues of nutrition, since they have been eloquently discussed by Derrick and E. P. Patrice Jelliffe in their many works.

xi

Throughout this book, since a nursing mother is a female, the personal pronoun *she* has been used. In referring to the infant, the choice between *he* or *she* has been made, using the male pronoun only to enhance clarity between reference to mother or child. The physician has been referred to as *he*, although I am thoroughly cognizant of the inordinate injustice perpetrated by this historical usage.

I should like to acknowledge the help and support of the many colleagues who encouraged me to investigate this subject and the hosts of nursing mothers who helped me learn what I am sharing here.

Extensive library research was done by Nancy Hess and Cathy Goodfellow, who worked as professional volunteers. Editing and tracking specific data were done by Timothy Lawrence, whom I also wish to thank. No writing is accomplished without diligent preparation of the manuscript. Loretta H. Anderson prepared many of the rough drafts. Carleen Wilenius was invaluable for her many skills with the manuscripts, not the least of which were final preparation and typing of many of the lengthy charts and bibliographies. I also wish to thank Rosemary E. Disney, who designed the cover art.

Ruth A. Lawrence

Contents

BREAST-FEEDING

a guide for the medical profession

CHAPTER 1

Breast-feeding in modern medicine

There is a reason behind everything in nature.
Aristotle

Until recently, breast-feeding has been a subject considered too imprecise and nonspecific to justify consideration by scientists and clinicians confronted with questions of infant nutrition. Decades have been spent in the laboratory deciphering the nutritional requirements of the growing neonate. A considerably greater investment in time, talent, and money has been put toward the development of an ideal substitute for human milk. On a parallel tract in the veterinary field, a careful study of the science of lactation in other species, especially bovine, has been made because of the commercial significance of a productive herd.

While expertise has produced refinements in the analysis of food constituents, it also has become possible to learn more about human milk. The traditional lip service paid to breast-feeding conceded that human milk is for human infants. A simple chart that showed the difference between human and cow's milk in protein, fat, and carbohydrate content and the calcium/phosphorus ratio has been used to support the statement. It was usually quickly pointed out that simple adjustments in cow's milk would actually mitigate these seeming differences. Students of pediatrics received no formal training in the management of breast-feeding and were thus ill prepared to counsel a mother who wished to nurse. Furthermore, if the process did not go smoothly and was not easily managed by the mother alone, the pediatrician was at a loss to help. Indeed, many physicians had been warned of the dangers of undernutrition associated with breast-feeding and the deviation from the "ideal" growth curve set by overfed bottle infants. When the natural process of human lactation presented a question or a concern to the physician, the advice was frequently to wean the infant to a formula that could be clinically measured and volumetrically controlled with scientific precision.

The world scientific literature, predominantly from countries other than the United States, actually has many tributes to human milk. Early writings on infant care in the 1800s and early 1900s pointed out the hazards of serious infection in bottle-fed infants. Mortality charts were clear in the difference in risk of death between breast- and bottle-fed infants.[8,9] Only in recent years have the reasons for this phenomenon been identified in terms comparable to those used to define other anti-infectious properties. The identification of specific immunoglobulins and specific influence of the pH and flora in the intestine of the breast-fed infant are examples. It became clear that the infant receives systemic protection transplacentally and local intestinal tract protection orally via the colostrum. It has been

1

further identified that the intestinal tract environment of a breast-fed infant continues to afford protection against infection by influencing the bacterial flora until the infant is weaned. It has been shown that breast-fed infants also have fewer respiratory infections.

Refinement in the biochemistry of nutrition has afforded an opportunity to restudy the constituents of human milk. A closer look at the amino acids in human milk has demonstrated clearly that the array is more physiologically suited for the human newborn. Forced by legislation mandating mass newborn screening for phenylalanine in all hospitals, physicians were faced with the problem of the newborn who had high phenylalanine or tyrosine levels in his blood. It became apparent that many traditional formulas provided an overload of these amino acids in the diet, which some infants were unable to handle well.

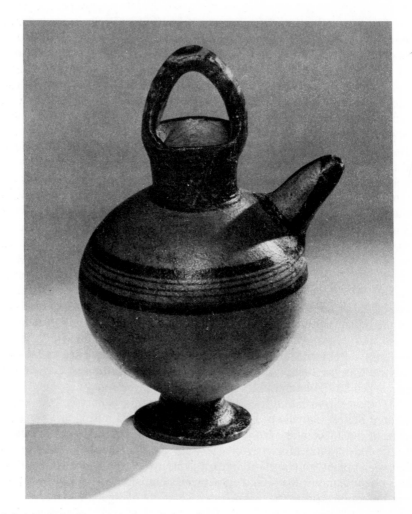

Fig. 1-1. Infant's feeding bottle from Cyprus. Circa 500 BC. Unglazed pottery. Although ancient Egyptian feeding flasks are almost unknown, specimens of Greek origin are fairly common in infant burials.

While one selectively chastises the modern woman for abandoning breast-feeding in the past two decades because of the ready availability of prepared formulas, paraphernalia of bottles and rubber nipples, and ease of sterilization, it should be pointed out that this is not a new problem. Meticulous combing of civilized history reveals that almost every culture had to deal with the mother who could not or would not nurse her infant. Blame cannot be placed solely at the feet of an uninformed and unsupportive medical profession or at the feet of the formula manufacturers.

Hammurabi's code from about 1800 BC contained regulations on the practice of wet nursing, that is, nursing another woman's infant, often for hire. Throughout Europe spouted feeding cups have been found in the graves of infants dating from about 2000 BC. Paralleling the information about ancient feeding techniques is the problem of abandoned infants. Well-known biblical stories report such events as do accounts from Rome during the time of the early popes. In fact, so many abandoned infants were discovered that foundling homes were started. French foundling homes in the 1700s were staffed by wet nurses who were carefully selected and their lives and activites controlled.

If one looks back to Spartan times,[19] it was required that a Spartan woman, even though she was the wife of a king, nurse her eldest son; plebians were to nurse all their children. Plutarch reported that a second son of King Themistes inherited the kingdom of Sparta only because he was nursed with his mother's milk. The eldest son had been nursed by a stranger and therefore was rejected. Hippocrates is said to have written on the subject of nursing, declaring, ''One's own milk is beneficial, other's harmful'' (Fig. 1-1).

In eighteenth century France, both before and during the revolution that swept Louis XVI from the throne and brought Napoleon to power, infant feeding included maternal nursing, wet nursing, artificial feeding with the milk of animals, and feeding of pap and panada. Panada is from the French panade, bread, and means a food consisting of bread, water or other liquid, and seasoning, boiled to the consistency of pulp (Fig. 1-2). The majority of infants, especially in Paris, were placed out with wet nurses. The reason given for this widespread practice was that maternal nursing was ''not the custom.'' Mothers wished to ''guard their beauty and freshness.'' In 1718, Dionis wrote ''today not only ladies of nobility, but yet the rich and the wives of the least of the artisans have lost the custom of nursing their infants.'' As early as 1705 there were laws controlling wet nursing. The laws required wet nurses to register, forbade them nursing more than two infants in addition to their own, and stipulated that there be a crib for each infant to prevent the nurse taking them to bed and chancing suffocation.*

A more extensive historical review would reveal other examples of social problems in achieving adequate care of infants. Long before our modern society there were women who failed to accept the biological role as nursing mothers, and society failed to provide adequate support for nursing mothers (Fig. 1-3).

According to Phillips,[14] breast-feeding was more common and of a longer duration in stable, hard-working eras and rarer in periods of ''social dazzle'' and

---

*It is interesting to note that at the National Convention of France of 1793, laws were passed to provide relief for infants of indigent families. The provisions are quite similar to our present-day welfare programs.[4]

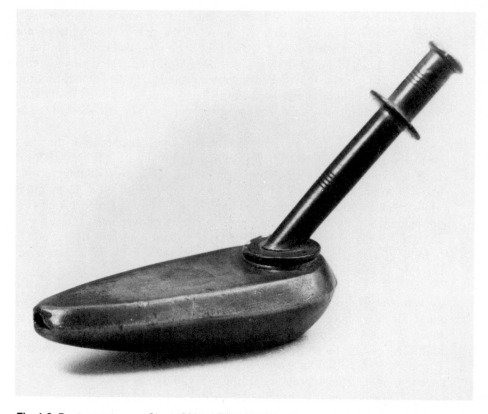

Fig. 1-2. Pewter pap spoon. Circa 1800 AD. Thin pap was placed in bowl. Tip of bowl was placed in child's mouth. Flow could be controlled by placing finger over open end of hollow handle. If contents were not taken as rapidly as desired, one could blow down handle.

lowered moral standards. Mothers in the cities have had greater access to alternatives, and rural women have had to continue to breast-feed in greater numbers.

Reasons given for the decrease in breast-feeding in this century have been reviewed by sociologists. Urbanization and technological advances have affected social, medical, and dietary trends throughout the world. The social influences include the changing pattern of family life—smaller, isolated families that are separated from the previous generation. In medicine, the emphasis has been on disease and its treatment, especially as it relates to laboratory study and hospital care. The science of nutrition developed a reliance on measurement and analysis, which encouraged the impression that prepared foods were superior because they could be measured and calculated to meet precise needs.

If recent statistics are reviewed, there are encouraging trends. The acceptance or rejection of breast-feeding is being influenced in the Western world to a greater degree by the knowledge of the benefits of human lactation. Cultural rejection, negative attitudes about convenience, and lack of support from health professionals are being replaced by interest in child rearing and preparation for childbirth. This has created a system that encourages a prospective mother to consider the options for herself and her infant. The attitude in the Western world toward the

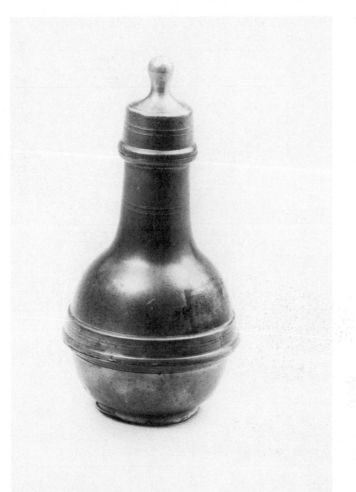

Fig. 1-3. Infant's feeding bottle. English. Circa 1780 AD. This pewter feeder is of type common to England, France, and Holland from 1600 to 1800.

female breast as a sex object to the exclusion of its ability to nurture has influenced young mothers in particular not to nurse. The emancipation of women, which began in the 1920s, was symbolized by short hair, short skirts, contraceptives, cigarettes, and bottle-feeding. In the second half of this century, women have sought to be well informed, and many wish the right to choose how they feed their infant. Within the boundaries of medical prudence, the medical profession should be prepared with adequate information to support the mother's desire to breast-feed.

FREQUENCY OF BREAST-FEEDING

Data collected recently[18] in the Ross National Mothers Survey MR 77-48, which included 10,000 mothers, revealed a general trend toward breast-feeding (Tables 1-1 and 1-2). In 1975, 33% of the mothers started out breast-feeding, and

Table 1-1. Estimated* percentages of infants receiving various types of milks and formulas†

Feeding	Age (mo)							
	0 to 1	1 to 2	2 to 3	3 to 4	4 to 5	5 to 6	6 to 9	9 to 12
Breast-fed	20	15	12	10	8	5	2	<1
Milk-based formulas‡	64	65	59	49	41	29	3	1
Milk-free formulas‡	10	10	10	10	8	6	2	1
Evaporated milk formulas	4	4	3	—	—	—	—	—
Evaporated milk and water	—	—	2	2	2	2	1	1
Fresh cow's milk	2	6	14	29	41	58	92	96

*Estimates based on any breast-feeding on a given day of the month in question. Estimates from 1974.
†From Fomon, S. J.: Pediatrics **56**:350, 1975, copyright American Academy of Pediatrics, 1975.
‡Commercially prepared.

Table 1-2. Percent of total infant feeding at 1 week of age*

	1975	1976	1977
Total prepared formula	69	64	61
With iron	35	33	32
Without iron	34	31	29
Total breast-feeding	33	39	43
Breast alone	30	34	38
Breast and supplement	3	5	5
Whole cow's milk/evaporated milk	1	1	†
Hypoallergenics	2	2	3
Sample size	10,052	11,441	19,442

*From Ross National Mothers Survey MR77-48, 1978.
†Less than 1%.

15% were still nursing at five to six months. In 1977, the figures indicated that 43% of the mothers left the hospital nursing, and 20% were still nursing at 5 to 6 months. Others studies have shown a regional variation, with a higher percentage of mothers nursing on the West Coast than in the East.

A study by Fitzpatrick and Kevany[5] in 1975 reported only 16% of all babies to be breast-fed at a few days of age in Dublin, Ireland. Sloper and co-workers[17] reported similar results from Oxford in the same year; 14% of the babies were breast-fed at discharge from the hospital, another 13% were receiving combined breast- and bottle-feedings.

DURATION OF BREAST-FEEDING

Coupled with concerns about the decreasing number of mothers nursing their infants when they leave the hospital is the concern about duration of breast-feeding. There is a sharp decline by age 6 months, in 1977 from 43% to 20%. Other studies that have looked at duration more closely have noted an appreciable decline shortly after discharge from the hospital.

Before one evaluates the duration of breast-feeding in the industrialized world, it is wise to consider that there are two types of breast-feeding, as Newton[13] points out—unrestricted breast-feeding and token breast-feeding.

Unrestricted breast-feeding usually means the infant is put to the breast immediately following delivery and nursed on demand thereafter. The infant is put to the breast without rules or limitations. There may be ten or twelve feedings a day in the early weeks, with the number gradually decreasing over the first year of life. Breast milk continues to be a major source of nourishment in infancy in these infants.

Token breast-feeding, in contrast, is characterized by constant restrictions on the time and duration of nursing. Usually the feedings are scheduled. Even the amount of mother-infant contact is limited initially, such as in hospitals where newborns are kept in a central nursery and only taken out for feedings. The infant is often offered water or glucose water by rubber-nippled bottle, which confuses the infant while he is trying to establish his sucking techniques. Feeding by the clock may mean the infant is too frantic from crying or not yet awake enough to suckle. The whole process is inhibited, and a secure milk supply may not be established.

If one examines the duration of breast-feeding there is a difference between unrestricted and token feeding groups. There are also cultural differences. In societies that have yet to be caught up in industrialization and continue to maintain ancient cultural patterns of child rearing, the duration is well beyond a year. A study of forty-six such societies reported by Ford[7] revealed that weaning at about 2 to 3 years of age occurred in three fourths of them. A fourth of the groups began weaning at 18 months of age, and one culture started at 6 months. A similar anthropological investigation of primitive child-rearing practices found a distinct correlation with the time of weaning and the behavior of the tribes.[7] Where weaning was delayed there were peaceful tribes. In contrast, tribes that abruptly weaned their infants at 6 months of age and practiced other rigid disciplinary practices were warlike.

In the United States and Europe at the beginning of this century over 50% of the infants were breast-fed beyond 1 year of age. The Plunket Society of New Zealand conducted three surveys to evaluate the extent and duration of breast-feeding.[3] These showed a progressive decline in the number of nursing mothers and in the duration of nursing (Fig. 1-4).

In 1966, less than one in three mothers in the United States were breast-feeding when they left the hospital. Only 5% of the nation's infants are breast-fed after 6 months of age. Fomon[6] has asserted that most breast-fed infants receive solid foods or cow's milk supplements early.

A Texas study by Halpern and colleagues[10] in 1972 followed 2310 infants, of whom 459 were breast-fed when dicharged from the hospital. By 4 weeks of age 32.9% had been stopped and by 26 weeks (6 months) 84% were no longer breast-fed (Table 1-3).

A study in Dublin by Fitzpatrick and Kevany[5] in 1977 looked at the duration of breast-feeding. Only six of nineteen infants (31.9%) were still wholly breast-feeding at 6 weeks, two were given some bottle-feedings and eleven (57.9%) had been weaned by 6 weeks (Fig. 1-5). A higher rate of success was experienced in mothers who had nursed a previous infant (Fig. 1-6). The rapid decline was

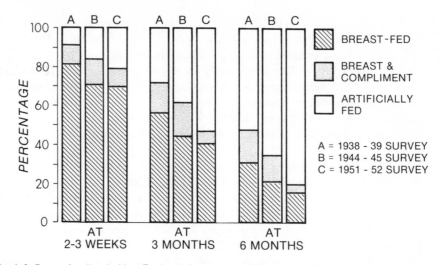

Fig. 1-4. Breast-feeding in New Zealand. A summary of the results of the Plunket Society's surveys of 1938 to 1939, 1944 to 1945, and 1951 to 1952. (From Deem, H., and McGeorge, M.: N.Z. Med. J. **57:**539, 1958.)

Table 1-3. Duration of breast-feeding among 459 mothers*

Duration of breast-feeding	Number of infants discontinuing breast-feeding	Number of infants still breast-feeding
1-2 wk	84 (18.3%)	459 (100%)
3-4 wk	67 (14.6%)	375 (81.7%)
5-8 wk	93 (20.3%)	308 (67.1%)
9-12 wk	28 (6.1%)	215 (46.8%)
13-16 wk	50 (10.9%)	187 (40.7%)
17-20 wk	33 (7.0%)	137 (29.8%)
21-25 wk	31 (6.8%)	104 (22.8%)
26 wk or longer	73 (16.0%)	73 (16.0%)
TOTAL	459 (100%)	

*From Halpern, S. R., et al.: South. Med. J. **65:**100, 1972, reprinted by permission.

attributed to lack of appropriate advice, including the early introduction of solid foods, and psychological support while in the hospital (Fig. 1-7). A similar study in Boston in 1960 had shown a mean duration of nursing to be 3½ months. Cole[1] conducted a two-part survey in a Boston suburb in 1977 that included 332 pregnant women and 140 new mothers—51% intended to breast-feed, 42% intended to bottle-feed, and 1% was undecided. There was a correlation with education of the mother and incidence of breast-feeding, with 44% of high school graduates, 62% of college graduates, and 65% of those with postgraduate education desiring to breast-feed (Table 1-4). Other researchers have made similar observations in the past decade, noting that 40% of the upper- and middle-class mothers breast-feed, compared to 15% in lower classes.

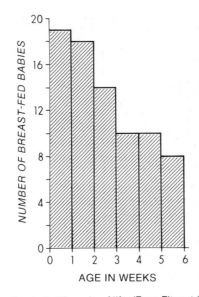

Fig. 1-5. Decline of breast-feeding in first 6 weeks of life. (From Fitzpatrick, C., and Kevany, J.: J. Irish Med. Assoc. **70:**3, 1977.)

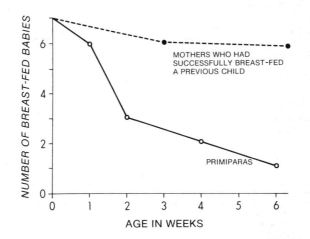

Fig. 1-6. Duration of breast-feeding in primiparas compared with mothers who have successfully breast-fed a previous child. (From Fitzpatrick, C., and Kevany, J.: J. Irish Med. Assoc. **70:**3, 1977.)

The length of breast-feeding for 140 women was studied (Table 1-5). By the time the infant was 4 weeks of age 80% of the women were still nursing, but only 58.6% were still breast-feeding beyond 4 months. The most frequent reasons for stopping were (1) not enough milk, (2) felt tired, and (3) infant's physician told mother to stop. This study also pointed out the pivotal role for the pediatrician in the successful maintenance of lactation as well as the importance of the postpartum environment.

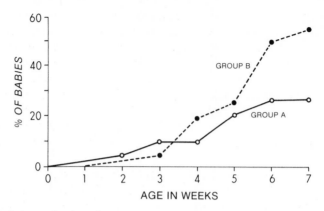

Fig. 1-7. Group A, breast-feeding; Group B, bottle-feeding. (From Fitzpatrick, C., and Kevany, J.: J. Irish Med. Assoc. **70:**3, 1977.)

Table 1-4. Mother's education and projected feeding choice* † ‡

Feeding choice	High school	Some college or degree	Graduate work or professional degree
Breast	44 (44%)	90 (62%)	55 (65%)
Bottle	55 (56%)	55 (38%)	29 (35%)
TOTAL	99	145	84

*From Cole, J. P.: Clin. Pediatr. **16:**352, 1977.
†Corrected chi-square = 10.33 with 2 df.
‡$p = 0.01$.

Table 1-5. Length of breast-feeding for 140 nursing women*

Infant's age when all breast-feeding stopped	Number	Percent	Cumulative %
Under 2 wk	7	5.0	5.0
2-4 wk	14	10.0	15.0
1-2 mo	8	5.7	20.7
2-3 mo	20	14.3	35.0
3-4 mo	2	1.4	36.4
In process of weaning	7	5.0	41.4
Still breast-feeding	82	58.6	100.0
TOTAL	140	100.0	100.0

*From Cole, J. P.: Clin. Pediatr. **16:**352, 1977.

MORBIDITY AND MORTALITY STUDIES IN BREAST-FED AND ARTIFICIALLY FED INFANTS

Assessing the mortality of breast-fed compared to bottle-fed infants is difficult to do today because many infants also receive supplements of cow's milk and solid foods. The risk of death in the first year of life has diminished in civilized countries in this century, since the advent of antibiotics and many other advances in pediatric care. Data from previous decades and other nations do show a significant difference, however.[8,9] Knobel[12] presented a complete table, including rates from cities in Germany, France, England, Holland, and the United States (Table 1-6). Mortality among breast-fed infants is clearly lower than that among bottle infants. Knobel pointed out that the early neonatal deaths in the first week or so of life were excluded.

In another study in 1922, Woodbury[20] reported mortality of infants by type of feeding. Mortality is less at all ages for breast-fed infants (Fig. 1-8). Overwhelming evidence of the impact of human milk on mortality is displayed in the widely publicized statistics currently available on third-world countries, where infant formulas are rapidly replacing human milk. The death rate is higher, malnutrition starts earlier and is more severe, and the incidence of infection is greater in formula-fed infants (Figs. 1-9 and 1-10). Data from the work of Scrimshaw and associates[16] show mortality of 950/1000 live births in the artificially fed infants and 120/1000 in breast-fed infants. The data were collected in Punjab villages from 1955

Table 1-6. Mortality rates and survivorship to age 1 year in breast-fed and artificially fed infants* †

Study area	Date	Mortality (per 1000)		Survivors to age 1 year (per 1000)		
		Breast-fed	Artificially fed	Breast-fed	Artificially fed	Difference
Berlin, Germany	1895-1896	57	376	943	624	319
Barmen, Germany	1905	68	379	932	621	311
Hanover, Germany	1912	96	296	904	704	200
Boston, Mass.	1911	30	212	970	788	182
Eight U.S. cities‡	1911-1916	76	255	924	745	179
Paris, France	1900	140	310	860	690	170
Cologne, Germany	1908-1909	73	241	927	759	168
Amsterdam, Holland	1904	144	304	856	696	160
Liverpool, England	1905	84	134	916	866	144
Eight U.S. cities§	1911-1916	76	215	924	785	139
Derby, England	1900-1903	70	198	930	802	128
Chicago, Ill.	1924-1929	2	84	998	916	82
Liverpool, England	1936-1942	10	57	990	943	47
Great Britain	1946-1947	9	18	991	982	9

*From Knodel, J.: Science **198**:1111, 1977, copyright 1977 by the American Association for the Advancement of Science.

†Most of these rates do not include deaths in the first few days or weeks of life; mortality is therefore underestimated and survival overestimated. Only the rates for the eight U.S. cities in 1911-1916 represent mortality from birth; deaths that occurred before any feeding are proportionately allocated to the two feeding categories. The rates for Berlin, Barmen, Hanover, Cologne, and the eight U.S. cities were derived by applying life table techniques to mortality given by single months of age.

‡Comparison of breast-fed infants with infants artificially fed from birth.

§Comparison of breast-fed infants with all infants artificially fed in the period of observation.

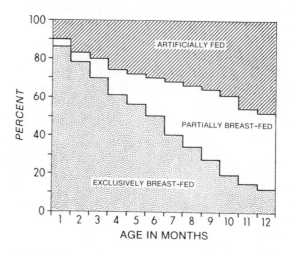

Fig. 1-8. Percentage of infants who are breast-fed, partially breast-fed, and artificially fed by age in months. (Modified from Woodbury, R. M.: Am. J. Hyg. **2:**668, 1922.)

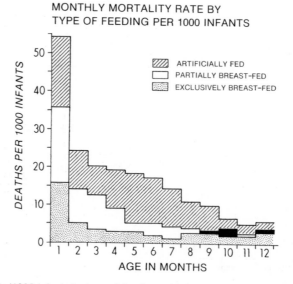

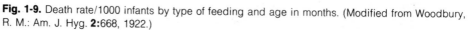

Fig. 1-9. Death rate/1000 infants by type of feeding and age in months. (Modified from Woodbury, R. M.: Am. J. Hyg. **2:**668, 1922.)

THE MESSAGE ON BREAST-FEEDING ISN'T NEW

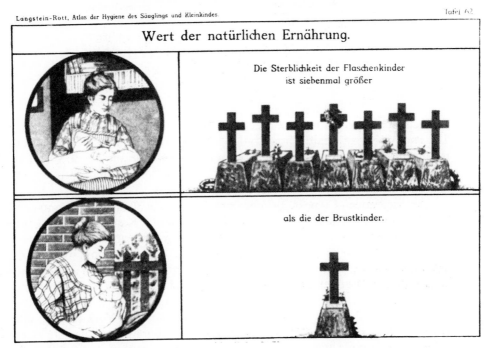

Fig. 1-10. Poster used in 1918 to educate parents on the value of breast-feeding. Title is *Value of Natural Feeding*. Text explains that mortality of bottle-fed infants (Flaschenkinder) is seven times higher than that of breast-fed infants (Brustkinder). (From Langstein, R.: Atlas der Hygiene des Sauglings und Kleinkindes, Berlin, 1918, Julius Springer Verlag.)

Table 1-7. Deaths and death rates by feeding regimen in seven Punjab villages, 1955-1959*

Feeding regimen	Newborn infants		Neonatal deaths†		Postneonatal deaths‡		Infant mortality§	
	Number	% of total	Number	Deaths/ 1000	Number	Deaths/ 1000	Number	Deaths/ 1000
No food given	16	2.1	16	1000.0	—	—	16	1000.0
Artificial feeding from birth	20	2.6	15	750.0	4	200.0	19	950.0
Breast-fed at birth	739	95.3	34	46.0	555	74.4	89	120.4
TOTAL	775	100.0	65	83.9	559	76.1	124	160.0

*From Scrimshaw, N. S., Taylor, C. E., and Gordon, J. E.: WHO monograph no. 29, Geneva, 1968.
†0 to 28 days inclusive.
‡29 days to 11 months inclusive.
§0 to 11 months inclusive.

Table 1-8. Incidence of infants hospitalized for severe diarrhea from three Arab villages in Israel, analyzed by feeding schedule*

Method of feeding	Hospitalization rate (%)
Breast-fed only (6 mo)	0.5
Breast-fed only (3 mo, <6 mo)	2.9
Mixed >3 mo	7.0
Bottle only (3 mo)	24.8

*From Kanaaneh, H.: J. Trop. Pediatr. **18**:302, 1972.

through 1959. The deaths were predominantly due to diarrheal disease (Table 1-7). The Pan American Health Organization has reported similar correlations between malnutrition, infection, and mortality. In Puffer and Serrano's[15] 1973 work in São Paulo the death rates among breast-fed infants were lower and the proportions due to diarrheal disease and malnutrition were also less.

The incidence of illness, or morbidity, among artificially fed infants in third-world countries is equally as dramatic as the mortality. Kanaaneh's[11] observations in Arab villages in Israel showed hospitalization rates to vary with method of feeding. Only 0.5% of breast-fed infants required hospitalization, whereas infants fed more than 3 months but less than 6 months at the breast had a 2.9% hospitalization rate, and infants who were bottle-fed had a 24.8% rate. This is a fiftyfold difference (Table 1-8).

Cunningham[2] undertook a study in rural upstate New York to determine the impact of feeding on the health of the infant. Of 326 infants studied, 162 were fed proprietary formula and 164 were breast-fed at birth, with only 4% still breast-fed at 1 year of age. Breast-feeding was associated with significantly less illness during the first year of life. Breast-feeding was associated with a higher level of parental education, but controlling for that factor, the difference in morbidity is even more significant.

In the United States, diarrheal disease is uncommon in breast-fed infants, and the treatment is usually to continue to breast-feed. Similarly, breast-fed infants have fewer episodes of respiratory illness and otitis media. When afflicted with such febrile illnesses, the breast-fed infant does not become dehydrated and rapidly toxic.

Despite the clear-cut data on mortality and morbidity from past generations and from cultures seemingly remote from industrialized and medically sophisticated societies, present-day pediatricians often discount the advantages, except psychological, of breast-feeding.

REFERENCES

1. Cole, J. P.: Breastfeeding in Boston suburbs in relation to personal-social factors, Clin. Pediatr. **16**:352, 1977.
2. Cunningham, A. S.: Morbidity in breast-fed and artificially fed infants, J. Pediatr. **90**:726, 1977.
3. Deem, H., and McGeorge, M.: Breastfeeding, N. Z. Med. J. **57**:539, 1958.
4. Drake, T. G. H.: Infant welfare laws in France in the 18th century, Ann. Med. Hist. **7**:49, 1935.
5. Fitzpatrick, C., and Kevany, J.: The duration of breast feeding, J. Irish Med. Assoc. **70**:3, 1977.
6. Fomon, S. J.: What are infants fed in the United States? Pediatrics **56**:350, 1975.
7. Ford, C. S.: A comparative study of human reproduction, anthropology publ. no. 32, New Haven, Conn., 1945, Yale University Press.

8. Grulee, C. G., Sanford, H. N., and Herron, P. H.: Breast and artificial feeding, J.A.M.A. **103:**735, 1934.
9. Grulee, C. G., Sanford, H. N., and Schwartz, H.: Breast and artificially fed infants, J.A.M.A. **104:**1986, 1935.
10. Halpern, S. R., Sellars, W. A., Johnson, R. B., et al.: Factors influencing breast-feeding: notes on observations in Dallas, Texas, South. Med. J. **65:**100, 1972.
11. Kanaaneh, H.: The relationship of bottle feeding to malnutrition and gastroenteritis in a pre-industrial setting, J. Trop. Pediatr. **18:**302, 1972.
12. Knodel, J.: Breast feeding and population growth, Science **198:**1111, 1977.
13. Newton, N.: Psychologic differences between breast and bottle feeding. In Jelliffe, D. B., and Jelliffe, E. F. P., editors: Symposium, the uniqueness of human milk, Am. J. Clin. Nutr. **24:**993, 1971.
14. Phillips, V.: Infant feeding through the ages, Keeping Abreast J. **1:**296, 1976.
15. Puffer, R. R., and Serrano, C. V.: Patterns of mortality in childhood, scientific publ. no. 262, Washington, D.C., 1973, Pan American Health Organization.
16. Scrimshaw, N. S., Taylor, C. E., and Gordon, J. E.: Interaction of nutrition and infection, WHO monograph no. 29, Geneva, 1968, World Health Organization.
17. Sloper, K., McKean, L., and Baum, J. D.: Patterns of infant feeding in Oxford, Arch. Dis. Child. **49:**749, 1974.
18. Stone, R. J.: Personal communication, Ross National Mothers Survey, MR 77-48, Columbus, Ohio, 1978, Ross Laboratories.
19. Taylor, J.: The duty of nursing children. In Ratner, H.: The nursing mother: historical insights from art and theology, Child Fam. **8**(4):19, 1949.
20. Woodbury, R. M.: The relation between breast and artificial feeding and infant mortality, Am. J. Hyg. **2:**668, 1922.

CHAPTER 2

Anatomy of the human breast

GROSS ANATOMY

The mammary gland, as the breast is medically termed, got its name from mamma, the Latin word for breast. Mammary glands begin to develop in the 6-week-old embryo, continuing their proliferation until milk ducts are developed by the time of birth. The breast is made up of glandular tissue, supporting connective tissue, and protective fatty tissue. Right after birth the newborn's breast may even be swollen and secreting a small amount of milk, known as witch's milk. This very common phenomenon among both male and female infants is caused by the stimulation of the infant's mammary glands by the same hormones produced by the placenta to prepare the mother's breast for lactation. This subsides quickly and from then on the mammary glands are inactive until shortly before the onset of puberty, when hormones begin to stimulate growth again.

The breast is located in the superficial fascia between the second rib and sixth intercostal cartilage and is superficial to the pectoralis major muscle. It tends to overlap this muscle inferiorly to become superficial to the external oblique and serratus anterior muscles. It measures 10 to 12 cm in diameter. It is located horizontally from the parasternal to midaxillary line. The central thickness of the breast is 5 to 7 cm (Fig. 2-1).

At puberty the breasts in the female enlarge to their adult size, one frequently being slightly larger than the other. In a nonpregnant woman, the mature breast weighs approximately 200 g, the left being somewhat larger than the right. During pregnancy there is some increased size and weight, thus near term the breast weighs between 400 and 600 g. During lactation the breast weighs between 600 and 800 g (Fig. 2-2).

The shape of the breast varies from woman to woman, just as body build and facial characteristics do. Commonly the breast is dome shaped or conical in adolescence, becoming more hemispherical and finally pendulous in the parous female. There is some projection of mammary glandular tissue into the axillary region. This is known as the tail of Spence. The presence of this mammary tissue becomes more obvious during the period of lactation. The three major structures are skin, subcutaneous tissue, and corpus mammae. The corpus mammae is the breast mass that remains after freeing the breast from the deep attachments and removing the skin, subcutaneous connective tissue, and adipose tissue.

The breast of the adult female develops from a line of glandular tissue, which is found in the fetus, known as the milk line. Hypermastia is the presence of accessory mammary glands, which are phylogenic remnants of the embryonic

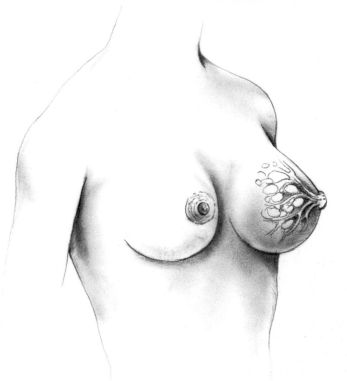

Fig. 2-1. Mammary gland in longitudinal cross section showing mature nonlactating duct system.

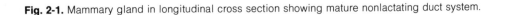

mammary ridge. Because of this origin, accessory nipples and glandular tissue may be found along these lines, which extend from the clavicular to the inguinal regions. Occasionally, supernumerary glands are found in the urogenital region, on the buttocks, or on the back, as well. The glands are derived from the ectoderm, whereas the connective tissue stroma is mesodermal in origin.

The accessory tissue may involve the corpus mammae, the areola, and/or the nipple.[3] From 2% to 6% of women have hypermastia. The response of hypermastia to pregnancy and lactation will depend on the tissue present. Hyperthelia is the presence of nipple tissue without breast tissue, and hyperadenia is the presence of mammary tissue without nipples. The swelling and secretion of this tissue may produce pain during lactation.

Corpus mammae

The mammary gland is a conglomeration of a variable number of independent glands. The morphology of the corpus mammae includes two major divisions, the parenchyma and the stroma.[1] The parenchyma includes the ductular-lobular-alveolar structures. It is composed of the alveolar gland with treelike ductular branching. The alveoli are approximately 0.12 mm in diameter. The ducts are approximately 2.0 mm in diameter. The lactiferous sinuses are 5 to 8 mm in

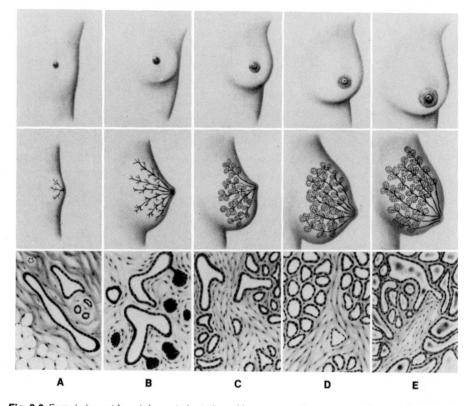

Fig. 2-2. Female breast from infancy to lactation with corresponding cross section and duct structure. **A, B,** and **C,** Gradual development of well-differentiated ductular and peripheral lobular-alveolar system. **D,** Ductular sprouting and intensified peripheral lobular-alveolar development in pregnancy. Glandular luminal cells begin actively synthesizing milk fat and proteins near term; only small amounts are released into lumen. **E,** With postpartum withdrawal of luteal and placental sex steroids and placental lactogen, prolactin is able to induce full secretory activity of alveolar cells and release of milk into alveoli and smaller ducts.

diameter, whereas the lobi, which are arranged like spokes converging on the central nipple, are fifteen to twenty-five in number. Each lobus is divided again into twenty to forty lobuli, and each lobulus is again subdivided into 10 to 100 alveoli for tubulosaccular secretory units. The stroma includes the connective tissue, fat tissue, blood vessels, nerves, and lymphatics.

The mass of tissue in the breast consists of the tubuloalveolar glands embedded in fat (the adipose tissue), giving the gland its smooth rounded contour. Each gland forms a lobe of the breast, and the lobes are separated by connective tissue septa. These septa attach to the skin. Each tubuloalveolar gland opens into a lactiferous duct, which leads into a more dilated area, the lactiferous sinus; there is a slight constriction before the sinus opens onto the surface of the nipple (Fig. 2-2).

Nipple and areola

The skin of the breast includes the nipple, the areola, and the general skin. The skin is the thin, flexible, elastic cover of the breast adherent to the fat-laden subcutaneous tissue. It contains hair, sebaceous glands, and apocrine sweat glands. The nipple, or papilla mammae, is a conical elevation located in the center of the areola at about the fourth intercostal space, slightly below the midpoint of the breast. The nipple contains fifteen to twenty-five milk ducts. Each of the tubuloalveolar glands that make up the breast opens onto the nipple by a separate opening. It also contains sensory nerve endings and is well supplied with sebaceous and apocrine sweat glands, but no hair. The nipple also contains smooth muscle fibers, which contract on tactile, thermal, or sexual stimulation, inducing greater firmness and prominence. The nipple is surrounded by the areola, or areola mammae, a circular pigmented area. It is usually pink before pregnancy, turning reddish brown during pregnancy, and always maintaining some pigmentation thereafter. It measures 15 to 16 mm in diameter, enlarging during pregnancy and lactation. Morgagni's tubercles containing the ductular openings of the Montgomery glands are present in the areola. The Montgomery glands are large sebaceous glands with miniature milk ducts opening into the skin of the areola. Sweat glands and smaller free sebaceous glands are also present in the areola. The corium of the areola lacks fat, but it contains smooth muscle and collagenous and elastic connective tissue fibers in radial and circular arrangements. The contraction of the smooth muscle fibers causes the nipple to erect. The Montgomery glands become enlarged and look like small pimples during pregnancy and lactation. They secrete a substance that lubricates and protects the nipples during nursing. After lactation these glands recede again to their former unobtrusive state. The areola and nipple are darker than the rest of the breast, ranging from a light pink in very fair-skinned women to very dark brown in others. The darker color of the areola may be some sort of visual signal to the newborn infant so that he will close his mouth on the areola, not on the nipple alone, to obtain milk. Local venostasis and hyperemia occur to enhance the process of erection of the nipple because the nipple and areola are rich in arterial venous anastomoses. Nipple erection is induced by tactile, sensory, or autonomic sympathetic stimuli. The dermis of the nipple and the areola contains a large number of multibranched free nerve fiber endings. The skin of the nipple is wrinkled, containing large papillae of the corium.

Each nipple contains fifteen to twenty-five lactiferous ducts surrounded by fibromuscular tissue (Figs. 2-3 to 2-5). These ducts end as small orifices near the tip of the nipple. Within the nipple the lactiferous ducts may merge. The ductular orifices therefore are sometimes fewer in number than the respective breast lobi. The milk ducts within the nipple dilate at the nipple base into the cone-shaped ampullae of milk sinuses. The ampullae function as temporary milk containers during lactation but contain only epithelial debris in the nonlactating state. The lining of the infundibular and ampullar parts of the lactiferous ducts consists of an eight to ten cell–layered squamous epithelium. The bulk of the nipple is composed of smooth musculature, which represents a closing mechanism for the milk ducts and sinuses of the nipple. The milk ducts in the nipple are embedded in stretchable and mobile connective tissue. The inner longitudinal muscular arrangements and the outer, more circular and radial arrangements do not obstruct the milk ducts. Tangential fibers also branch off from the more circular muscular fibers of the nipple bases to the outer circular muscular range. The functions of the muscular fibroelastic system of the areola and nipple include decreasing the surface area of the areola, producing nipple erection, and emptying the lactiferous sinuses and

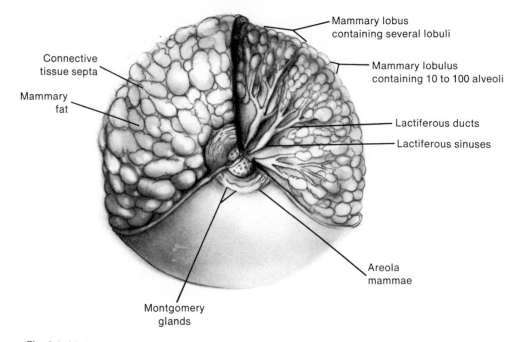

Fig. 2-3. Morphology of mature breast with dissection to reveal mammary fat and duct system.

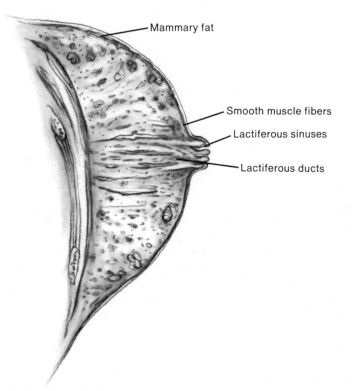

Fig. 2-4. Morphology of mature breast in cross section to reveal lactiferous duct system.

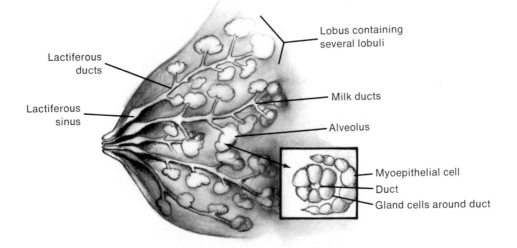

Lobus containing several lobuli

Lactiferous ducts

Milk ducts

Lactiferous sinus

Alveolus

Myoepithelial cell

Duct

Gland cells around duct

Fig. 2-5. Simplified schematic drawing of duct system with cross section of myoepithelial cells around duct opening. Myoepithelial cells contract to eject milk.

ducts during nursing. When the nipple erects, the system causes the nipple to become smaller and firmer, and thus the milk sinuses are emptied.

The mammary tissues are enveloped by the superficial pectoral fascia, and the breast is fixed by fibrous bands to the overlying skin and the underlying pectoral fascia, which are known as Cooper's ligaments. The glandular part of the breast is surrounded by a fat layer that seldom extends beyond the lower border of the pectoralis major. The breast is supported by the muscles attached to the ribs, the collar bone, and the bones of the upper arm near the shoulder.

Blood supply

The blood supply to the breast is from branches of the intercostal arteries and the perforating branches of the internal thoracic artery; the third, fourth, and fifth are usually most prominent. The major blood supply to the breast is provided by the internal mammary artery and the lateral thoracic artery. There is a small supply obtained from the intercostal arteries and the arterial branches of the axillary and subclavian arteries, but this contribution is minimal, since 60% of the total breast tissue receives blood from the internal mammary artery. All the mammary branches of this artery lead transversely to the nipple and anastomoses with branches coming from the lateral thoracic artery.[3] Anastomoses with intercostal arteries are less common, but the blood supply to the nipple is extensive. Many areas of the breast are supplied by two or three different arterial sources. The veins end in the internal thoracic and the axillary veins. Some veins may reach the external jugular vein (Fig. 2-6).

Lymphatic drainage

The lymph drainage of the breast has been the subject of considerable study because of the frequency of breast cancer, but it has significance for the lactating breast as well. Because of the proximity to the skin and superficial fascia, the

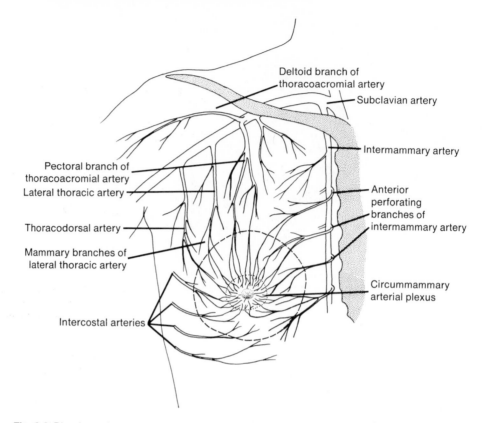

Deltoid branch of
thoracoacromial artery

Subclavian artery

Intermammary artery

Pectoral branch of
thoracoacromial artery

Lateral thoracic artery

Anterior
perforating
branches of
intermammary artery

Thoracodorsal artery

Mammary branches of
lateral thoracic artery

Circummammary
arterial plexus

Intercostal arteries

Fig. 2-6. Blood supply to mammary gland. Major blood supply from anterior perforating branches of internal mammary artery.

lymphatic drainage can be quite extensive. The main drainage is to axillary nodes and to the parasternal nodes along the internal thoracic artery inside the thoracic cavity. The lymphatics of the breast originate in the lymph capillaries of the mammary connective tissue, which surrounds the mammary structures. The lymph supply to the breast is extensive. The lymph drainage of the breast consists of the superficial, or cutaneous section, the areola, and the glandular, or deep-tissue section. A major portion of the lymphatic drainage is toward the axilla. Other points of drainage are to pectoral nodes between the pectoralis major and minor muscles and to the subclavicular nodes in the neck deep to the clavicle. There is some transmammary lymph drainage to the opposite breast as well as subdiaphragmatic lymphatics that lead ultimately to the liver and intra-abdominal nodes (Fig. 2-7).

Innervation of the mammary gland

The nerves of the breast are from branches of the fourth, fifth, and sixth intercostal nerves and consist of sensory fibers and sympathetic fibers innervating the smooth muscles in the nipple and blood vessels. The sensory innervation of the nipple and areola is extensive and consists of both autonomic and sensory nerves. The innervation of the corpus mammae is minimal by comparison and predomi-

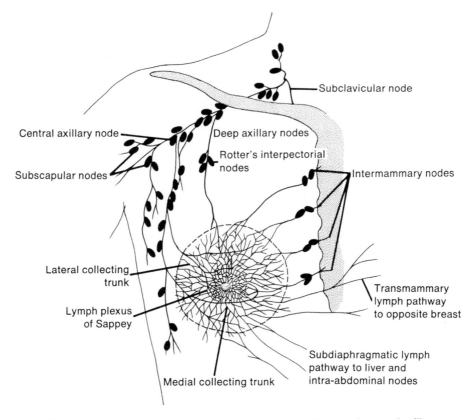

Fig. 2-7. Lymphatic drainage of mammary gland. Major drainage is toward axilla.

nately autonomic. There are no parasympathetic or cholinergic fibers supplying any part of the breast. There are no ganglia found in mammary tissue. Norepinephrine-containing nerve fibers are abundant among the smooth muscle cells of the nipple and at the interface between the media and adventitia of the breast arteries. Physiological observations demonstrate that the efferent nerves to these structures are sympathetic adrenergic.

The majority of the mammary nerves follow the arteries and arterioles and supply these structures. A few fibers from the the perivascular networks course along the wall of the ducts. They may correspond to sensory fibers for sensing milk pressure. No innervation of mammary myoepithelial cells has been identified. It can therefore be concluded that secretory activities of the acinar epithelium depend on hormonal stimulation such as that of prolactin and other hormones and are not stimulated via the nervous system directly.

Stimulation of the sensory nerve fibers or sensory receptors does induce the release of adenohypophyseal prolactin and neurohypophyseal oxytocin via an afferent sensory reflex pathway whereby stimuli reach the hypothalamus. Sympathetic mammary stimulation causes the contraction of the small muscles of the areola and the nipple. The locally released norepinephrine induces stimulation of the myoepithelial adrenergic receptors, causing muscular relaxation. In the ab-

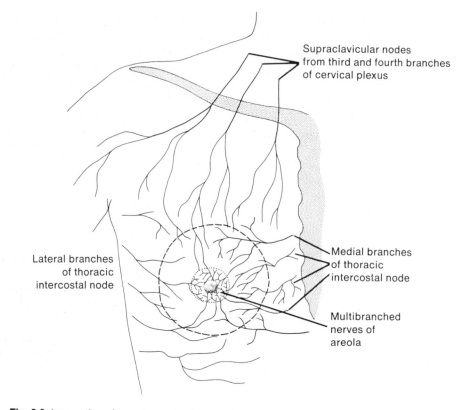

Fig. 2-8. Innervation of mammary gland supraclavicular nerves and lateral and medial branches of intercostal nerves provide sensory innervation. Sympathetic and motor nerves are provided by supracervical and intercostal nerves.

sence of parasympathetic activity, a minor physiological catamine inhibitory effect on the mammary myoepithelium may exist, which is overcome by oxytocin release during suckling, inducing myoepithelial contraction.

The supraclavicular nerves supply the sensory fibers for innervation of the upper cutaneous parts of the breast. Branches of the intercostal nerves provide the major sensory innervation of the mammary gland. The sympathetic sensory and motor fibers are derived from the supraclavicular and intercostal nerves, respectively. Sympathetic fibers only run along the mammary gland–supplying arteries to innervate the glandular body. There is relatively restricted innervation to the epidermal parts of the nipple and areola. Thus the skin in these areas responds only to major stimuli such as sucking. The relatively large number of dermal nerve endings provides a high mammary responsiveness toward stimuli for elicitation of the sucking reflex. The neuroreflex induces adequate release of both prolactin and oxytocin. It appears that, in addition to the hormonal actions, breast nerves can also influence the mammary blood supply and milk secretion. Abnormalities of sensory or autonomic nerve distributions in the areola and nipple, therefore, could impair adequate lactation, especially in the functioning of the let-down reflex and the secretion of prolactin and oxytocin.

In summary, the somatic sensory cutaneous nerve supply of the breast includes the supraclavicular nerves and the thoracic intercostal nerves. The autonomic motor nerve supply of the breast is derived from the sympathetic fibers of the intercostal nerves, which supply the smooth musculature of the areola and the nipple. The autonomic motor nerve supply of the breast is also derived from sympathetic fibers of the accompanying arteries, which innervate the smooth musculature of the inner glandular blood vessel walls to produce constriction. The nerve supply to the area of the areola and the nipple includes free sensory nerve endings, tactile corpuscles to the papillae of the corium of the nipple and areola, and the fibers around the larger lactiferous duct and in the dermis of the areola and peripheral breast. All cutaneous nerves run radially to the glandular body toward the nipple. The nerve supply to the inner gland is sparse and contains only sympathetic nerves accompanying blood vessels (Fig. 2-8).

MICROSCOPIC ANATOMY

In their structure and mode of development, the mammary glands somewhat resemble the sweat glands. During embryonic life, their differentiation is similar in the two sexes. The male experiences little additional development postnatally. The female, in contrast, experiences extensive structural change paralleling her age and the functional state of the reproductive system.

The greatest development in the female is reached by the twentieth year. Gradual changes are correlated with the menstrual cycle, and major changes accompany pregnancy and lactation.

Resting mammary gland

The mammary gland is a compound tubuloalveolar gland containing fifteen to twenty-five irregular lobes radiating from the nipple.[2] Each lobe has a lactiferous duct (2 to 4 mm in diameter) lined by stratified squamous epithelium. The duct opens on the nipple and has an irregular angular outline. Beneath the areola each duct has a local dilation, the lactiferous sinus, and finally emerges at the end of the nipple as a 0.4 to 0.7 mm opening. Each lobe is subdivided into lobules of various orders; the smallest are elongated tubules, the alveolar ducts, covered by small saccular evaginations, the alveoli. The interlobular connective tissue is dense; however, it is more cellular, has fewer collagenous fibers, and contains almost no fat. Greater distensibility is permitted by the looser connective tissue.

The secretory portions of the gland, the alveolar ducts and the alveoli, have cuboidal or low-columnar secretory cells, resting on basal laminae and myoepithelial cells. These myoepithelial cells enclose the alveoli in a loosely meshed network with their many starlike branchings. The myoepithelial cells are stimulated by prolactin and sex steroids. The presence of myoepithelial cells has been used as evidence that the mammary gland is related to the sweat gland.

In the resting phase, epithelial structures consist of the ducts and their branches. The presence of a few alveoli budded off from the ends of ducts is still under discussion. This variance may be due to the effect of the menstrual cycle. The swelling and engorgement accompanying the menstrual cycle are associated with hyperemia and some edema of the connective tissue. Most significant is the fact that the gland does not have a single duct but rather, many. Each lobe is a separate compound alveolar gland whose primary ducts join into larger and larger ducts. These ducts drain into a lactiferous duct. Each lactiferous duct drains separately at the tip of the nipple.

The epidermis of the nipple and areola is invaded by unusually long dermal papillae whose capillaries richly vascularize the surface and impart the pinkish hue. Bundles of smooth muscle, longitudinally placed along the lactiferous ducts and circumferentially within the nipple and at its base, permit the erection of the nipple. In the areola are the areolar Montgomery glands, which are intermediate in their structure between sweat glands and true mammary glands. The periphery of the areola also has sweat glands and sebaceous glands (Fig. 2-4).

Mammary gland in pregnancy

Changes in levels of circulating hormones result in profound changes in the ductular-lobular-alveolar growth during pregnancy. During the first trimester there is rapid growth and branching from the terminal portion of the duct system. As the epithelial structures proliferate, the adipose tissue seems to diminish. During this time there is increasing infiltration of the interstitial tissue with lymphocytes, plasma cells, and eosinophils. The rate of hyperplasia levels off. In the last trimester any enlargement is the result of enlargement of the parenchymal cells and the distention of the alveoli with early colostrum, which is rich in protein and relatively low in lipid. There is a gradual accumulation of fat droplets in the secretory alveolar cells. The interlobular connective tissue is noticeably decreased and alveolar proliferation extensive. The histological appearance of the gland is quite variable. The functional state appears to vary from dilated, thin-walled lumen to narrow-lumened, thick-walled glandular tissue. Epithelial cells vary, being flat to low columnar in shape with indistinct boundaries. Some cells protrude into the lumen of the alveoli; others are short and smooth. The lumen of the alveoli is crowded with fine granular material and lipid droplets similar to those protruding from the cells.

The former concepts of mammary gland secretion indicated that the mode of release was apocrine secretion. Apocrine secretion is the process by which the cell undergoes partial disintegration. A fat-filled portion projects into the lumen; the fat globule constricts at the base, and the cell replaces itself. Electron microscopy has shown that the cell has two distinct secretory products, formed and released by different mechanisms. The protein constituents of milk are formed and released identically to those of other protein-secreting glands, classed as merocrine glands. Secretory materials are passed out through the cell apex without appreciable loss of cytoplasm in merocrine glands. The fatty components of milk arise as lipid droplets free in the cytoplasmic matrix. The droplets increase in size and move into the apex of the cell. They project into the lumen, covered by a thin layer of cytoplasm. The droplets are ultimately cast off, enveloped by a detached portion of the cell membrane and a thin rim of subjacent cytoplasm. This is referred to as apocrine, since it involves the loss of some cytoplasm (Fig. 2-2).

Lactating mammary gland

The lactating mammary gland is characterized by a large number of alveoli. The alveoli of the lactating gland are made up of cuboidal epithelial and myo-epithelial cells. Only a small amount of connective tissue separates the neighboring alveoli. Under special preparations lipid can be seen as small droplets within the cells. These droplets become larger and are discharged into the lumen.

The functioning of the mammary gland depends on the interplay of multiple and complex nervous and endocrine factors. Some are involved in the development of the mammary glands to a functional state (mammogenesis), others to the establishment of milk secretion (lactogenesis), and finally others are responsible for the maintenance of lactation (galactopoiesis).

The division and differentiation of mammary epithelial cells and presecretory alveolar cells into secretory milk-releasing alveolar cells takes place in the third trimester. Stimulation of RNA synthesis promotes galactopoiesis and apocrine milk secretion into the alveoli. The DNA and RNA content of the cellular nuclei increases during pregnancy and is highest at lactation (Fig. 2-2).

Postlactation regression of the mammary gland

If milk is not removed from the breast, the glands become greatly distended, and milk production gradually ceases. Part of the decrease is due to the lack of stimulation of sucking, which initiates the neurohormonal reflex for maintenance of prolactin secretion. Perhaps a stronger effect is the engorgement of the breast with compression of blood vessels, causing diminished flow. The diminished flow results in decreased oxytocin to the myoepithelium. The alveoli are greatly distended and the epithelium flattened. The secretion remaining in the alveolar spaces and ducts is absorbed. There is a gradual collapse of the alveoli and an increase in perialveolar connective tissue. The glandular elements gradually return to the resting state. Adipose tissue increases. There are increased macrophages. The gland does not return completely to the prepregnancy state, in that the alveoli formed do not totally involute. Some appear as scattered, solid cords of epithelial cells.

Microscopically, there is increased autophagic and heterophagic processes in the first few days after weaning. Lysosomal enzymes increase, whereas non-lysosomal enzymes decrease.

Although the process of regression has been studied carefully in animals, little study has been done in the human. It is probable that slow weaning, which usually takes 3 months, has a very different timetable than abrupt weaning, in which marked involution has been intense and rapid over a matter of days or weeks.

REFERENCES

1. Crafts, R. C.: A textbook of human anatomy, New York, 1966, Ronald Press Co.
2. Bloom, W., and Fawcett, D. W.: A textbook of histology, ed. 10, Philadelphia, 1975, W. B. Saunders Co.
3. Vorherr, H.: The breast: morphology, physiology, and lactation, New York, 1974, Academic Press, Inc.

CHAPTER 3

Physiology of lactation

HORMONAL CONTROL OF LACTATION

Lactation is an integral part of the reproductive cycle of all mammals, including the human. The hormonal control of lactation can be described under three main headings: mammogenesis, or mammary growth; lactogenesis, or initiation of milk secretion; and finally galactopoiesis, or the maintenance of established milk secretion.

Under the influence of sex steroids, especially the estrogens, the mammary glandular epithelium proliferates, becoming multilayered. Buds and papillae then form. The growth of the mammary gland is a gradual process, which starts during puberty. It has been shown to depend on pituitary hormones. Lobuloalveolar development and ductal proliferation also depend on an intact pituitary gland.

Mammogenesis: mammary growth

Prepubertal growth. The primary and secondary ducts that develop in the fetus in utero continue to grow in both the male and female in proportion to growth in general. Shortly before puberty, a more rapid expansion of the duct system begins in the female. The growth of the duct system seems to depend predominantly on estrogen and does not occur in the absence of ovaries. The complete growth of the alveoli requires stimulation by progesterone as well.

Studies of hypophysectomized animals have shown failure of full mammary growth even with adequate estrogen and progesterone. It has been shown that it is the secretion of prolactin and somatotropin by the pituitary gland that effects mammary growth. Adrenocorticotropic hormone (ACTH) and thyrotropic hormone (TSH) acting on the adrenal gland and the thyroid gland also play a minor role in growth of the mammary gland.

Pubertal growth. When the hypophyseal-ovarian-uterine cycle is established, a new phase of mammary growth begins, which includes extensive branching of the system of ducts and proliferation and canalization of the lobuloalveolar units at the distal tips of the branches. Organization of the stromal connective tissue forms the interlobular septa. The ducts, ductules (terminal intralobular ducts), and alveolar structures are all formed by double layers of cells. One layer, the epithelial cells, circumscribes the lumen. The second layer, the myoepithelial cells, surrounds the inner epithelial cells and is bordered by a basement lamina.

Menstrual cycle growth. The cyclical changes of the adult mammary gland can be associated with the menstrual cycle and the hormonal changes that control that cycle. Estrogens stimulate parenchymal proliferation, with formation of epithelial sprouts. This hyperplasia continues into the secretory phase of the cycle. Anatomically, when the corpus luteum provides increased amounts of estrogens and progesterone, there is lobular edema, thickening of the epithelial basal membrane, and secretory material in the alveolar lumen. Lymphoid and plasma cells infiltrate the stroma. Clinically, there is increased mammary blood flow in this luteal phase. This is experienced by women as fullness, heaviness, and turgescence. The breast may become nodular due to interlobular edema and ductular-acinar growth.

After the onset of menstruation and the reduction in sex steroid levels, there is limited milk-secretory prolactin action. Postmenstrual changes occur rapidly, with degeneration of glandular cells and proliferation tissue, loss of edema, and decrease in breast size. The ovulatory cycle actually enhances mammary growth in the early years of menstruation (until about age 30) because the postmenstrual regression of the glandular-alveolar growth after each cycle is not complete. These changes of ductal and lobular proliferation, which occur during the follicular phase before ovulation, continue in the luteal phase and regress after the menstrual phase, exemplifying the sensitivity of this target organ to variations in the balance of hormones.

Growth during pregnancy. Hormonal influences on the breast cause profound changes during pregnancy (Fig. 3-1). Early in pregnancy a marked increase in ductular sprouting, branching, and lobular formation is evoked by luteal and placental hormones. Placental lactogen, prolactin, and chorionic gonadotropin have been identified as contributors to the accelerated growth. The dichorionic

GESTATION

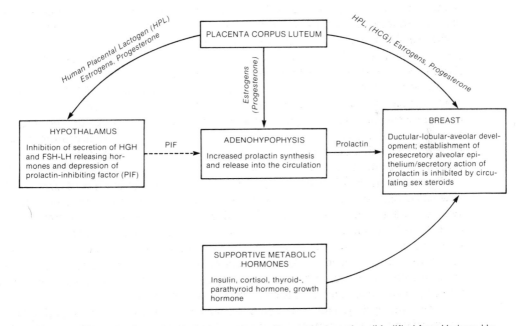

Fig. 3-1. Hormonal preparation during pregnancy of breast for lactation. (Modified from Vorherr, H.: The breast, morphology, physiology and lactation, New York, 1974, Academic Press, Inc.)

ductular sprouting has been attributed to estrogen, and lobular formation has been attributed to progesterone.

From the third month of gestation, secretory material that resembles colostrum appears in the acini. Prolactin from the anterior pituitary gland stimulates the glandular production of colostrum. By the second trimester, placental lactogen begins to stimulate the secretion of colostrum. The effectiveness of hormonal stimulation on lactation has been demonstrated by the fact that a mother who delivers after 16 weeks of gestation will secrete colostrum, although she has had a nonviable infant.

An estrogen-mediated increase in prolactin secretion in pregnancy may produce as much as a tenfold to twentyfold increase in plasma prolactin. This effect may be partially controlled by lactogen from the placenta, which inhibits the production of prolactin. Hormonal regulation of the growth and proliferation of the mammary gland cells has been carefully studied in many species.

There is a complex sequence of events governed by hormonal action, which prepare the breast for lactation (Fig. 3-1). Estradiol 17β stimulates the ductal system of epithelial cells to elongate during pregnancy. Progesterone, in turn, induces the specific epithelial cells of the tubular invaginations to produce distinct ducts, which branch from the main tubules. The end result of the combined actions of estrogen and progesterone is a richly branched arborization of the gland. Highly differentiated secretory alveolar cells develop at the ends of these ducts, under the influence of prolactin.

Serum growth factor, which is present in normal human serum, and insulin can stimulate the stem cells of the gland to proliferate. This proliferation is enhanced by estradiol 17β. These dividing cells are further directed to the formation of alveoli by corticosteroid hormones. There are at least two types of cells identified in the epithelial layer of the gland, stem cells and secretory alveolar cells. At this point in the pregnancy prolactin influences the production of the constituents of milk.

Lactogenesis: initiation of milk secretion

The breast tissue, which has been prepared during pregnancy, responds to the release of prolactin by producing the constituents of milk (Fig. 3-2).

Prolactin. Human prolactin is a significant hormone in pregnancy and lactation.[4] Prolactin also has a range of actions in various species that is greater than any other known hormone. Prolactin has been identified in many animal species whether they nurse their young or not. Because of the original association with lactation, the term describes its action, "support or stimulation of lactation." Prolactin, however, has been shown to control nonlactating responses in other species and has been identified with over eighty different physiological processes. Study of prolactin was hampered until 1970, when it became possible to separate prolactin from human growth hormone and to measure prolactin levels. Prior to 1971 growth hormone and prolactin in humans were considered to be the same hormone. Growth hormone, however, is present in the human pituitary gland in amounts 100 times that of prolactin.

The levels of prolactin are essentially the same in the human male and female. Moreover, both male and female experience a rise in prolactin levels during sleep. At puberty the increase in estrogens causes a slight but measurable increase in

POSTPARTUM

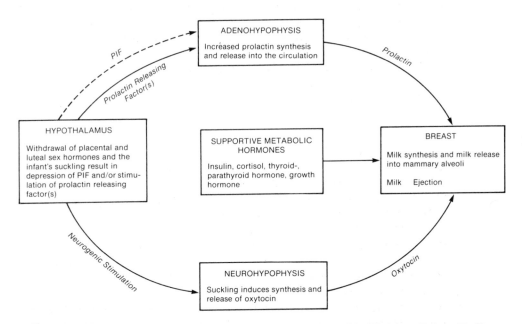

Fig. 3-2. Hormonal preparation of breast postpartum for lactation. (Modified from Vorherr, H.: The breast, morphology, physiology and lactation, New York, 1974, Academic Press, Inc.)

prolactin. There is an increase in prolactin in the proliferative phase of the menstrual cycle but not during the secretory phase. There is also a normal diurnal variation in levels in both male and female. A number of factors, including some that are significant for the nursing mother, increases prolactin levels. Psychogenic influence and stress increase prolactin levels. Anesthesia, surgery, exercise, nipple stimulation, and sexual intercourse also produce increased amounts in both the lactating and nonlactating female. Prolactin levels increase as serum osmolality increases.

Prolactin-inhibiting factor. The prolactin-inhibiting factor (PIF) controls the secretion of prolactin from the hypothalamus. Prolactin thus is unusual among the pituitary hormones, since it is inhibited by a hypothalamic substance. Catecholamine levels in the hypothalamus control the inhibiting factor. The inhibiting factor is poured into the circulation as a result of dopaminergic impulses. Drugs and events that decrease catecholamines also decrease the inhibiting factor, causing a rise in prolactin. Dopamine itself can act directly on the pituitary gland to decrease prolactin secretion. Agents that increase prolactin by decreasing catecholamines and thus the PIF level include the phenothiazines and reserpine. Thyrotropin-releasing hormone is a strong stimulator of prolactin secretion, but its physiological role is not clear, since thyrotropin levels do not rise during normal nursing. In the postpartum period, a dose of thyrotropin-releasing hormone will cause a marked increase in prolactin. Even the nonnursing postpartum mother will experience engorgement and milk release when stimulated with thyrotropin-releasing hormone. Ergot, which is frequently prescribed for the postpartum patient, inhibits prolactin secretion either by direct inhibition or by its effect on the hypothalamus.

Following are factors affecting prolactin release in normal humans[5]:

Physiological stimuli
    Nursing in postpartum women—breast stimulation
    Sleep
    Stress
    Sexual intercourse
    Pregnancy

Pharmacological stimuli
    Neuroleptic drugs
    TRH
    Estrogens
    Hypoglycemia

Pharmacological suppressors
    L-dopa
    Ergot preparations (2-Br-α-ergocryptine)

In pregnancy, prolactin levels begin to rise in the first trimester and continue to rise throughout gestation. In the nonnursing mother, prolactin levels drop to normal in 2 to 3 weeks, independent of therapy to suppress lactation.

At delivery, with the expulsion of the placenta, there is an abrupt decline in estrogens and progesterone. The withdrawal of estrogen triggers the onset of lactation. Estrogens enhance the effect of prolactin on mammogenesis but an-

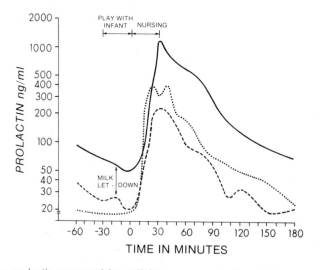

Fig. 3-3. Plasma prolactin measured by radioimmunoassay, before, during, and after period of nursing in three mothers, 22 to 26 days postpartum. Prolactin rose with suckling and not with infant contact. (Modified from Josimovich, J. B., Reynolds, M., and Cobo, E.: Lactogenic hormones, fetal nutrition, and lactation. In Josimovich, J. B., Reynolds, M., and Cobo, E.: Problems of human reproduction, vol. 2, New York, 1974, John Wiley & Sons.)

tagonize prolactin in inhibiting secretion of milk. After delivery, there are low estrogen and high prolactin levels. Suckling provides a continued stimulus for prolactin release. If prolactin, essential for lactation, is diminished by hypophysectomy or medication, lactation ceases. Prolactin levels do eventually diminish to more normal levels months after parturition, although lactation may continue. Suckling stimulates the release of adenohypophyseal prolactin and neurohypophyseal oxytocin. These hormones stimulate milk synthesis and production of milk-ejection metabolic hormones, which are also necessary in the process of milk synthesis. Thus suckling, emptying the breast, and receiving adequate precursor nutrients are essential to effective lactation (Fig. 3-3).

The most effective and specific stimulus to prolactin release is nursing. The stimulation is a result of nipple or breast manipulation, especially suckling, not a psychological effect of the presence of the infant (Fig. 3-3). The prolactin-release reflex during nipple stimulation is suppressed in some adult women, only being evidenced during pregnancy and lactation.

In the nursing mother, Tyson and associates[14] have described three types of prolactin response to nursing at the breast (Table 3-1). Stage one occurs during the first week postpartum. Prolactin levels are still elevated, thus suckling causes only small increases. The second stage is observed from the second week to the second month postpartum; baseline levels are two to three times normal and increase to ten to twenty times normal following suckling. During stage three (from the third month until weaning) prolactin levels are back to normal and suckling produces no rise in levels. It is interesting to note that milk production continues to be adundant despite only modest levels of prolactin.

Human placental lactogen and pituitary growth hormone. There are three main hormones recognized in the lactogenic process: human placental lactogen (HPL), pituitary growth hormone, or human growth hormone (HGH), and prolactin. The progressive rise in prolactin during pregnancy parallels the rise in HPL, becoming measurable at 6 weeks of gestation and increasing to 6000 ng/ml at term. This

Table 3-1. Prolactin levels*

	Range (ng/ml)	Average (ng/ml)
Male and female (throughout menstrual life)	<25	10
Term pregnancy	200 to 500	200
Amniotic fluid	Up to 10,000	
Lactating women		
Stage one†	200	
Stage two‡	2 times normal (resting)	
	10 to 20 times normal (during suckling)	
Stage three§	Normal (no rise with suckling)	

*Modified from Tyson, J. E.: Med. Clin. North Am. **61**:153, 1977.
†Stage one—first week postpartum.
‡Stage two—second week to third month postpartum.
§Stage three—beyond third month postpartum.

parallel action contributed to the belief that prolactin and HPL were the same. Although the principal function of HPL and prolactin in the human is a lactogenic one, no lactation appears prior to delivery.[10]

HPL is derived from the chorion and has an anabolic action with growth hormone–like activities. It has been associated with mobilization of free fatty acid and inhibiton of peripheral glucose utilization and lactogenic action.[12]

HGH is secreted from the anterior pituitary eosinophilic cells. These cells have been identified by staining techniques that distinguish them from those that produce prolactin. Toward the end of pregnancy, the cells that produce prolactin are noticeably more numerous, whereas those that produce HGH are "crowded out."

Galactopoiesis: maintenance of established lactation

The maintenance of established milk secretion is called galactopoiesis. An intact hypothalamic-pituitary axis regulating prolactin and oxytocin levels is essential to the initiation and maintenance of lactation.[6] The process of lactation requires milk synthesis and milk release into the alveoli and the lactiferous sinuses. When the milk is not removed, effecting the diminution of capillary blood flow, the lactation process can be inhibited. Lack of sucking stimulation means lack of prolactin release from the pituitary gland. Basal prolactin levels that are enhanced by the spurts that result from sucking are necessary to maintain lactation in the first weeks postpartum. Without oxytocin, however, a pregnancy can be carried to term but the female will fail to lactate.[1]

Sensory nerve endings, located mainly in the areola and nipple, are stimulated by suckling. The afferent neural reflex pathway via the spinal cord to the mesencephalon and then to the hypothalamus, produces secretion and release of prolactin and oxytocin. Hypothalamic suppression of PIF secretion causes adrenohypophyseal prolactin release. When prolactin is released into the circulation, it stimulates milk synthesis and secretion.

Hormonal regulation of prolactin and oxytocin. The release of prolactin is inhibited by PIF.[7] The PIF has not been described, but it is closely associated with dopamine. There is also evidence of either serotonin release of prolactin or catecholamine-serotonin control of prolactin release. TSH has also been shown to stimulate the release of prolactin. In addition, the release of prolactin is related to stress and sleep states. The amount of prolactin is proportional to the amount of nipple stimulation.

When suckling occurs, oxytocin is released. It enters the circulation and rapidly causes ejection of milk from alveoli and smaller milk ducts into larger lactiferous ducts and sinuses. This is the pathway of the let-down, or ejection, reflex. Oxytocin also causes contraction of the myometrium and involution of the uterus.

Neuroendocrine control of milk ejection. Milk ejection involves both neural and endocrinological stimulation and response. A neural afferent pathway and an endocrinological efferent pathway are required.[9]

The ejection reflex depends on the existence of receptors located in the canalicular system of the breast. When the canalicules are dilated or stretched, the reflex release of oxytocin is triggered. There are tactile receptors for both oxytocin and reflex prolactin release located in the nipple. Neither the negative and positive pressures exerted by suckling nor thermal changes trigger the milk-ejection reflex. There is some minor effect of negative pressures, but tactile stimulation is the most important factor.

The release of oxytocin by neurohypophyseal responses during lactation has been evoked both by infant's suckling and mechanical dilation of the mammary ducts. This release of oxytocin was demonstrated to be independent of vasopressin release. Conversely, further study[6] demonstrated that the stimulation of vasopressin release could occur independent of oxytocin release.*

Human myoepithelium is specifically stimulated by oxytocin, and this sensitivity and specificity increases throughout pregnancy. Suckling can induce milk secretion, which is under control of the adenohypophysis. In this case, oxytocin released by the neurohypophysis because of the suckling stimulus would cause both milk ejection and release of the anterior pituitary hormones responsible for milk secretion as well. This is probably the mechanism behind relactation and induced lactation in the woman who has never been pregnant. Mammary growth and lactogenesis may be induced by suckling, massage, and breast stimulation in many species.[3]

Suckling brings about functional changes in the offspring. When an infant sucks on an artificial nipple, he quickly decreases the amount of body movement, increases his mouthing activity, and decreases crying. The suckling experience may affect infant behavior and mother-infant interaction. Nonnutritive sucking is observed in many species. In the human infant, nutritive sucking is shown to be a continuous stream of regular sucks with few, if any, pauses. Nonnutritive sucking has bursts of activity alternating with no sucking. Suckling can be altered by extraneous stimuli such as aural, visual, or olfactory stimulation.

Effects of suckling on the mother include the stimulation of afferent nerves for the removal of milk.[8] Reduction in sucking stimulus produces a reduction in prolactin and in milk synthesis. The lactating glands are good at adjusting the milk supply to demand, probably due to both a local and an endocrinological mechanism. Variations in milk secretion are rapidly reflected in anatomical changes in the mammary gland. Mammary tissue shows regression after the first week or so, if unstimulated. Tissue regression proceeds at a rate parallel to the demand for secretory tissue. Thus, when the suckling infant signals his needs, the breast will respond.

There are effects on maternal behavior that have been attributed to lactation. Maternal behavior is more easily defined in many other species, in which early nursing is initiated by the mother, who stimulates the neonate to suckle by grooming him. She then presents her mammary gland to the offspring so that the nipple is located with minimal effort. It has been shown that lactating females have a lessened response to stress. In the human, however, there is a strong voluntary nature to nursing behavior.

If one explores the possible spinal and brain stem pathways by which the suckling stimulus reaches the forebrain, the spinothalamic tract is the most likely. The areas of the forebrain influenced by the sucking stimulus include the hypothalamic structures that mediate oxytocin and prolactin release.

SYNTHESIS OF HUMAN MILK

The function of the mammary gland is unique in that it produces a material that makes tremendous demands on the maternal system without producing any

---

*It has been shown that alcohol has an effect on the CNS in inhibiting milk ejection. This effect is dose related.

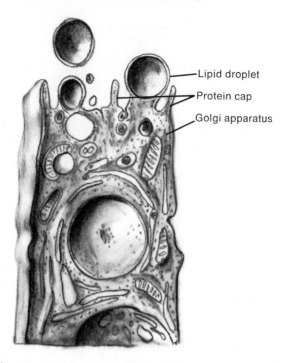

Lipid droplet
Protein cap
Golgi apparatus

Fig. 3-4. Apocrine secretory mechanism for lipids, proteins, and lactose in milk.

physiological advantage to the maternal organism. Because lactation is anticipated, the body prepares the breast anatomically and physiologically.[11] When
lactation begins there is a marked alteration in the metabolism of the mother.
There is a redistribution of the blood supply and an increased demand for
nutrients, which requires an increased metabolic rate to accommodate the production. The mammary gland may have to produce milk at the metabolic expense of
other organs. The supply of materials to the lactating breast for milk production
and energy metabolism requires extensive cardiovascular changes in the mother.
There is increased mammary blood flow, increased blood flow into the gastrointestinal tract and liver, and a high cardiac output. The mammary blood flow,
cardiac output, and milk secretion are suckling dependent. Suckling induces the
release of anterior pituitary hormones that act directly on breast tissue.

Milk is isosmotic with plasma in all species. Human milk differs from many
other milks in that the concentration of major monovalent ions is lower and lactose
is higher. If one looks at other milks, the higher the ions, the lower the lactose,
and vice versa. Many of the disparities in the intermediary metabolism between
species of animals can be linked to evolutionary adaptions involving the digestive
process. Nonruminants rely on glucose, derived from carbohydrate in the diet.
Ruminants, because of extensive fermentation in the rumen, absorb little glucose.
The microbial fermentation products, which include acetate, propionate, and
butyrate, play a significant part as energy and carbon sources for tissue metabolism. Amino acids are primary substitutes for glucose in ruminants.

The biosynthesis of milk involves a cellular site where the metabolic processes

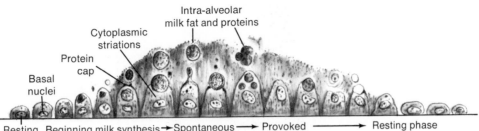

Fig. 3-5. Diagram of cycle of secretory cells from resting stage to secretion and return to resting stage. (Modified from Vorherr, H.: The breast, morphology, physiology and lactation, New York, 1974, Academic Press, Inc.)

occur. The epithelial cells of the gland contain stem cells and highly differentiated secretory alveolar cells at the terminal ducts. The stem cells are stimulated by HGH and insulin. Prolactin synergizes the insulin effect to stimulate the cells to secretory activity.

The cells of the acini and smaller milk ducts are active in milk synthesis and the secretion of the milk into the alveoli and smaller milk ducts. Most milk is synthesized during the process of suckling; its production is stimulated by prolactin. Cortisol plasma levels are increased during suckling as well. The secretory cells are cuboidal, changing to a cylindrical shape just prior to milk secretion, while cellular water uptake is increased. The cell's single nucleus is at the base in the dormant cell but migrates to the apex just prior to milk secretion.

The cytoplasm is finely granular in the resting phase, but striated as milk secretion begins. As secretion commences, the enlarged cell with its thickened apical membrane becomes clublike in shape. The tip pinches off, leaving the cell intact. The protein is thus free in the secreted solution, retaining a cap of membrane (Fig. 3-4).

Milk is therefore secreted by apocrine and merocrine mechanisms. There is minimal glandular mitosis in the lactating breast (Fig. 3-5).[15]

Function of the cellular components of the lactating breast

The schematic representation of the mammary secretory cell has been described by Davis and Bowman[2] (Fig. 3-6).

Nucleus. The nucleus is essential to the duplication of genetic material and the transcription of the genetic code. The nucleus is also considered a regulatory organelle in cell metabolism, transmitting the design of the enzymatic profile of the cell. The DNA and RNA content of the cellular nuclei increases during pregnancy and is highest at the time of lactation.

Cytosol. The cytosol, which consists of the cytoplasm minus the mitochondrial and microsomal fractions, is also called the particle-free supernatant. The cytosol contains enzymes that involve key intermediates and cofactors essential to the process of milk synthesis.

Mitochondrial proliferation. Mitochondria are increased in the epithelial cell at the onset of the lactation process. Mitochondrial proliferation has been observed

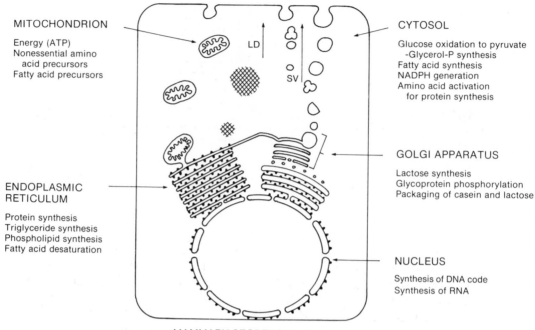

MITOCHONDRION

Energy (ATP)
Nonessential amino
acid precursors
Fatty acid precursors

CYTOSOL

Glucose oxidation to pyruvate
-Glycerol-P synthesis
Fatty acid synthesis
NADPH generation
Amino acid activation
for protein synthesis

GOLGI APPARATUS

Lactose synthesis
Glycoprotein phosphorylation
Packaging of casein and lactose

**ENDOPLASMIC
RETICULUM**

Protein synthesis
Triglyceride synthesis
Phospholipid synthesis
Fatty acid desaturation

NUCLEUS

Synthesis of DNA code
Synthesis of RNA

MAMMARY SECRETORY CELL

Fig. 3-6. Schematic representation of cytological and biochemical interrelationships of secretory cell of mammary gland. *LD,* Lipid droplet; *SV,* secretory vesicle.

in all cells with a high metabolic rate and high oxygen utilization. As with other cells, the mitochondria are key to the respiratory activity of the cell. Mitochondria control some cellular metabolism through differential permeability to certain anions. The citrate in the mitochondria is a major source of carbon for fatty acid biosynthesis. Mitochondria also supply the carbon for synthesis of nonessential amino acids.

Microsomal fraction. The microsomal fraction of the cell, which includes the Golgi apparatus, the endoplasmic reticulum, and the cell membranes, is involved in lipid synthesis. The role of the microsomal fraction is also to assemble the constituent parts such as amino acids, glucose, and fatty acids into the final products of protein, carbohydrate, and fat for secretion.

Intermediary metabolism of the mammary gland

Following is a summary of the process of milk synthesis[15]:

Protein—de novo synthesis → Apocrine secretion
Fat—de novo synthesis → Apocrine secretion
Lactose—synthesis from glucose → Merocrine secretion
Ions ↔ Diffusion plus active transport
Water ↔ Diffusion
Primary alveolar milk diluted → Plasma isotonicity
by water from extracel-
lular fluid

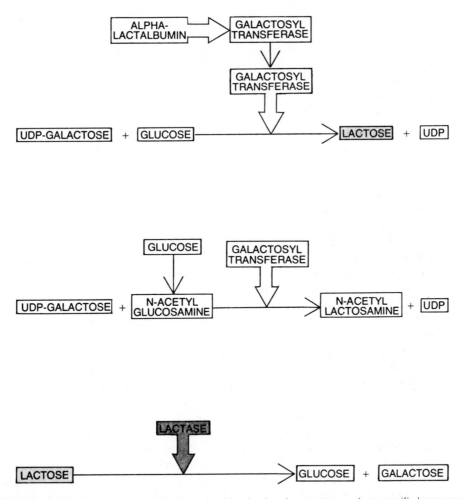

Fig. 3-7. Synthesis of lactose in mammary gland begins late in pregnancy when specific hormones and protein α-lactalbumin are present. Latter modifies enzyme galactosyl transferase, "specifying" it so that it catalyzes synthesis of lactose from glucose and galactose *(top)*. In nonlactating gland glucose and galactose *(bottom)*. (From Kretchmer, N.: Lactose and lactase, Sci. Am. **227:**71, copyright © 1972 by Scientific American, Inc. All rights reserved.)

Glucose. Glucose metabolism is a key function in milk production. Glucose serves as the main source of energy for other reactions as well as a critical source of carbon. Glucose is critical to the volume of milk produced. Glucose is also used in the production of lactose. The synthesis of lactose combines glucose and galactose, the latter originating from glucose-6-phosphate.

Lactose synthesis is carried out by the following equation, as described by Turkington[13]:

$$\text{UDP-galactose} + N\text{-acetylglucosamine} \rightarrow N\text{-Acetyllactosamine} + \text{UDP} \qquad \textbf{(1)}$$

$$\text{UDP-galactose} + \text{glucose} \rightarrow \text{Lactose} + \text{UDP} \qquad \textbf{(2)}$$

UDP is uridine diphosphogalactose. The catalyst in equation 1 is a galactosyl transferase, N-acetyllactosamine synthetase.

Most of the intracellular glucose is derived from blood sugar. A specific whey protein, α-lactalbumin, catalyzes the lactose synthesis (Fig. 3-7). It is a rate-limiting enzyme, which is inhibited by progesterone during pregnancy. In the absence of α-lactalbumin, little lactose is present. With the drop in progesterone and estrogen levels after the removal of the placenta at delivery, there is an increase in prolactin. The synthesis of α-lactalbumin becomes greater, and large amounts of lactose are produced from glucose. Progesterone regulates the onset of lactose synthesis, causing the initiation of production just as the infant is in need of nutrition.

Fat. Fat synthesis takes place in the endoplasmic reticulum. The alveolar cells are able to synthesize short-chain fatty acids, which are derived predominantly from acetate. Long-chain fatty acids, derived chiefly from blood plasma, are used in milk fat. Triglycerides are utilized from the plasma, as well as synthesized from intracellular glucose oxidized via the pentose pathway. Synthesis of fat from carbohydrate plays a predominant role in fat production in human milk.

Two enzymes, lipoprotein lipase and palmitoyl-CoA L-glycerol-3-phosphate palmitoyl transferase, increase markedly after delivery. The lipase acts at the walls of the capillaries to catalyze the lipolysis and uptake of glycerol into the epithelial cells. The transferase catalyzes the process of synthesizing glycerides to triglycerides. It is believed that the marked increase of the lipase and transferase is stimulated by prolactin. Hormonal control of the glycerol precursors and the enzymatic release of fatty acids, leading to the formation of triglycerides, has been associated not only with prolactin but also with insulin, which stimulates the uptake of glucose into the mammary cells.

Esterification of fatty acids takes place in the endoplasmic reticulum. The triglycerides subsequently accumulate into fat droplets in several cisternae. The small droplets sit on the base of the cell and coalesce to larger droplets that move toward the apex of the cell. The fat droplets are engulfed in the apical membrane, and project into the alveolar lumen. The droplets are discharged by apocrine secretion. Apocrine secretion involves the bulging of the cell apex to envelop the fat globules, protein, and a small amount of cytoplasm; with the pinching off, the globule becomes detached into the lumen. The membrane of the fat globule contains all the normal plasma enzymes. The fat droplets contain predominantly polar lipid and phosphatidyl choline.

Fatty acid synthesis involves a source of substrates and associated enzymes for their conversion to acetyl-CoA and NADPH in the cytoplasm of the cell and the conversion of acetyl-CoA to malonyl-CoA. The newly synthesized fatty acid is then released from the fatty acid synthetase complex.

Protein. Most proteins in milk are formed from free amino acids in the secretory cells of the mammary gland. The definitive data confirming the origin of milk proteins were accumulated in the past two decades. The vast majority of proteins present in normal milk are specific to mammary secretions and are not identified in any quantity elsewhere in nature.[6]

The formation of milk protein and mammary enzymes is induced by prolactin and further stimulated by insulin and cortisol. De novo synthesis of protein uses both essential and nonessential plasma amino acids. Nuclear ribonucleic acids,

Table 3-2. Alveolar epithelial membrane permeability

Cell ↔ alveolar lumen	Cell → alveolar lumen
Glucose	Lactose
Water	Sucrose
Sodium	Citrate
Potassium	Proteins
Calcium	Fat
Chloride	
Iodine	
Phosphate	
Sulfate	

induced by prolactin, stimulate synthesis of messenger and transfer RNA. The messenger RNA conveys the genetic information to the protein-synthesizing centers of the cells. The transfer RNA interprets the message to assemble the amino acids in the appropriate sequence of polypeptide chains of the specific milk proteins. The newly synthesized proteins are secreted into the milk during lactation. Casein, α-lactalbumin, and β-lactoglobulin from plasma amino acids are synthesized on the ribosomes of the endoplasmic reticulum, where they are condensed and appear as visible secretory granules moving toward the cellular apex. Proteins are discharged predominantly by apocrine secretion. There is, however, some merocrine secretion, in which proteins and other cellular constituents are secreted, leaving the cell membrane intact. Protein caps or signets, protruding into alveolar lumen, have been described on the outside of the apical membrane. Protein and lactose secreted into the lumen cannot be reabsorbed (Table 3-2).

The synthesis of proteins in the mammary gland follows the general pathway of all proteins under genetic control. Induction of synthesis is under hormonal control. This process involves synthesis from amino acids via the detailed system controlled by RNA and under genetic control of DNA.

Ions and water. Sodium, potassium, chloride, magnesium, calcium, phosphate, sulfate, and citrate pass the membrane of the alveolar cell in both directions. Water also passes in both directions, predominantly, from the alveolar cells, but also from the interstitial fluid. Plasma water passage depends on the amount of intracellular glucose available for lactose. The aqueous phase of milk is isosmotic to plasma. The major osmole of the aqueous phase of milk is lactose. The concentrations of sodium and chloride are less than those in plasma.

Human milk differs from that of many other species in that the monovalent ions are in low concentration and lactose is in high concentration.[8] The osmolarity is the same, that is, isosmotic with plasma, thus the higher the lactose, the lower the ions. It is presumed that the intracellular concentration of potassium is held high and that of sodium low by a pump on the basal membrane. The sodium and potassium ions are distributed according to the electrical potential gradient. Milk is electrically positive compared to intracellular fluid. The ratio of sodium to potassium is 1:3 in both milk and intracellular fluid. It is thought by Vorherr[15] that lactose secretion is responsible for the potential difference across the apical membrane, thus keeping sodium and potassium ion concentration low.

The variation from species to species in the concentration of lactose and ions is due to the rate of lactose synthesis, the permeability of the membrane, and the number of fixed negative charges on the membrane. The potential difference is higher in the human mammary gland than in any other species evaluated to date.

Citrate is the main buffer system of milk. It is formed within the secretory cell, but how it is secreted into the milk is not clear. It is suggested that citrate and lactose are secreted by a similar route. Following the dilution of milk in the gland with isosmotic lactose, the equilibrium is restored across the apical membrane in experimental models by sodium, potassium, and chloride entering the milk. No citrate, calcium, or protein enters in excess of normal secretion rate. Inorganic phosphate is the other major buffer system, but how it is secreted is also unknown.

Calcium, much of which is bound to casein, enters the Golgi apparatus, where it is essentially trapped, then enters the alveolar milk by unidirectional flow.

Milk enzymes. Some milk enzymes enter the alveolar milk from the mammary blood capillaries via the intercellular fluid. Others come from the breakdown of the mammary secretory cells. The milk enzymes, xanthine oxidase, aldolase, and alkaline phosphatase, are contained in the fat globule, membrane, and milk serum. The most significant enzyme, lipase, splits triglycerides. Amylase, catalase, peroxidase, and alkaline and acid phosphate are not known to contribute to the infant's digestion of human milk.

Cellular components. Human milk has been called a live fluid by many and "white blood" in many ancient rites. Breast milk contains about 4000 cells/ml, which have been identified with leukocytes.[15] The cell number is particularly high in colostrum. The cells in greatest number are the macrophages, which secrete lysozyme and lactoferrin. Lymphocytes, neutrophils, and epithelial cells are also present. Lymphocytes produce IgA and interferon.

REFERENCES

1. Cowie, A. T.: Comparative physiology of lactation, Proc. R. Soc. Med. **65:**1084, 1972.
2. Davis, C. L., and Bowman, D. E.: General metabolism associated with the synthesis of milk. In Larson, B. L., and Smith, V. R., editors: Lactation, vol. II. Biosynthesis and secretion of milk/maintenance, New York, 1974, Academic Press, Inc.
3. Fournier, P. J. R., Desjardins, P. D., and Friesen, H. G.: Current understanding of human prolactin physiology and its diagnostic and therapeutic applications: a review, Am. J. Obstet. Gynecol. **118:**337, 1974.
4. Frantz, A. G.: Prolactin, Physiol. Med. **298:**201, 1978.
5. Josimovich, J. B., Reynolds, M., and Cobo, E.: Lactogenic hormones, fetal nutrition, and lactation. In Josimovich, J. B., Reynolds, M., and Cobo, E., editors: Problems of human reproduction, vol. 2, New York, 1974, John Wiley & Sons.
6. Larson, B. L., editor: Lactation, vol. IV. The mammary gland/human lactation/milk synthesis, New York, 1978, Academic Press, Inc.
7. Larson, B. L., and Smith, V. R., editors: Lactation, vol. II. Biosynthesis and secretion of milk/diseases, New York, 1974, Academic Press, Inc.
8. Larson, B. L., and Smith, V. R., editors: Lactation, vol. III. Nutrition and biochemistry of milk/maintenance, New York, 1974, Academic Press, Inc.
9. Meites, J.: Neuroendocrinology of lactation, J. Invest. Dermatol. **63:**119, 1974.
10. Sherwood, L. M.: Human prolactin, N. Engl. J. Med. **284:**774, 1971.
11. Smith, V. R.: Lactation, vol. I. The mammary gland/development and maintenance, New York, 1974, Academic Press, Inc.

12. Spellacy, W. N., and Buhi, W. C.: Pituitary growth hormone and placental lactogen levels measured in normal term pregnancy and at the early and late postpartum periods, Am. J. Obstet. Gynecol. **105**:888, 1969.
13. Turkington, R. W.: Human prolactin, editorial, Am. J. Med. **53**:389, 1972.
14. Tyson, J. E.: Mechanisms of puerperal lactation, Med. Clin. North Am. **61**:153, 1977.
15. Vorherr, H.: The breast, morphology, physiology and lactation, New York, 1974, Academic Press, Inc.

CHAPTER 4

Biochemistry of human milk

The constituents of milk include a tremendous array of molecules whose descriptions have only recently been refined as qualitative and quantitative laboratory techniques have been perfected. Resolution of lipid chemicals has advanced dramatically in recent years, but new compounds have been identified in carbohydrate and protein as well. Some of the compounds recently identified may well be intermediary products in the process that occurs within the mammary cells and only incidental in the final product.[57]

Human and bovine milk are known in the greatest detail.[23] There is, however, much information about five other species, including water buffalo, goat, sheep, horse, and pig. There are miscellaneous scattered data on the milk of 150 more species and no data at all on another 4000 species. Jenness and Sloan[29] have compiled a summary of 140 species from which a sampling has been extracted (Table 4-1). Jenness and Sloan have further pointed out that the constituents of milk can be divided into the following groups, according to their specificity:

1. Constituents specific to both organ and species (example: most proteins and lipids)
2. Constituents specific to organ but not to species (example: lactose)
3. Constituents specific to species but not to organ (example: albumen and some immunoglobulins)

NORMAL VARIATIONS IN HUMAN MILK

In defining the constituents of human milk, it is important to recognize that the composition varies with the stage of lactation, the time of day, the sampling time during a given feeding, maternal nutrition, and individual variation. Many early interpretations of the content of human milk were based on spot samples or even pooled samples from multiple donors at different times and stages of lactation. Samples obtained by pumping may vary from those obtained by the suckling infant, in view of the variation in content between the various methods of pumping.

An example of variation is the fat content. Fat content changes during a given feeding, increasing at the end of the feeding. Fat content rises from early morning to midday; the volume increases from two to five times, according to studies by Hall.[22] In the later part of the first year of lactation, the fat content diminishes (Fig. 4-1). Recent work by Atkinson and co-workers[3] has suggested that the nitrogen content of the milk of mothers who deliver prematurely is higher. For a given volume of milk, the premature infant would receive 20% more nitrogen than the full-term infant, if both were fed their own mother's milk.

An additional consideration in reviewing information available on the levels of various constituents is the technique used to derive the data. In 1977, Hambraeus[24] reported that there was less protein in human milk than originally calculated. The present techniques of immunoassay measure the absolute amounts, whereas earlier figures were derived from calculations from the nitrogen content. About 25% of the nitrogen in human milk is nonprotein nitrogen. Cow's milk has only 5% nonprotein nitrogen.

A major concern regarding variation in content of human milk is related to the mother's diet. Maternal diet is of particular concern when the mother is malnourished or eats an unusually restrictive diet. Malnourished mothers have

Table 4-1. Constituents of milk of specific mammals*

Mammalian species in taxonomic position	Total solids (g/100 g)	Fat (g/100 g)	Casein (g/100 g)	Whey protein (g/100 g)	Total protein (g/100 g)	Lactose (g/100 ml)	Ash (g/100 g)
Man	12.4	3.8	0.4	0.6		7.0	0.2
Baboon	14.4	5.0			1.6	7.3	0.3
Orangutan	11.5	3.5	1.1	0.4		6.0	0.2
Black bear	44.5	24.5	8.8	5.7		0.4	1.8
California sea lion	52.7	36.5			13.8	0.0	0.6
Black rhinoceros	8.1	0.0	1.1	0.3		6.1	0.3
Spotted dolphin	31.0	18.0			9.4	0.6	—
Domestic dog	23.5	12.9	5.8	2.1		3.1	1.2
Norway rat	21.0	10.3	6.4	2.0		2.6	1.3
Whitetail jackrabbit	40.8	13.9	19.7	4.0		1.7	1.5

*Modified from Jenness, R., and Sloan, R. E.: Composition of milk. In Larson, B. L., and Smith, V. R., editors: Lactation, vol. III. Nutrition and biochemistry of milk/maintenance, New York, 1974, Academic Press, Inc.

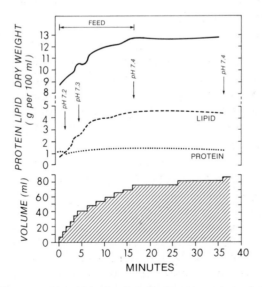

Fig. 4-1. Changes in milk composition during feeding. Continuous analysis of milk of one woman with 5-week-old infant. Infant fed at left breast while milk pumped from right breast. (Modified from Hall, B.: Lancet **1:**779, April 5, 1975.)

approximately the same proportions of protein, fat, and carbohydrate, but they produce less milk. Water-soluble vitamins, ascorbic acid, thiamin, and B_{12} levels are quickly affected by deficient diets.

COLOSTRUM

The consistently identifiable stages of human milk are colostrum, transitional milk, and mature milk, and their relative contents are significant for the newborn infant and his physiological adaption to extrauterine life.

The residual mixture of materials present in the mammary glands and ducts at delivery and immediately after is progressively mixed with newly secreted milk, forming colostrum. Human colostrum is known to differ from mature milk in composition, both in the nature of its components and in their relative proportions. The first postpartum week's mammary secretion consists of a yellowish, thick fluid, colostrum. Its specific gravity is 1.040 to 1.060. The mean energy value is 67 kcal/100 ml compared to the 75 kcal/100 ml of mature milk. The volume varies between 2 and 10 dl/feeding/day in the first 3 days. The volume also varies with the parity of the mother. Women who have had other pregnancies, particularly those who have nursed infants previously, have colostrum more readily available at delivery, and the volume increases more rapidly. The yellow color is due to β-carotene. The ash content is high, and the concentrations of sodium, potassium, and chloride are greater than in mature milk. Protein, fat-soluble vitamins, and minerals are present in greater percentages than in transitional or mature milk.

Colostrum facilitates the establishment of bifidus flora in the digestive tract. Colostrum also facilitates the passage of meconium. Meconium contains an essential growth factor for *Lactobacillus bifidus* and is the first culture medium in the sterile intestinal lumen of the newborn infant. Human colostrum is rich in antibodies, which may provide protection against various infections.

A survey of the fatty acid components by Read and Sarrif[48] showed the lauric acid and myristic acid content to be low in concentration the first few days. When the lauric and myristic acid increased, C_{18} acids decreased. Palmitoleic acid increased at the same rate as the myristic acid. From this it was concluded that the early fatty acids are derived from extramammary sources, but the breast quickly begins to synthesize fatty acids for the production of transitional and mature milk (Table 4-2). The total fat content may have a predictive value, since it was shown by Hytten[26] that 90% of the women whose milk contained 20 g or more of fat per feeding on the seventh day were successfully breast-feeding 3 months later.

Table 4-2. Fat distribution in milk in milligrams

Fat distribution	Colostrum (1 to 5 days)	Transitional (6 to 10 days)	Mature (after 30 days)	Cow's milk
Lipid phosphorus	2	3	4	4
Total cholesterol	27	29	20	14
Lecithin	—	—	78	57
Total fats	2900	3600	3800	3700

From Macy, I. G., and Kelly, H. J.: Human milk in infant nutrition. In Kon, S. K., and Cowie, A. T., editors: Milk: the mammary gland and its secretion, vol. II, New York, 1961, Academic Press, Inc., p. 265.

Women who only had 5 to 10 g of fat on the seventh day had an 80% drop-out rate by 3 months.

Colostrum's high protein and low fat are in keeping with the needs and reserves of the newborn. Although the content of total nitrogen or any amino acid in breast milk in 24 hr is grossly related to the volume produced, the concentration in milligrams per 100 ml is not so related. The relative distribution of nitrogen of the individual amino acids in each 100 ml of milk differs in each mother. The colostrum may actually reflect a transitional blood picture, which is associated with nitrogen metabolism of the postpartum period. The postpartum period is one of involution of body tissue and catabolism of protein.

The mineral and vitamin reserves of the newborn infant are related to the maternal diet. A fetal supply of vitamin C, iron, and amino acids is adequate, since infant blood levels exceed those of the mother. Colostrum is rich in fat-soluble vitamin A, carotenoids, and vitamin E. The average vitamin A level on the third day can be three times that of mature milk. Similarly, carotenoids may be ten times the level in mature milk and vitamin E two to three times greater than mature milk.

TRANSITIONAL MILK

The milk produced between the colostrum and mature milk stages is transitional milk; its content gradually changes. The transitional phase is considered to be approximately from 7 to 10 days postpartum to 2 weeks postpartum. The concentration of immunoglobins and total protein decreases, while the lactose, fat, and total caloric content increase. The water-soluble vitamins increase, and the fat-soluble vitamins decrease to the levels of mature milk.

MATURE MILK
Water

In almost all milks, water is the constituent in the largest quantity with the exception of some arctic and aquatic species who produce milks with high fat content (e.g., the northern fur seal, 54% fat and 65% total solids) (Table 4-1). All other constituents are dissolved, dispersed, or suspended in water. Water contributes to the temperature-regulating mechanism of the newborn because 25% of his heat loss is from evaporation of water from the lungs and skin. The lactating woman has a greatly increased obligatory water intake. If the water intake is restricted during lactation, other water losses through urine and insensible loss are decreased before water for lactation is diminished. Since lactose is the regulating factor in amount of milk produced, the secretion of water into milk is partially regulated by lactose synthesis. Recent investigations by Almroth[1] show that the water requirement of infants in a hot humid climate can be provided entirely by the water in human milk.

Lipids

By percentage of concentration, the second most common constituent in milk is the lipid fraction, which is extractable by suitable solvents. Complete extraction in human milk is difficult because of the lipids bound to protein. From 30% to 55% of the kilocalories are derived from fats; this represents a concentration of 3.5 to 4.5 g/100 ml. Milk fat is dispersed in the form of droplets or globules maintained in solution by an adsorbed layer or membrane. The protective membrane of the fat globules is made up of phospholipid complexes. The rest of the phospholipids found in human milk are dispersed in the skim milk fraction. The principal classes of milk lipids are readily separated by chromatography. Triglycerides, diglycerides, monoglycerides, free fatty acids, phospholipids, glycolipids, sterols, and sterol esters are found in human milk. Vitamin A esters, vitamin D, vitamin K, alkylglyceryl ethers, and glyceryl ether diesters are also in the lipid fraction but do not fall into the classes listed.

Renewed interest in defining the constituents of human milk lipid has devel-

Table 4-3. Composition of milks obtained from different mammals and the growth rate of their offspring*

Species	Days required to double birth weight	Content of milk (%)			
		Fat	Protein	Lactose	Ash
Man	180	3.8	0.9	7.0	0.2
Horse	60	1.9	2.5	6.2	0.5
Cow	47	3.7	3.4	4.8	0.7
Reindeer	30	16.9	11.5	2.8	
Goat	19	4.5	2.9	4.1	0.8
Sheep	10	7.4	5.5	4.8	1.0
Rat	6	15.0	12.0	3.0	2.0

*From Hambraeus, L.: Pediatr. Clin. North Am. **24:**17, 1977.

Table 4-4. Fatty acid composition of human milk lipids as of December 1976*

Type	Number	Identity
Saturates		
Normal, even	10	4:0−22:0
Normal, odd	7	11:0−23:0
Monobranched	49	10:0−18:0†
Multibranched	5	12:0, 13:0, 15:0, 16:0‡
Monoenes		
cis §	59	10:1−18:1, 20:1
trans	3	16:1, 18:1, 20:1
Dienes	22	12:2−22:2 all even *cis, cis; cis, trans; trans, trans;* positional isomers
Polyenes		
Tri	6	18:3, 20:3, 22:3 geometric and positional isomers
Tetra	2	20:4, 22:4
Penta	2	20:5, 22:5
Hexa	1	22:6
Cyclic		
Hexane	1	11, terminal hexane
TOTAL	167	

*From Jensen, R. G., Hagerty, M. M., and McMahon, K. E.: Am. J. Clin. Nutr. **31:**990, 1978.
†Signifies *n*-acids with methyl branches.
‡Signifies *n*-acids with three or four methyl branches.
§Designated as *cis,* but not usually determined.

oped in recent years, as investigators look for the causes of obesity, atherosclerosis, and other degenerative diseases and their relationship to infant nutrition (Table 4-3). There are a number of reports of historical value that are plagued with the technical problems of sampling. Since the fat content of a feeding varies with time, spot samples give spurious results. Jensen and associates[30] have reviewed the literature exhaustively and describe the fractionated lipid constituents in detail (Table 4-4).

The average fat content of pooled 24 hr samples has been reported from various sources to vary in mature milk from 2.10% to 3.33%. Maternal diet affects the constituents of the lipids but not the total amount of fat. A minimal increase in total lipid content was observed when an extra 1000 kcal of corn oil was fed to lactating mothers. A diet rich in polyunsaturated fats will cause an increased percentage of polyunsaturated fats in the milk without altering the total fat content. When the mother is calorie deficient, depot fats are mobilized and milk resembles depot fat. When excessive nonfat kilocalories are fed, levels of saturated fatty acids increase as lipids are synthesized from tissue stores.

Fatty acid patterns of human milk were recently studied by Guthrie and colleagues[18] to determine the impact of the modern diet on milk. The USDA has reported that the average American diet now includes 156 g of fat, up from 141 g in 1947. The significant change is from animal to vegetable fat, which is now 39% of total dietary fats, due especially to the switch from butter and lard. The original studies on human milk lipids were done from 1940 to 1950. The analysis by Guthrie and co-workers[18] in 1977 shows over 56% of the fatty acids are monoenoic and polyenoic C_{18} fatty acids (i.e., 18 carbons). Oleic ($C_{18:1}$), linoleic ($C_{18:2}$), linolenic ($C_{18:3}$), and palmitic ($C_{16:0}$) acids are present in the highest amounts. The results show a change in fatty acid content to more long-chain fatty acids and a twofold to threefold increase in linoleic acid (Table 4-5).

Table 4-5. Lipid and fatty acid composition of human milk compared to literature values*

Fatty acid	Current study, Guthrie et al. (1977)	Previous studies		
		Macy et al. (1953)†	Insull and Ahrens (1958)‡	Glass et al. (1967)§
12:0 Lauric	3.8 (1.6)‖	5.5	7.0	3.1
14:0 Myristic	5.2 (1.7)	8.5	8.8	5.1
16:0 Palmitic¶	22.5 (2.6)	23.2	21.0	20.2
16:1 Palmitoleic¶	4.1 (1.3)	3.0	2.2	5.7
18:0 Stearic	8.7 (1.4)	6.9	7.2	5.9
18:1 Oleic	39.5 (3.8)	36.5	35.8	46.4
18:2 Linoleic	14.4 (4.1)	7.8	6.4	13.0
18:3 Linolenic	2.0 (0.7)	—	—	1.4
Number of samples	110	200	11	7
Total lipid (g/dl)	3.1 ± 2.2	—	3.5	—

*From Guthrie, H. A., et al.: J. Pediatr. **90**:39, 1977.
†Macy, I. G., et al.: The composition of milks, publ. no. 254, Washington, D.C., National Research Council.
‡Insull, W., and Ahrens, E. H.: Biochem. J. **72**:27, 1958.
§Glass, R. L., Trooplin, H. A., and Jenness, R.: Comp. Biochem. Physiol. **22**:415, 1967.
‖Percentage of total fatty acid (mean ± SD).
¶n = 99; smaller number due to technical error in separating $C_{16:0}$ and $C_{16:1}$ in eleven samples.

P/S is the ratio of polyunsaturated to saturated fats; polyunsaturates include $C_{18:2}$ and $C_{18:3}$, or linoleic and linolenic acid. Bovine P/S ratio is 4. The P/S ratio has shifted as a result of recent dietary changes to 1.3 from 1.35 in human milk. The P/S is significant in facilitating calcium and fat absorption. Calcium absorption is depressed by a 4:5 P/S ratio.

The breast can dehydrogenate saturated and monounsaturated fatty acids in milk synthesis. A study by Read and co-workers[49] of four groups of nursing mothers from different ethnic groups revealed that a high dietary intake of carbohydrate was associated with high lauric and myristic acid levels and low linoleic and palmitic acid levels in the milk. If the diet is high in linoleic acid and the dietary carbohydrate is moderate, then there is a high level of linoleic acid in the breast milk. Other fatty acids in the diet had little effect on the milk fatty acid produced. Palmitic acid appeared to be derived from extramammary lipid.

At least 167 fatty acids have been identified in human milk (Table 4-6); possibly others are there in trace amounts. Bovine milk has been identified to have 437 fatty acids. Marked change in fatty acid composition would be the result of major dietary changes.

Essential fatty acid requirements for humans have been studied by many investigators.[50] Diets free from added fats or linoleic acid induce deficiency symp-

Table 4-6. Lipids of human milk and infant formulas—composition of glyceryl ethers from neutral lipids (N) and phospholipids (P) in human milk lipids*

	Colostrum†		Transition milk‡		Mature milk§		Transition milk‖		Mature milk‖	
Alkylchain	N	P	N	P	N	P	N	P	N	P
12:0			0.2	0.4						
14:0	0.5	0.7	0.5	0.7	0.9	0.8	1.5	0.7	Trace	Trace
15:0	0.5	0.4	0.5	0.4	0.5	0.6	0.9	1.1	Trace	Trace
16:0	33.8	32.5	26.0	27.7	24.8	25.3	71.6	84.9	75.8	77.4
16:1	1.5	1.7	1.1	1.6	3.2	4.6				
17:0	0.7	1.1	1.2	3.8	1.4	1.8	0.8	0.5	0.6	0.3
17:1	0.6	1.0	Trace	1.1	1.6	1.5	3.5	1.0	3.3	2.7
18:0	21.2	19.1	21.5	17.8	21.8	19.0	1.8	2.6	1.8	1.2
18:1	29.7	29.2	38.3	34.1	37.5	34.7	19.9	8.0	18.5	16.7
19:0	0.1	0.1	0.1	0.1	0.1	0.1		0.5		0.7
19:1	0.3	0.3	0.1	0.2	0.4	0.5		0.7		0.1
20:0	1.6	2.1	1.4	1.8	0.9	1.6				0.2
20:1	1.2	2.4	1.4	2.1	1.7	2.4				0.1
21:0 and 1	0.1	0.1	0.1	0.3	0.3	0.5				0.2
22:0	1.3	1.4	1.0	1.2	0.7	0.9				Trace
22:1	3.0	3.7	3.1	2.9	2.7	2.8				0.2
23.0 and 1	0.3	Trace	0.2	0.2	0.1	0.6				
24:0	0.5	0.4	0.3	0.6	Trace	0.4				
24:1	3.1	3.8	3.0	1.4	1.9					

*From Jensen, R. G., Hagerty, M. M., and McMahon, K. E.: Am. J. Clin. Nutr. **31**:990, 1978.
†From 1 to 2 days.
‡From 3 to 7 days.
§From 8 days to 3 months.
‖2-Methoxy substituted glyceryl ethers.

toms in infants. These symptoms include skin lesions, insufficient weight gains, and poor wound healing. Low-fat diets in newborn rats have affected cerebral function. The American Academy of Pediatrics has recently recommended that infant formulas contain a minimum of 3.3 g of fat/kcal (30% of total kilocalories) and 300 mg of linoleic acid (18.2)/100 kcal (about 1.7% of total kilocalories). It did not set a limit on linoleic content of diet, since some human milks have 8% to 10% of the fat as linoleic acid (Table 4-7). Studies of vegetarians (Table 4-8) have shown extremely high levels of linoleic acid, four times that of cow's milk. Some researchers include other long-chain fatty acids such as $C_{20:2}$, $C_{20:3}$, $C_{20:4}$, and $C_{22:3}$ as essential nutrients because they are structural lipids in the brain and nervous tissue.

Table 4-7. Fatty acid composition of some commercial infant formulas*

Manufacturer	Source of fat	Fatty acid (wt %)									
		4:0–8:0	10:0	12:0	14:0	16:0	18:0	18:1	18:2	18:3	Miscellaneous
Gerber MBF†	Sesame, beef hearts				0.7	14.4	7.3	43.0	32.7	0.7	1.2
Loma Linda‡											
Soyalac powder	Soy					9.8	3.3	23.2	55.7	7.4	
Soyalac, conc, liquid	Soy					9.1	3.5	21.8	57.8	7.8	
Soyalac, 87%, H₂O	Soy					8.0	3.3	22.7	59.7	6.3	
Mead Johnson†											
Enfamil 20	Soy and coconut	1.9	1.1	10.0	4.1	11.1	3.8	21.1	41.1	5.9	
Pregestamil	MCT§ and corn			20.0	(>2.9)	1.4	0.4	3.9	7.1		
Premature formula‖	Corn				0.3	10.0	3.0	30.5	56.2		
Prosobee	Soy				0.3	10.6	4.7	24.4	50.3	8.5	
Ross†											
Similac powder, liquid 60/40	Coconut and corn	4.2	3.6	29.7	11.7	10.3	2.8	15.2	22.5		
Similac, conc, liquid RTF, Isomil	Coconut and soy	4.2	3.6	29.7	11.7	9.5	2.8	13.6	21.3	3.6	
Advance conc, liquid and RTF	Soy and corn	0.01	0.1	0.5	0.4	10.7	4.7	24.5	53.7	4.7	0.7
Syntex† ¶	Soy				0.1	8.0	4.0	28.0	54.0	5.0	0.8
Wyeth SMA†	Oleo, coconut, safflower and soy	2.0	1.4	14.5	6.0	12.8	7.4	38.9	13.1	1.1	2.8

*Jensen, R. G., Hagerty, M. M., McMahon, K. E.: Am. J. Clin. Nutr. **31**:990, 1978.
†Data supplied by manufacturers.
‡Analyzed by Jensen et al.
§Medium chain TGs.
‖Source of fat to be changed to 40% medium chain TGs, 40% corn oil, and 20% coconut oil as of April 1977.
¶Includes Mullsoy, Neomullsoy, and carbohydrate-free formulations.

Table 4-8. Breast milk fatty acids in vegans and omniovore controls* †

Methyl esters	Vegans			Controls		
	Mean	SE	Range	Mean	SE	Range
$C_{12:0}$ Lauric	39	12.5	21-76	33	7.1	19-51
$C_{14:0}$ Myristic	68	17.0	50-118	80	5.3	68-90
$C_{16:0}$ Palmitic	166‡	14.4	139-204	276	10.5	246-293
$C_{18:0}$ Stearic	52‡	5.9	37-66	108	8.5	84-123
$C_{16:1}$ Palmitoleic	12‡	0.9	11-15	36	5.3	25-46
$C_{18:1}$ Oleic	313	25.0	277-383	353	11.1	331-383
$C_{18:2\omega6}$ Linoleic	317‡	44.5	202-397	69	8.1	56-91
$C_{18:3\omega3}$ Linolenic	15‡	2.4	9-20	8	0.5	7-9

*Modified from Sanders, T. A. B., et al.: Am. J. Clin. Nutr. **31**:805, 1978.
†Mean values expressed as milligrams per gram total methyl esters detected for four vegans and four omniovore controls.
‡Statistical significance of difference between means shown when p < 0.05.

Different periods of brain development have been described biochemically by Sinclair and Crawford.[53] First there is cell division, with the formation of neurons and glial cells, and second, myelination. They showed in the rat brain that 50% of polyenoic acids of the gray matter lipids were laid down by the fifteenth day of life. The fatty acids characteristic of myelin lipids appeared later. Gray matter is largely composed of unmyelinated neurons, whereas white matter contains a very high proportion of myelinated conducting nerve fibers. Normal brain function depends on both.

The fatty acids characteristic of gray matter ($C_{20:4}$ and $C_{22:6}$) accumulate prior to the appearance of fatty acids characteristic of myelin ($C_{20:1}$ and $C_{24:1}$) in the developing brain. Arachidonic ($C_{20:4}$) and docosahexaenoic ($C_{22:6}$) acids are synthesized from linoleic and linolenic respectively, but the latter two must be obtained in the diet.

The essential fatty acids, linoleic and linolenic acids, may have greater significance in the quality of the myelin laid down. Dick[10] has made a very interesting observation in the geographical distribution of multiple sclerosis worldwide. He notes that the disease is rare in countries where breast-feeding is common. He postulates that the development of myelin in infancy is critical to preventing degradation later. Dick is presently investigating the difference between human milk and cow's milk in relation to myelin production in multiple sclerosis.

Experimental allergic encephalitis is a demyelinating condition, which can be produced by shocking animals that have been sensitized to central nervous system (CNS) antigens. Newborn rats deficient in essential fatty acids are more susceptible to experimental allergic encephalitis, which has recently been described as resembling multiple sclerosis pathologically.

Widdowson[58] analyzed the body fats of children from Britain and Holland. At birth, body fat was 1.3% linoleic acid for both groups of children. British infants received cow's milk formulas that contained 1.8% linoleic acid. The Dutch infants received corn-oil formulas that were 58.2% linoleic acid. The Dutch infants had body fat that was 25% linoleic acid at 1 month of age and 32% to 37% at 4 months of age. The infant receiving cow's milk formulas had 3% or less linoleic acid in their body fat. The Dutch infants also had lower serum cholesterol levels. The children are now approximately 10 years old and appear to be entirely normal.

Cholesterol. Cholesterol has been a factor of great concern because of the apparent association with risk factors for atherosclerosis and coronary heart disease. At present, commercial formulas have high P/S ratios and low cholesterol levels compared to human milk. Dietary manipulation does not change the cholesterol level in the breast milk.[46] When the dietary cholesterol level was controlled, a fall in the infant's plasma cholesterol levels was, however, associated with an increase in the amount of linoleic acid in the milk.[45]

No long-range effect of serum cholesterol level has been identified, although Osborn[42] described the pathological changes in 1500 young people (newborns to age 20). He observed the spectrum of pathological changes from mucopolysaccharide accumulations to fully developed atherosclerotic plaques. Lesions were more frequent and severe in children who had been bottle-fed. Lesions were uncommon or mild in the breast-fed children. Investigations done on rats indicated that animals given high levels of cholesterol early in life were better able to cope with cholesterol in later life and maintained a lower cholesterol level.

The validity of the results of several studies done on human infants with controlled cholesterol intakes has been questioned. The mean serum cholesterol levels for the breast-fed infants were significantly higher (147 mg/100 ml) than those of bottle-fed infants (130 mg/100 ml). A year later, when all the infants were on regular diets, the levels were similar. The cholesterol content of human milk varies markedly from 104 to 208 mg/L. There is insufficient information to determine the value or risk of cholesterol in human milk as compared to low-cholesterol milks. It appears that cholesterol absorption can be inhibited by certain substances such as orotic acid. Orotic acid is high in bovine milk and yogurt and is presumably absent in human milk. From the data available, the purpose of cholesterol in human milk has not as yet been determined, beyond the belief that the composition of human milk must be best for human infants.[59]

Lipases. Milk fat is almost completely digestible. The emulsion of fat in breast milk is greater than in cow's milk, resulting in smaller globules. Milk lipases play an active role in creating the emulsion, which yields a finer curd and facilitates the digestion of triacylglycerols. The newborn easily digests and completely uses the well-emulsified small fat globules of human milk. Free fatty acids are important sources of energy for the infant. The lipase in human milk makes the free fatty acids available in a large proportion even before the digestive phase of the intestine. The lipolytic milk-enzyme activity is similar to the activity of pancreatic lipase, breaking down triglycerides to free fatty acids and glycerol. The enzyme is present in the fat fraction and is inhibited by bile salts. There are additional lipases in the skim milk fraction, and these are stimulated by bile salts. The lipase stimulated by bile salts has greater activity and splits all three ester bonds of the triglyceride. This lipase is also stable in the duodenum and contributes to the hydrolysis of the triacylglycerols in the presence of the bile salts.[25]

When fresh human milk is refrigerated or even placed in a deep freeze, lipolysis takes place, as demonstrated by the appearance of free fatty acids and a lowering of the pH of the milk. Apparently, even in the absence of bile salts, some lipolysis can take place. Since the fat of human milk contains a high proportion of palmitic acid in the number 2 position, it will be absorbed as a 2-monoglyceride from the intestine. This has been shown to have a more rapid absorption time but, in addition, does not bind calcium and interfere with calcium absorption, as the free palmitic acid of cow's milk does. The palmitic acid of cow's milk is in the number 1 and 3 positions.

Protein

All milks have been evaluated for their protein contents, which vary from species to species, 0.9% in human milk to 20% in some rabbit species. Proteins of milk include casein, serum albumen, and α-lactalbumen, β-lactoglobulins, immunoglobulins and other glycoproteins. Eight of twenty amino acids present in milk are essential and are derived from plasma. The mammary alveolar epithelium synthesizes some nonessential amino acids (Table 4-9).

Casein. It is well known that milk consists of casein, or curds, and whey proteins, or lactalbumins. The term casein includes a group of milk-specific proteins characterized by ester-bound phosphate, high-proline content, and low solubility at pH of 4.0 to 5.0. Caseins form complex particles or micelles, which are usually complexes of calcium caseinate and calcium phosphate. When milk clots or curdles due to heat, pH changes, or enzymes, the casein is transformed into an insoluble calcium caseinate–calcium phosphate complex. There are phys-

Table 4-9. Nonprotein contents and amino acid components of human milk (compared to cow's milk, in milligrams)*

Constituents	Colostrum (1-5 days)	Transitional (6-10 days)	Mature (after 30 days)	Cow's milk
Nonprotein components				
Creatine	—	—	3.3	3.1
Creatinine	—	—	2.2	0.9
Urea	—	23.3	32.2	15.1
Uric acid	—	—	4.6	1.9
Dispensable amino acids				
Alanine	—	—	35	75
Aspartic acid	—	—	116	166
Cystine	—	55	29	29
Glutamic acid	—	—	230	680
Glycine	—	—	0	11
Proline	—	—	80	250
Serine	—	—	69	160
Tyrosine	—	125	62	190
Indispensable amino acids				
Arginine	126	64	51	124
Histidine	57	38	23	80
Isoleucine	121	97	86	212
Leucine	221	151	161	356
Lysine	163	113	79	257
Methionine	33	24	23	87
Phenylalanine	105	63	64	173
Threonine	148	79	62	152
Tryptophan	52	28	22	50
Valine	169	105	90	228

*From Macy, I. G., and Kelly, H. J.: Human milk and cow's milk in infant nutrition. In Kon, S. K., and Cowie, A. T., editors: Milk: the mammary gland and its secretion, vol. II, New York, 1961, Academic Press, Inc.

iochemical differences between human and cow caseins. Casein has a species-specific amino acid composition.

METHIONINE/CYSTEINE RATIO. The cysteine content is high in human milk, whereas it is very low in cow's milk. Instead, the methionine content is high in bovine milk, thus the methionine/cysteine ratio is two to three times greater in cow's milk than in most mammals and seven times that in human milk. Human milk is the only animal protein in which the methionine/cysteine ratio is close to 1. Otherwise, this ratio is only seen in plant proteins. Two significant characteristics of amino acid composition of human milk are the ratio between the sulfa-containing amino acids methionine and cysteine and the low content of the aromatic amino acids phenylalanine and tyrosine. The newborn or premature infant is ill-prepared to handle phenylalanine and tyrosine due to low levels of the specific enzymes required to metabolize them.

TAURINE. A third sulfur-containing amino acid has been found in high concentrations in human milk, which is virtually absent in cow's milk and prepared formulas. Free taurine and glutamic acid have been measured in breast milk in high concentration. Taurine has been associated in the body at all ages with bile acid conjugation; in the newborn bile acids are almost exclusively conjugated with taurine. It has been suggested by the work of Sturman and associates[56] that taurine may also be a neurotransmitter or neuromodulator in the brain and retina. Taurine is found in very high concentrations in the milk of cats.[47] Kittens deprived of taurine by feeding with purified taurine-free casein diets after weaning develop retinal degeneration and blindness. The taurine levels were more severely depleted in the brain tissue, but its significance has not been identified yet.[55] Both humans and cats are unable to synthesize taurine to any degree. The process requires cystathionase and cysteinesulfinic acid decarboxylase, which are enzymes that convert methionine, cysteine, or cystine to taurine. The requirement for taurine of the developing neonate is just being explored.

Whey proteins. When clotted milk stands, the clot contracts, leaving a clear fluid called "whey," which contains water, electrolytes, and proteins. The ratio of whey proteins to casein is 1.5 for breast milk and 0.2 for cow's milk, that is, 40% of human milk protein is casein and 60% lactalbumin, and cow's milk is 80% casein and 20% lactalbumen.[59]

Human milk forms a flocculent suspension with 0 curd tension. The curds are easily digested. The total amount of protein has been recently measured to be 0.9%, which is lower than the previously reported figure of 1.2%. The discrepancy is due to recalculation of the data in which the total amount of protein was determined by measuring the nitrogen content and multiplying by 6.25. Actually, it was pointed out by Macy and Kelly[39] in 1961 that 25% of the nitrogen content is nonprotein nitrogen, whereas in bovine milk 5% of the nitrogen is from nonprotein nitrogen. Hambraeus[24] has recently reported the composition of the nonprotein fraction to be urea, creatine, creatinine, uric acid, small peptides, and free amino acids (Table 4-10).

Closer examination of the whey proteins shows α-lactalbumin and lactoferrin to be the chief fractions, with no measurable β-lactoglobulin. β-Lactoglobulin is the chief constituent of cow's milk. The term lactalbumin includes a mixture of whey proteins found in bovine milk and should not be confused with α-lactalbumin, which is a specific protein that is part of the enzyme lactose synthetase. The α-lactalbumin content parallels lactose levels in different species. Human milk is high in both lactose and α-lactalbumin.

LACTOFERRIN. Lactoferrin is an iron-binding protein that is part of the whey fraction of proteins in human milk. It is in very low amounts in bovine milk. Lactoferrin has been observed to inhibit the growth of certain iron-dependent bacteria in the gastrointestinal tract. It has been suggested that lactoferrin protects against certain gastrointestinal infections in breast-fed infants. Giving iron to newborn infants appears to inactivate the lactoferrin by saturating it with iron.

Immunoglobulins. The immunoglobulins in breast milk are distinct from those of the serum. The main immunoglobulin in serum is IgG, which is present in the amount of 1210 mg/100 ml. IgA is found in the serum at 250 mg/100 ml, a fifth the level of IgG. The reverse is true of human colostrum and milk, in which there are 1740 mg of IgA/100 ml in colostrum and 100 mg/100 ml in milk, and 43 mg of IgG/100 ml and 4 mg of IgG/100 ml are found in colostrum and milk, respectively. The IgA and IgG in human milk are derived from serum and from synthesis in the mammary gland. The IgA is secretory IgA, the principle immunoglobulin in colostrum and milk. sIgA contains an antigenic determinant associated with a secretory component. It is synthesized in the gland from two molecules of serum IgA linked by disulfide bonds. The sIgA levels are very high in colostrum the first few days and then decline rapidly, disappearing almost completely by the fourteenth day. Secretory IgA is very stable at low pH and resistant to proteolytic enzymes. It is present in the intestine of breast-fed infants and provides a protec-

Table 4-10. Composition of protein nitrogen and nonprotein nitrogen in human milk and cow's milk* †

	Human milk		Cow's milk	
Protein nitrogen		1.43 (8.9)		5.03 (31.4)
Casein nitrogen		0.40 (2.5)		4.37 (27.3)
Whey protein nitrogen		1.03 (6.4)		0.93 (5.8)
α-Lactalbumin	0.42 (2.6)		0.17 (1.1)	
Lactoferrin	0.27 (1.7)		Traces	
β-Lactoglobulin	—		0.57 (3.6)	
Lysozyme	0.08 (0.5)		Traces	
Serum albumin	0.08 (0.5)		0.07 (0.4)	
IgA	0.16 (1.0)		0.005 (0.03)	
IgG	0.005 (0.03)		0.096 (0.6)	
IgM	0.003 (0.02)		0.005 (0.03)	
Nonprotein nitrogen		0.50		0.28
Urea nitrogen	0.25		0.13	
Creatine nitrogen	0.037		0.009	
Creatinine nitrogen	0.035		0.003	
Uric acid nitrogen	0.005		0.008	
Glucosamine	0.047		?	
α-Amino nitrogen	0.13		0.048	
Ammonia nitrogen	0.002		0.006	
Nitrogen from other components	?		0.074	
TOTAL NITROGEN		1.93		5.31

*Courtesy Forsum, E., and Lönnerdal B.: Protein evaluation of breast milk and breast milk substitutes with special reference to the nonprotein nitrogen. Unpublished data.
†Values refer to grams of nitrogen per liter; values within parentheses to grams of protein per liter.

tive defense against infection by keeping viruses and bacteria from invading the mucosa. The protective qualities are further described in Chapter 5.

Lysozyme. Lysozyme is a specific protein found in high concentration in egg whites and human milk but in low concentration in bovine milk. It has been identified as a nonspecific antimicrobial factor. This enzyme is bacteriolytic against Enterobacteriaceae and gram-positive bacteria. It has been found in concentrations up to 0.2 mg/ml. Lysozyme is stable at 100° C and at an acid pH. Lysozyme contributes to the development and maintenance of specific intestinal flora of the breast-fed infant. It will be further described in Chapter 5.

Carbohydrate

The predominant carbohydrate of milk is lactose, or milk sugar. It is present in high concentration (6.8 g/100 ml in human milk and 4.9 g/100 ml in bovine milk). Lactose is a disaccharide compound of two monosaccharides, galactose and glucose. Lactose is synthesized by the mammary gland. There are a number of other carbohydrates present in milk. They are classified as monosaccharides, neutral and acid oligosaccharides, and peptide- and protein-bound carbohydrates. There is a small amount of glucose (14 mg/100 ml) and galactose (12 mg/100 ml) present in breast milk also. There are other complex carbohydrates present in free form

Table 4-11. Amounts of disaccharides that can be hydrolyzed in vitro by the entire small intestinal mucosa at maximal velocities* in 24 hours†

Gesta-tional age (lunar months)	Num-ber of cases	Disaccharide (g/24 hours)			Lactose	
		Maltose	Sucrose	Isomaltose	Younger than 1 day	Older than 1 day
Between 2 and 3 months	3	0.05 (0.002−0.08)	0.02 (0.0008−0.035)	0.02 (0.0005−0.03)	0.01 (0.002−0.03)	
Between 3 and 4 months	2	1 (0.5−1.5)	0.72 (0.27−1.17)	0.40 (0.19−0.62)	0.12	
4 months and 25 days	1	5.2	2.7	1.9	0.8	
6 months	1	10	6.4	3.9	0.3	
Between 7 and 8 months	6	30 (10.5−43.5)	13 (6.6−25)	8.9 (4.4−15.7)	3.8 (3−4.7)	6.4 (2.8−8.3)
Between 8 and 9 months	8	60 (43−79)	34 (28.4−45)	21.3 (16.2−28)	5.8 (4.1−8)	23.4 (13.2−33.4)
9 months and 6 days	1	68	37	26.2		14.4
10 months	3	107 (90−123)	72 (59−87)	46 (38.5−51)		62 (57−67)

*The observed velocity of the in vitro reactions was converted to apparent maximal velocities as calculated by Auricchio et al.

†From Aurricchio, S., Rubino, A., and Murset, E.: Pediatrics **35**:944, 1965, copyright American Academy of Pediatrics, 1965.

or bound to amino acids or protein, such as *N*-acetylglucosamine. The concentration of oligosaccharides is about ten times greater than in cow's milk. This difference arises, no doubt, from biosynthetic control mechanisms yet to be described. These carbohydrates and glycoproteins possess bifidus factor activity. There is also fucose, which is not present in bovine milk and may be important to the early establishment of *L. bifidus* as gut flora. The nitrogen-containing carbohydrates are 0.7% of milk solids.

Observations have documented the fact that the enzyme for digesting lactose, lactase, is only seen in mammals, and, moreover, it gradually disappears from the intestinal tract in infancy. The tapering occurs after age 3 and is complete by age 5. It is considered abnormal to maintain measurable levels of lactase in adult life. Studies[4,52] of enzyme levels in the premature and newborn intestinal tract show lactase to be one of the last to appear and thus would make the use of lactose by a premature under 30 weeks gestation minimal (Table 4-11).

Lactose does appear to be specific, however, for newborn growth. It has been shown to enhance calcium absorption and has been suggested as being critical to

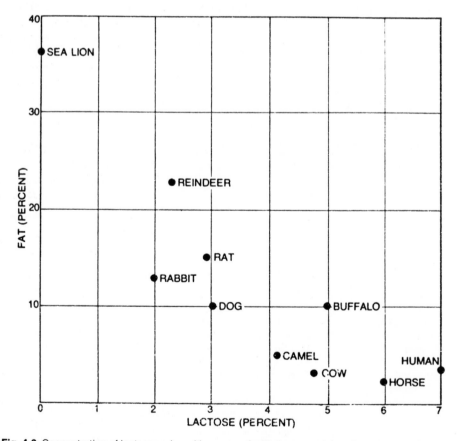

Fig. 4-2. Concentration of lactose varies with source of milk. In general, less lactose, more fat, which can also be utilized by newborn animal as energy source. (From Kretchmer, N.: Lactose and lactase, Sci. Am. **227:**73, copyright © 1972 by Scientific American, Inc. All rights reserved.)

the prevention of rickets, in view of the relatively low calcium levels in human milk.[38] Lactose is a readily available source of galactose, which is essential to the production of the galactolipids, including cerebroside. These galactolipids are essential to CNS development.

Interesting correlations have been made between the amount of lactose in a species milk and the relative size of the brain (Fig. 4-2). Excessive lactose does not make a brain bigger. It should also be noted that porpoises and dolphins have practically no lactose in their milks (0.6% to 1.3%), although they have high total solids (31.0% to 41.0%). These mammals have been considered by some to be very intelligent. The fact that lactose is only found in milk and not in other animal and plant sources enhances the significance of its high level in human milk. Lactose levels are quite constant throughout the day in a given mother's milk. Even in poorly nourished mothers the levels of lactose do not vary. Since lactose is influential in controlling volume, the total output for the day may be diminished, but the concentration of lactose in human milk will be 6.2 to 7.2 g/100 ml (Table 4-12).

Nucleotides

Nucleotides are compounds derived from nucleic acid by hydrolysis and consist of phosphoric acid combined with a sugar and a purine or pyrimidine derivative. The level and components of acid-soluble nucleotides of several species, including humans, have been studied, since recent work has shown a characteristic nucleotide composition in the milk that differed from that of the mammary gland. Johke[31] reviewed the existing knowledge on nucleotides in milk. The

Table 4-12. Fat, lactose, protein, and calcium content of mature human milk from some well-nourished and poorly nourished communities*

Community	Study	Fat (g/100 ml)	Lactose (g/100 ml)	Protein (g/100 ml)	Calcium (mg/100 ml)
Well nourished					
America	Macy (1949)	4.5	6.8	1.1	34.0
Britain	Kon and Mawson (1960)	4.78	6.95	1.16	29.9
Alexandria, Egypt (healthy women)	Hanafy, et al. (1972)	4.43	6.65	1.09	—
Brazil (high-economic status)	Carneiro and Dutra (1973)	3.9	6.8	1.3	20.8
Poorly nourished					
India	Belavady and Gopalan (1959)	3.42	7.51	1.06	34.2
South Africa (Bantu)	Walker, Arvidsson, and Draper (1952)	3.90	7.10	1.35	28.7
Brazil (low economic status)	Carneiro and Dutra (1973)	4.2	6.5	1.3	25.7
Ibadan, Nigeria	Naismith (1973)	4.05	7.67	1.22	—
Pakistan	Lindblad and Rahimtoola (1974)	2.73	6.20	0.8-0.9	28.4
Chimbu, New Guinea Highlands	Venkatachalam (1962)	2.36	7.34	1.01	—

*Modified from Jelliffe, D. B., and Jelliffe, E. F. P.: Human milk in the modern world, Oxford, 1978, Oxford University Press.

large numbers of purine and pyrimidine nucleotides present in various tissues have a number of functions in the cell. They are part of nucleic acid synthesis and metabolism and are also part of milk synthesis. It is well known that ATP supplies utilizable energy for biosynthetic reactions.

Human milk has been recorded to have 6.1 to 9.0 μmol of free nucleotides/100 ml, according to Johke.[31] The levels in colostrum and mature milk are similar. The conspicuous difference in quality and quantity of nucleotides between the mammary gland and its secretion would indicate that nucleotides are secreted from the epithelial cells of the gland into the milk. There are distinct species differences in composition and content of nucleotides as well.[53] CMP and uracil are the nucleotides in the highest concentration in human milk, but it also contains UDP-N-acetyllactosamine and other oligosaccharides. Human milk contains only a trace of orotic acid and no GDP-fucose. Orotic acid is the chief nucleotide of bovine milk.[34] Nucleotide levels fall rapidly in bovine milk to minimal levels in mature bovine milk.

Nucleotides are important in the process of protein synthesis, which is enhanced in the newborn infant by a dietary supply of nucleotides. A statistically significant increase in weight was observed by György[19] and his colleagues when weanling rats who had been fed a low-protein diet (10% casein) were given added nucleotides as compared with controls without supplements of nucleotides. A high-protein diet (20%) did not produce significant growth increase when nucleotides were added. How this applies to human infants who receive low-protein and high-nucleotide levels in breast milk needs further elaboration.

Minerals

The total ash content of milk is species specific and parallels the growth rate and body structure of the offspring. There are a number of metallic elements and organic and inorganic acids in milk. They may be present as ions, un-ionized salts, and weakly ionized salts. Some are bound to other constituents. Sodium, potassium, calcium, and magnesium are the major cations. Phosphate, chloride, and citrate are the major anions. High-lactose milks, in general, contain less total ash than low-lactose milks, which have high total salt content. This maintains osmolality close to that of serum. The high mineral content is associated with a rapid growth rate as well.

Potassium and sodium. Potassium levels are much higher than sodium, which is similar to the proportions in intracellular fluids (Table 4-13). Although sodium, potassium, and chloride are present as free ions, the other constituents appear as complexes and compounds. Ions can pass through the secretory cell membrane in both directions and in and out of the lumen. Intracellular sodium, chloride, and potassium are in equilibrium with the ions of the plasma and alveolar milk. An apical pumping mechanism has been calculated for chloride release, whereas sodium, potassium, and intracellular chloride pass into milk due to their electrochemical gradients. The cellular pumping mechanism maintains the ionic concentrations in the extracellular fluid and alveolar milk.

Sodium levels in cow's milk are 3.6 times those in human milk (human, 7 mEq/L or 16 mg/100 ml; bovine, 22 mEq/L or 50 mg/100 ml). Hypernatremic dehydration has been associated with cow's milk feedings. Experiments with newborn rats on high salt intakes have shown that hypertension can develop.

Table 4-13. Minerals in human milk and cow's milk (per 100 ml)

Minerals	Colostrum	Transitional	Mature	Cow's milk
Calcium (mg)	39.0	46.0	35.0	130.0
Chlorine (mg)	85.0	46.0	40.0	108.0
Copper (μg)	40.0	50.0	40.0	14.0
Iron (μg)	70.0	70.0	100.0	70.0
Magnesium (mg)	4.0	4.0	4.0	12.0
Phosphorus (mg)	14.0	20.0	15.0	120.0
Potassium (mg)	74.0	64.0	57.0	145.0
Sodium (mg)	48.0	29.0	15.0	58.0
Sulfur (mg)	22.0	20.0	14.0	30.0
Total ash (mg)	—	—	200.0	700.0

Table 4-14. Principal salt constituents in bovine and human milks*

Constituent	Bovine (mg/100 ml)	Human (mg/100 ml)
Calcium	125	33
Magnesium	12	4
Sodium	58	15
Potassium	138	55
Chloride	103	43
Phosphorus	96	15
Citric acid	175	20–80
Sulfur	30	14
CO_2	20	—

*From Jenness, R., and Sloan, R. E.: Composition of milk. In Larson, B. L., and Smith, V. R., editors: Lactation, vol. III. Nutrition and biochemistry of milk/maintenance, New York, 1974, Academic Press, Inc.

Table 4-15. Statistical analysis by Student's 't' test of blood urea levels in sixty-one healthy infants aged 1 to 3 months*

Infant group	Number	Blood urea, mean ± SE (mg/100 ml)	Individual values >40 mg/100 ml	
			Number	Total observations (%)
A: breast-fed	12	22.7 ± 1.6†	0	0§
B: artificial milk alone	16	47.4 ± 2.0‡	12	75‖
C: artificial milk + solid foods	33	51.9 ± 1.8	29	88

*From Davies, D. P., and Saunders, R.: Arch. Dis. Child. **48:**563, 1973.
†When compared with group B and group C: $p < 0.001$ (t = 9·7) and $p < 0.001$ (t = 11·5), respectively.
‡When compared with group C: $p > 0.05$ (t = 1·6).
§When compared with group B and group C: $p < 0.001$ (t = 6·9) and $p < 0.001$ (t = 15·5), respectively.
‖When compared with group C: $p > 0.05$ (t = 1·1).

Potassium concentrations are 13 mEq or 51 mg/ml in human milk and 35 mEq or 137 mg/ml in bovine milk.

Most attention has been paid to the role of sodium in hypertension. Potassium has a reciprocal relationship with sodium in many biological functions. Potassium administration can lower elevated blood pressures in some adults.

At a constant sodium intake, decreasing the Na/K ratio in the diet by increasing potassium lowers blood pressure. The dietary Na/K ratio has an important role in determining severity, if not the development, of salt-induced hypertension. The mechanism of potassium's antihypertensive effect is unclear. But the higher potassium and lower sodium levels of breast milk appear to be physiologically beneficial.

Total ash. Cow's milk has three times the total ash content of human milk (Table 4-14). All the minerals that appear in cow's milk also appear in human milk. Phosphorus level is six times greater in cow's milk; calcium level is four times higher.

The renal solute load of cow's milk is considerably higher than that of breast milk. This is magnified by the metabolic breakdown products of the high protein content, which are in increased amounts, also. This is shown in the high urea levels in formula-fed infants (Table 4-15). Although the mean urea levels in breast milk are 37 mg/100 ml and only 15 mg/100 ml in cow's milk, the blood urea levels in breast-fed infants are about 22 mg, whereas infants fed formula were 47 mg and those fed formula plus solids were 52 mg/100 ml (Table 4-15). The plasma osmolarity of infants fed breast milk is lower and approximates the physiological level of plasma (Table 4-16).

Calcium/phosphorus ratio. The ratio of calcium to phosphorus is considerably lower in cow's (1.4) than in human milk (2.2). Many investigators have studied calcium and phosphorus values in human milk and found some variation from mother to mother and study to study. The Ca/P ratio varied from 1.8 to 2.4, with the absolute values for calcium varying from 20 to 34 mg/100 ml and phosphorus from 14 to 18 mg/100 ml. Data compiled by Forfar[16] demonstrate the variation. Fetal and newborn plasma concentrations for calcium decline sharply from 10.4 mg/100 ml at birth to 8.5 mg/100 ml by day four. Unlike calcium, phosphorus concentrations rise in the postnatal period. The drop in serum calcium levels in the bottle-fed infants was more marked than in the breast-fed infants. Infant serum phosphorus concentrations rise during the postnatal period. Those infants fed cow's milk have a greater rise than those fed human milk. When gestation is prolonged or the mother has preeclampsia, the concentrations are even higher at birth. Barltop and Hillier[5] studied the calcium and phosphorus content of transitional and mature human milk and the corresponding infants' plasma levels (Table 4-17). No relationship between the milk composition and the plasma levels was seen on the sixth day of life. Although the Ca/P ratio has been stressed in the past, these researchers failed to find a statistical correlation between the calcium and phosphorus contents of plasma and corresponding breast milk Ca/P. This suggested that Ca/P ratio is not critical in the low mineral loads present in breast milk. There are extensive data to demonstrate the stress of high phosphorus and low calcium in serum of infants fed milk with a high mineral content. Lealman and colleagues[37] recently published a study of 138 infants on breast milk or cow's milk formulas. Infants fed cow's milk formulas showed changes by the sixth day of receiving the low calcium and high phosphorus levels. The total calcium require-

Table 4-16. Daily protein intake (g/kg) and mean plasma osmolality*

	Group A§	Group B‖	Group C#
Protein intake			
Day 7	2.1	4.6	6.8
Day 14	2.6	6.7	8.5
Day 28	ND†	ND†	ND†
Plasma osmolality			
Day 7	290.8	289.6	296.8
Day 14	287.2	291.7	298.8
Day 28	289.7	293.6	296.7

*From Davies, D. P.: Arch. Dis. Child. **48**:575, 1973.
†ND, not determined.
§Preterm infants fed breast milk containing 5.9% of total calories as protein.
‖Preterm infants fed formula B containing 15.4% of total calories as protein.
#Preterm infants fed formula C containing 21.1% of total calories as protein.

Table 4-17. Comparison of calcium and phosphorus content*

	Calcium (mg/100 ml)	Phosphorus (mg/100 ml)	Ca/P
Cord blood	10.2	5.5	—
Breast-fed, fourth day of life	9.5	5.3	—
Bottle-fed, fourth day of life	8.0	6.0	—
Transitional breast milk	28.0	15.5	2.0
Mature breast milk	27.6	16.2	1.8

*Modified from Barltrop, D., and Hillier, R.: Acta Paediatr. Scand. **63**:347, 1974.

ments for maximum growth have been questioned by those who believe the total amount of calcium is too low in breast milk. The fact that rickets has not been seen in infants totally breast-fed by well-nourished mothers is supportive circumstantial evidence. Fomon[15] has calculated the calcium needs for growth of premature infants to adequate stature at 1 year of age. His data clearly show breast milk to be an inadequate source of calcium for the premature infant. For each 100 g weight gain, the premature needs 617 mg of calcium, which would mean, assuming 65% dietary absorption, 190 mg/day of calcium, or a 600 ml intake of human milk for a 1200 g baby. A 1200 g infant would usually consume 180 ml/day of fluids.

Magnesium and other salts. Magnesium is present as a free ion and in complexes with casein and phosphate in caseinate micelles or citrate complexes. Cow's milk has three times as much magnesium as human milk (12 mg/100 ml compared to 4 mg/100 ml). Lealman and associates[37] studied the magnesium levels in the plasma of infants who received either breast milk or cow's milk formula. Breast-fed infants showed an increase in magnesium levels in the first week of life, whereas the others did not, and some infants even showed a drop.

Citrate is found in milks of many species and is three to four times higher in cow's milk than in human milk (Tables 4-14 and 4-17). The distribution of ions and salts differs in various milks and depends on the relative concentrations of casein and citrate.

Most of the sulfur in milk is in the sulfur-containing amino acids, with only about 10% present as sulfate ion. There are some organic acids present, and they appear as anions in milk.

Trace elements

IRON. Because of the great emphasis on iron in the modern diet and especially in the diet of the infant in the first year of life, the iron in human milk has been closely scrutinized. It has been determined that normal infants need 1500 mg of exogenous elemental iron in the first year of life, which can be translated into 8 to 10 mg/day. Prepared infant formulas currently supply 10 to 12 mg/day. Human milk contains more than cow's milk, however, in that human milk has 100 μg/100 ml and cow's 70 μg/100 ml. This does not meet the requirements just given. Historically, however, breast-fed infants have not been anemic.

Studies by Picciano and Guthrie[44] on fifty women and 350 samples of breast milk showed a variation between <0.1 and 1.6 μg of iron/ml. Results indicated a variation that would require multiple samples from an individual to obtain a representative estimate. Age, parity, and lactation history influenced the levels. A fully breast-fed infant would receive 0.05 mg of iron/kg/day, according to this study.

Iron absorption from human milk is more efficient and has been noted to be 49% of iron available, whereas only 10% of cow's milk iron and 4% of iron in iron-fortified formulas was absorbed. Hematological values of bottle-fed infants were abnormal, whereas those of breast-fed infants were not. The breast-fed infants had high ferritin levels, indicating a long-term adequacy of iron assimilation (Table 4-18). Studies in adults given tagged iron in human milk and in cow's milk show better absorption from the human milk solution (Table 4-19). Other factors that influence iron absorption include higher amounts of vitamin C. Lactose, which promotes iron absorption, is in higher concentration in breast milk, especially if compared to prepared formulas, which may not contain lactose. Phosphorus may interfere with iron absorption, as may high protein levels. There is still considerable doubt as to whether or not it is physiologically sound to increase the hemoglobin of an infant with exogenous iron. All species of mammals have low iron content in their milks. All mammals investigated so far have a drop in their hemoglobin levels after birth and a gradual rise to adult levels for that species. The requirement for iron is an unsettled question.

ZINC. Zinc has been identified as essential to the human. The chief roles described to date are as part of the enzyme structure or as activators of enzyme activity. Zinc deficiency has been described as well, most recently in newborns and prematures on hyperalimentation regimens. The chief clinical symptoms are failure to thrive and typical skin lesions. Milk has been identified as a food with bioavailable zinc. Johnson and Evans[32] studied the relative zinc availability in human breast milk, formulas, and cow's milk. Human milk had 2 μg/ml as compared to cow's milk, which had 4.1 μg/ml, and fortified formulas, which had 3 to 5 μg/ml. The bioavailability of zinc fed to rats in various milk solutions was 59.2% for human milk, 42% for cow's milk, and 26.8% to 39% for formulas.

Picciano and Guthrie[44] studied milk from fifty mothers in 350 samples. They found zinc levels to average 3.95 μg/ml and to be consistent regardless of time of day, duration of lactation, or other variables. They estimated breast-fed infants receive 0.35 mg of zinc/kg/day. Eckhert and co-workers[11] studied zinc binding in human and cow's milk to determine bioavailability. By gel chromatography they

Table 4-18. Age, weights, and hematological values for infants exclusively breast-fed*

Data	Patients				Normals
	1	2	3	4	
Age (mo)	8	9	8	18	—
Weight (kg)					
At birth	4.1	3.6	2.8	3.8	—
At time of study	11.0	10.2	9.0	12.0	—
Final weight ÷ Birth weight	2.68	2.83	3.21	3.15	—
Hemoglobin (g/dl)	11.3	12.5	11.3	12.2	>10.5
Mean corpuscular volume (cu/μm^3)	78	82	74	80	76 ± 3
Iron (μg/100 ml)	80	77	158	73	>70
Total iron-binding capacity (μg/100 ml)	320	—	502	408	—
% Saturation	20	—	31	18	>16
Free erythrocyte porphyrins (μg/100 ml)	51	42	53	37	<70

*From McMillan, J. A., Landaw, S. A., and Oski, F. A.: Pediatrics **58**:686, 1976, copyright American Academy of Pediatrics, 1976.

Table 4-19. Elemental iron and ^{59}Fe radioactivity level in milks fed to ten adult subjects*

Milk	Iron (mg/86 ml of milk)	^{59}Fe Added (μg)	Total elemental iron (μg)	cpm ingested	μg/cpm ingested†
Cow's milk					
Subjects 1 to 5	74.8	0.59	75.39	2.0 × 10^6	3.8 × 10^{-5}
Subjects 6 to 10	34.4	0.60	35.00	2.5 × 10^6	1.4 × 10^{-5}
Human milk					
Subjects 1 to 5	67.1	0.45	67.55	1.5 × 10^6	4.5 × 10^{-5}
Subjects 6 to 10	51.2	0.46	51.66	2.09 × 10^6	2.45 × 10^{-5}

*From McMillan, J. A., Landaw, S. A., and Oski, F. A.: Pediatrics **58**:686, 1976, copyright American Academy of Pediatrics, 1976.
†Assayed at day 36. Activity was adjusted to 10 μCi on the day of ingestion of each milk solution.

showed cow's milk zinc to be associated with high–molecular weight fractions and zinc in human milk to be associated with low–molecular weight fractions. The low–molecular weight ligand was readily absorbed. Breast milk has been therapeutic in the treatment of acrodermatitis enteropathica, an inherited zinc metabolism disorder, whereas cow's milk formulas are ineffective.

COPPER, SELENIUM, ALUMINUM, AND TITANIUM. Little is known about trace elements in human milk, although some work has been done by Archibald[2] on bovine milk. Picciano and Guthrie[44] studied copper levels in human milk and noted that the content varied considerably among women and within the same woman. The range was 0.09 to 0.63 μg/ml. Copper levels were higher in the morning. Dietary supplements did not alter results. Age, parity, and lactation history showed that older mothers and mulitparas had higher levels. The fully breast-fed infant would receive 0.05 mg of copper/kg/day.

High zinc/copper ratios as they relate to dietary intakes have been associated with coronary heart disease.[33] The zinc/copper ratios of human milk are lower than in cow's milk. Using figures from Picciano and Guthrie[44] (0.14 to 3.95:0.09 to 0.63), the ratio in human milk is 14:9. The ratio of zinc to copper in bovine milk (1000 to 6000:30 to 170) is at least 30:1.

Selenium concentrations in human milk are consistent in samples collected from many parts of the world, according to work by Hadjimarkos and Shearer.[20] The mean value was 0.020 ppm, which was similar to the value from many parts of the United States, where the range was 0.007 to 0.033 ppm. There was a parallel between the selenium content of bovine grazing crops in the area and bovine milk levels. Alterations in bovine diet produce more marked change in the selenium in the milk produced. Bovine levels range from 0.016 to 1.27 ppm. The significance is not clear, although questions have been raised surrounding the detrimental effects of high selenium on dentition.

FLUORINE. Fluorine has been widely accepted as a significant dietary factor in decreasing dental caries.[43] The effect has been associated with the conversion of the enamel hydroxyapatite to fluorapatite with a reduction in acid solubility. It has been suggested that the presence of fluorine during the formation of hydroxyapatite creates less soluble, more resistant, crystals. Fluorine levels in human milk are lower than in cow's milk. Ericsson and associates[13] have found lower values in human milk than previously reported. Cow's milk contains 0.03 to 0.10 mg/L and human milk contains 0.025 mg/L. Fluoridation of the water supply has shown variable results, but only a minimal effect on breast milk levels of fluorine.

The significant development of deciduous and permanent teeth is after birth and depends on fetal stores as well as fluorine available in the diet. Studies comparing breast-fed and bottle-fed infants show a distinct difference, with fewer dental caries and better dental health in breast-fed infants. The role of fluorine and other factors, such as selenium, which predispose the breast-fed infant to healthier teeth have yet to be defined completely. Nursing-bottle caries add to the total dental caries of the bottle-fed infant.

pH and osmolarity

The pH range in human milk is 6.7 to 7.4 with a mean of 7.1. The mean pH of cow's milk is 6.8. The caloric content of both human and cow's milk is 65 kcal/100 ml or 20 kcal/oz. The specific gravity is 1.031 and 1.032, respectively. The pH of the milk ingested has an effect on the infant and the development of metabolic acidosis, especially in episodes of dehydration.

The osmolarity of human milk approximates that of human serum or 286 mosmol/kg of water, whereas that for cow's milk is higher, 350 mosmol.[7] The renal solute load of human milk is considerably lower than that of cow's milk. Renal solute load is roughly calculated by totalling the solutes that must be excreted by the kidney. It consists primarily of nonmetabolizable dietary components, especially electrolytes, ingested in excess of body needs, and metabolic end products, mainly from the metabolism of protein. It can be estimated by adding the dietary intake of nitrogen and three minerals, sodium, potassium, and chloride. Each gram of protein is considered to yield 4 mosmol (as urea) and each milliequivalent of sodium, potassium, and chloride is 1 mosmol, according to Fomon.[14] The renal solute load of cow's milk is 221 mosmol compared to 79 mosmol for human milk (Tables 4-16 and 4-20).

Table 4-20. Dietary intake of protein, sodium, chloride, and potassium and estimated renal solute load from various feedings*

Feedings	Caloric density (kcal/100 ml)‡	Dietary intake					Estimated renal solute load†		
		Quantity (ml)‡	Protein (g)	Na (mEq)	Cl (mEq)	K (mEq)	Urea (mosmol)§	Na + Cl + K (mosmol)	Total (mosmol)
Milks									
Whole cow milk	67	1000	33	25	29	35	132	89	221
Boiled skim milk	33	1000	46	35	40	49	184	124	308
Human milk	67	1000	12	7	11	13	48	31	79
Formulas									
SMA	100	1000	22	10	18	21	90	49	139
Similac	100	1000	24	17	24	28	97	69	166
Strained foods									
Pears	69	100	0.3	0.2	0.2	1.6	1	2	3
Applesauce	84	100	0.2	0.3	0.2	2.6	1	3	4
Beef with vegetables	104	100	6.5	13.3	10.6	3.7	26	28	54
Chicken with vegetables	100	100	7.2	5.7	4.6	1.8	29	12	41

*From Fomon, S. J.: Infant nutrition, ed. 2, Philadelphia, 1974, W. B. Saunders Co.
†This simplified estimate of renal solute load is appropriate for use with respect to fullsize but not low–birth–weight infants.
‡For strained foods, 100 g rather than 100 ml.
§Assumed to account for 70% of nitrogen intake (Ziegler and Fomon, 1971).

Vitamins

Vitamin A. Vitamin A content is 75 μg/100 ml or 280 international units (IU) in mature human milk and 41 μg/100 ml or 180 IU in cow's milk (Table 4-21). Thus the supply of vitamin A and its precursors, carotenoids, is considered adequate to meet the estimated daily requirement, which varies from 500 to 1500 IU/day if the infant consumes at least 200 ml of breast milk per day. There is twice as much vitamin A in colostrum as in mature milk.

Vitamin D. Vitamin D has always been included in the fat-soluble vitamin group because, indeed, that is the form in which it has been identified in nature. Human milk has been shown to have vitamin D in both the fat and the aqueous fractions. Lakdawala and Widdowson[36] have reported concentrations of 1.78 μg/100 ml in the first few days and 1.00 μg/100 ml thereafter, as compared to 0.05 mg/100 ml previously reported in the fat fraction. It was the water-soluble conjugate of vitamin D with sulfate that was measured. The site of sulfation in the human has not been identified, although vitamin D is sulfated in the liver in rats. The level of 40 IU/100 ml or 1.00 μg/100 ml may provide adequate amounts in the fully breast-fed infant to meet the requirements of 400 IU or 10 mg/day. Levels of vitamin D are also higher in colostrum than in mature milk.

Vitamin E. Vitamin E has been the subject of much interest. Levels in colostrum are 1.5 mg/100 ml, whereas transitional milk has 0.9 mg/100 ml and mature milk 0.25mg/100 ml. Cow's milk has 0.07 mg/100 ml (Table 4-21). Correspondingly, serum levels in breast-fed infants rise quickly at birth and maintain a normal level, whereas cow's milk–fed infants have depressed levels. Vitamin E includes a group of fat-soluble compounds α-, β-, γ-, and δ-tocopherol and their unsaturated derivatives α-, β-, γ-, and δ-tocotrienol. An international unit of vitamin E is equal to 1.0 mg of synthetic α-tocopherol or 0.74 mg of natural α-tocopherol acetate. Vitamin

Table 4-21. Vitamins and other constituents of human milk and cow's milk (per 100 ml)

Milk elements	Colostrum	Transitional	Mature	Cow's milk
Vitamins				
Vitamin A (μg)	151.0	88.0	75.0	41.0
Vitamin B$_1$ (μg)	1.9	5.9	14.0	43.0
Vitamin B$_2$ (μg)	30.0	37.0	40.0	145.0
Nicotinic acid (μg)	75.0	175.0	160.0	82.0
Pantothenic acid (μg)	183.0	288.0	246.0	340.0
Biotin (μg)	0.06	0.35	0.6	2.8
Folic acid (μg)	0.05	0.02	0.14	0.13
Vitamin B$_{12}$ (μg)	0.05	0.04	0.1	0.6
Vitamin C (mg)	5.9	7.1	5.0	1.1
Vitamin D (IU)	—	—	5.0	2.5
Vitamin E (mg)	1.5	0.9	0.25	0.07
Vitamin K (μg)	—	—	1.5	6.0
Ash (g)	0.3	0.3	0.2	0.7
Calories (kcal)	57.0	63.0	65.0	65.0
Specific gravity	1050.0	1035.0	1031.0	1032.0
Milk (pH)	—	—	7.0	6.8

E is required for muscle integrity, resistance of erythrocytes to hemolysis, as well as for other biochemical and physiological functions. The requirement for vitamin E is related to the polyunsaturated fatty acid (PUFA) content of the cellular structures and of the diet. Satisfactory plasma levels are 1 mg/100 ml, and this can be maintained by feedings with a vitamin E/PUFA ratio of 0.4 mg/g. Ordinarily, this would be supplied by 4 IU of vitamin E/day. Since human milk contains 1.8 mg/L or 40 μg of vitamin E/g of lipid, it supplies more than adequate vitamin E.

Vitamin K. Vitamin K is in human milk at the level of 15 μg/100 ml, whereas cow's milk is 60 μg/100 ml. Vitamin K is essential for the synthesis of blood clotting factors, which are normal in the serum at the time of birth. Vitamin K is produced by the intestinal flora but takes several days in the previously sterile gut to be effective. It is recommended that all infants receive vitamin K at birth, regardless of feeding plans, to prevent hemorrhagic disease of the newborn due to vitamin K deficiency in the first few days of life.

Vitamin C. Human milk is an outstanding source of water-soluble vitamins and reflects maternal dietary intake. Increased vitamin C has been measured in the milk within 30 min of a bolus of vitamin C being given to the mother. Human milk contains 43 mg/100 ml (fresh cow's milk contains up to 21 mg). Vitamin C is part of several enzyme and hormone systems as well as intracellular chemical reactions. It is essential to collagen synthesis.

At a recent symposium[12] on vitamin C, it was pointed out that the body requirements for vitamin C increase during stress. Most species manufacture their own vitamin C, including the calf; therefore there is little in cow's milk. The common housefly, for example, makes 10 g of vitamin C for every 70 kg of housefly weight, according to the discussion by Enloe and colleagues.[12] It is probably appropriate for pregnant women and nursing mothers to increase their intake of vitamin C.

Vitamin B complex

VITAMIN B₁. Vitamin B_1, or thiamin, levels increase with the duration of lactation, but are lower in human milk (160 mg/100 ml) than in cow's milk (440 mg/100 ml). Thiamin is essential for the utilization of carbohydrates in the pyruvate metabolism (cofactor in pyruvic acid decarboxylation) for fat synthesis. Insufficient thiamin produces insufficient carbohydrate oxidation with accumulation of intermediary metabolites such as lactic acid.

VITAMIN B₂. Vitamin B_2, or riboflavin, is significant for the newborn in whom intestinal tract bacterial synthesis is minimal. Riboflavin is involved in oxidative intracellular systems and is essential for protoplasmic growth. There are 360 μg/100 ml in human milk and 1750 μg/100 ml in cow's milk.

NIACIN. Niacin (nicotinamide) is an essential part of the pyridine nucleotide coenzymes and is part of the intracellular respiratory mechanisms. There are 1470 μg/100 ml in human milk and 940 μg/100 ml in cow's milk.

VITAMIN B₆. Vitamin B_6 (pyridoxine) forms the enzyme group of certain decarboxylases and transaminases involved in metabolism of nerve tissue. There are 100 μg/100 ml in human milk and 640 μg/100 ml in cow's milk.

PANTOTHENIC ACID. Pantothenic acid is part of coenzyme A, a catalyst of acetylation reactions. The reaction of coenzyme A with acetic acid to form acetyl-CoA is prime to intermediary metabolism. There is 1.84 mg of pantothenic acid/ml of breast milk and 3.46 mg/100 ml in cow's milk.

FOLACIN. Folacin (folic acid) is part of the conversion of glycine to serine. It is also involved in the methylation of nicotinamide and homocystine to methionine. It is essential for erythropoiesis. There is 52 μg of folic acid/100 ml of breast milk and 55 μg/100 ml in cow's milk. Folic acid has also been identified as a critical element to deficiency states during pregnancy, being associated with abruptio placentae, toxemia, and intrauterine growth failure as well as megaloblastic anemia.

VITAMIN B$_{12}$. Vitamin B$_{12}$ is found in human milk in low concentration, 0.3 μg/100 ml, whereas cow's milk has 4.0 μg/ml. Well-nourished mothers on balanced diets appear to have adequate amounts for their infants. Vitamin B$_{12}$ functions in trans-methylations such as synthesis of choline from methionine, serine from glycine, and methionine from homocysteine. It is involved in pyrimidine and purine metabolism. B$_{12}$ also affects the metabolism of folic acid. Megaloblastic anemia is a common symptom of deficiency. B$_{12}$ occurs exclusively in animal tissue, bound to protein, and there is very little or none in vegetable protein. The minimum daily requirement for infants according to Fomon and associates[15] is 0.3 μg/day in the first year of life, when growth is rapid.

Enzymes

By and large, researchers have tended to dismiss the significance of enzymes in breast milk by saying that they are all destroyed by the gastric juices. Unfortunately, little effort has been applied to studying their activities in humans, although considerable data have been collected on the enzymatic activities of many milks. Jenness and Sloan[29] report forty-four enzymes detected so far in bovine, human, and some other milks. Xanthine oxidase, lactoperoxidase, UDP-galactose: glucose, galactosyl transferase, ribonuclease, lipase, alkaline phosphatase, acid phosphatase, and lysozyme have been isolated in crystalline form.

The most information has been accumulated about the activity of lipase, which has been demonstrated to be active in the duodenum. Stewart and co-workers[54] have studied the content of alkaline phosphatase in human milk, which is known to be in higher concentration than in cow's milk. They studied 199 samples from twenty donors. There is some correlation with the fat content, but none to nitrogen content or total solids. There is no relationship to age, nationality, or other characteristics of the donor except for a tendency to increase over time. Adding phosphatase to cow's milk formulas has improved the tolerance of infants to cow's milk.

Lysozyme has also been isolated from human milk. It is a thermostabile enzyme known as a nonspecific antimicrobial factor, that is, bacteriolytic toward Enterobacteriacea and gram-positive bacteria. Breast milk has 3000 times more lysozyme than cow's milk. Lysozyme also hydrolyzes mucopolysaccharides.

REFERENCES

1. Almroth, S. G.: Water requirements of breast-fed infants in a hot climate, Am. J. Clin. Nutr. **31:**1154, 1978.
2. Archibald, J. G.: Trace elements in bovine milk, Dairy Sci. Abstr. **20:**212, 1958.
3. Atkinson, S. A., Bryan, M. H., and Anderson, G. H.: Human milk: differences in nitrogen concentration in milk from mothers of term and premature infants, J. Pediatr. **93:**67, 1978.
4. Auricchio, S., Rubino, A., and Mürset, E.: Intestinal glycosidase activities in the human embryo, fetus, and newborn, Pediatrics **35:**944, 1965.

5. Barltrop, D., and Hillier, R.: Calcium and phosphorus content of transitional and mature human milk, Acta Paediatr. Scand. **63:**347, 1974.
6. Committee on Nutrition, American Academy of Pediatrics: Commentary on breast-feeding and infant formulas, including proposed standards for formulas, Pediatrics **57:**278, 1976.
7. Dale, G., et al.: Plasma osmolality, sodium, and urea in healthy breast-fed and bottle-fed infants in Newcastle upon Tyne, Arch. Dis. Child. **50:**731, 1975.
8. Davies, D. P.: Plasma osmolality and protein intake in preterm infants, Arch. Dis. Child. **48:**575, 1973.
9. Davies, D. P., and Saunders, R.: Blood urea: normal values in early infancy related to feeding practices, Arch. Dis. Child. **48:**563, 1973.
10. Dick, G.: The etiology of multiple sclerosis, Proc. R. Soc. Med. **69:**611, 1976.
11. Eckhert, C. D., et al.: Zinc binding: a difference between human and bovine milk, Science **195:**789, 1977.
12. Enloe, C. F., and Hartley, H. L., moderators: To dose or megadose: a debate about vitamin C, Nutr. Today **13**(2):6, 1978.
13. Ericsson, Y., Hellström, I., and Hofvander, Y.: Pilot studies on the fluoride metabolism in infants on different feedings, Acta Paediatr. Scand. **61:**459, 1972.
14. Fomon, S. J.: Infant nutrition, ed 2, Philadelphia, 1974, W. B. Saunders Co.
15. Fomon, S. J., Ziegler, E. E., and Vazquez, H. D.: Human milk and the small premature infant, Am. J. Dis. Child. **131:**463, 1977.
16. Forfar, J. O.: Calcium, phosphorus, magnesium metabolism. In Forfar, J. O., editor: Aspects of neonatal metabolism, Clin. Endocrinol. Metabol. **5**(1):123, 1976.
17. Glass, R. L., Troolin, H. A., and Jenness, R.: Comparative biochemical studies of milks, IV. Constituent fatty acids of milk fats, Comp. Biochem. Physiol. **22:**415, 1967.
18. Guthrie, H. A., Picciano, M. F., and Sheehe, D.: Fatty acid patterns of human milk, J. Pediatr. **90:**39, 1977.
19. György, P.: Biochemical aspects. In Jelliffe, D. B., and Jelliffe, E. F. P., editors: The uniqueness of human milk, Am. J. Clin. Nutr. **24:**970, 1971.
20. Hadjimarkos, D. M., and Shearer, T. R.: Selenium in mature human milk, Am. J. Clin. Nutr. **26:**583, 1973.
21. Hall, B.: Activation of human milk lipase, Biochem. Soc. Trans. **3:**90, 1975.
22. Hall, B.: Changing composition of human milk and early development of an appetite control, Lancet **1:**779, 1975.
23. Hambraeus, L., Forsum, E., Lonnerdal, B.: Nutritional aspects of breast milk and cow's milk formulas. In Hambraeus, L., Hanson, L., and Macfarlane, H., editors: Symposium on food and immunology, Stockholm, 1975, Almqvist and Wiksell, p. 116.
24. Hambraeus, L.: Proprietary milk versus human milk in infant feeding: a critical approach from nutritional point of view, Pediatr. Clin. North Am. **24:**17, 1977.
25. Hernell, O., and Olivecrona, T.: Human milk lipases, II. Bile-salt–stimulated lipase, Biochim. Biophys. Acta **369:**234, 1974.
26. Hytten, F. E.: Clinical and chemical studies in human lactation, VII. The effect of differences in yield and composition of milk on the infant's weight gain and duration of breast-feeding, Br. Med. J. **1:**1410, 1954.
27. Insull, W., and Ahrens, E. H.: The fatty acids of human milk from mothers on diets taken ad libitum, Biochem. J. **72:**27, 1959.
28. Jelliffe, D. B., and Jelliffe, E. F. P.: Human milk in the modern world, Oxford, 1978, Oxford University Press.
29. Jenness, R., and Sloan, R. E.: Composition of milk. In Larson, B. L., and Smith, V. R., editors: Lactation, vol. III. Nutrition and biochemistry of milk/maintenance, New York, 1974, Academic Press, Inc.
30. Jensen, R. G., Hagerty, M. M., McMahon, K. E.: Lipids of human milk and infant formulas: a review, Am. J. Clin. Nutr. **31:**990, 1978.
31. Johke, T.: Nucleotides of mammary secretions. In Larson, B. L., editor: Lactation, vol. IV. Mammary gland/human lactation/milk synthesis, New York, 1978, Academic Press.
32. Johnson, P. E., Evans, G. W.: Relative zinc availability in human breast milk, infant formulas, and cow's milk, Am. J. Clin. Nutr. **31:**416, 1978.
33. Klevay, L. M.: Ratio of zinc to copper in milk and mortality due to coronary artery disease. An

association. In Hemphill, D. D., editor: Trace substances in environmental health, vol. VIII, Columbia, Mo., University of Missouri Press.

34. Kobata, A., Suzuoki, Z., and Kida, M.: The acid soluble nucleotides of milk. I, Quantitative and qualitative differences of nucleotide constituents in human and cow's milk, J. Biochem. **51:**277, 1962.

35. Kretchmer, N.: Lactose and lactase, Sci. Am. **227:**73, 1972.

36. Lakdawala, D. R., and Widdowson, E. M.: Vitamin D in human milk, Lancet **1:**167, 1977.

37. Lealman, G. T., et al.: Calcium, phosphorus, and magnesium concentrations in plasma during first week of life and their relation to type of milk feed, Arch. Dis. Child. **51:**377, 1976.

38. Lengemann, F. W.: The site of action of lactose in the enhancement of calcium utilization, J. Nutr. **69:**23, 1959.

39. Macy, I. G., and Kelly, H. J.: Human milk and cow's milk in infant nutrition. In Kon, S. K., and Cowie, A. T., editors: Milk: the mammary gland and its secretion, vol. II, New York, 1961, Academic Press, Inc., p. 265.

40. Macy, I. G., Kelly, H. J., and Sloan, R. E.: The composition of milks, publ. no. 254, Washington, D. C., 1953, National Research Council.

41. McMillan, J. A., Landaw, S. A., and Oski, F. A.: Iron sufficiency in breast fed infants and the availability of iron from human milk, Pediatrics **58:**686, 1976.

42. Osborn, G. R.: Relationship of hypotension and infant feeding to aetiology of coronary disease, Coll. Int. Cont. Natl. Res. Sci. **169:**193, 1968.

43. Oseid, B. J.: Breast-feeding and infant health, Clin. Obstet. Gynecol. **18**(2):149, 1975.

44. Picciano, M. F., and Guthrie, H. A.: Copper, iron and zinc contents of mature human milk, Am. J. Clin. Nutr. **29:**242, 1976.

45. Picciano, M. F., Guthrie, H. A., and Sheehe, D. M.: The cholesterol content of human milk, Clin. Pediatr. **17:**359, 1978.

46. Potter, J. M., and Nestel, P. J.: The effect of dietary fatty acids and cholesterol on the milk lipids of lactating women and the plasma cholesterol of breast-fed infants, Am. J. Clin. Nutr. **29:**54, 1976.

47. Rassin, D. K., Sturman, J. A., and Gaull, G. E.: Taurine in milk: species variation, Pediatr. Res. **11:**449, 1977.

48. Read, W. W. C., and Sarrif, A.: Human milk lipids, I. Changes in fatty acid composition of early colostrum, Am. J. Clin. Nutr. **17:**177, 1965.

49. Read, W. W. C., Lutz, P. G., and Tashjian, A.: Human milk lipids, II. The influences of dietary carbohydrates and fat on the fatty acids of mature milk. A study in four ethnic groups, Am. J. Clin. Nutr. **17:**180, 1965.

50. Read, W. W. C., Lutz, P. G., and Tashjian, A.: Human milk lipids, III. Short-term effects of dietary carbohydrate and fat, Am. J. Clin. Nutr. **17:**184, 1965.

51. Sanders, T. A. B., et al.: Studies of vegans: the fatty acid composition of plasma choline phosphoglycerides, erythrocytes, adipose tissue, and breast milk, and some indicators of susceptibility to ischemic heart disease in vegans and omnivore controls, Am. J. Clin. Nutr. **31:**805, 1978.

52. Sheehy, T. W., and Anderson, P. R.: Fetal disaccharidases, Am. J. Dis. Child. **121:**464, 1971.

53. Sinclair, A. J., and Crawford, M. A.: The accumulation of arachidonate and docosahexaenoate in the developing rat brain, J. Neurochem. **19:**1753, 1972.

54. Stewart, R. A., Platou, E., and Kelly, V. J.: The alkaline phosphatase content of human milk, J. Biol. Chem. **232:**777, 1958.

55. Sturman, J. A., Rassin, D. K., and Gaull, G. E.: Taurine in developing rat brain: transfer of ^{35}S-taurine to pups via the milk, Pediatr. Res. **11:**28, 1977.

56. Sturman, J. A., et al.: Taurine in the developing kitten: nutritional importance, Pediatr. Res. **11:**450, 1977.

57. Vorherr, H.: The breast: morphology, physiology, and lactation, New York, 1974, Academic Press, Inc.

58. Widdowson, E. M., et al.: Body fat of British and Dutch infants, Br. Med. J. **i:**653, 1975.

59. Wing, J. P.: Human versus cow's milk in infant nutrition and health: update 1977, Curr. Prob. Pediatr. **8**(1): entire issue, Nov. 1977.

60. Ziegler, E. E., and Fomon, S. J.: Fluid intake, renal solute load, and water balance in infancy, J. Pediatr. **78:**561, 1971.

CHAPTER 5

Host-resistance factors and immunological significance of human milk

As the newborn infant prepares for existence outside the uterus, various organ systems adjust and adapt. It had been suggested that protection against infection was provided by the mother transplacentally, and it has been established that the neonate is immunologically immature at birth.

The neonate does not have sufficient innate defenses to protect himself against the highly contaminated environment he enters from the usually sterile environment of the uterus. The incidence of infection in the newborn infant is significant. It has been estimated that up to 10% of newborns are infected during delivery or in the first few months of life. It is generally believed that the newborn cannot muster the same level of defense against infection that an adult is capable of. The diminished phagocytic function of newborn cells is an example. This maturational defect is attributed to both cellular and extracellular factors.

Maternal antibody is transmitted to the fetus by different pathways in different species. An association has been recognized between the number of placental membranes and the relative importance of the placenta and the colostrum as sources of antibodies. By this analysis it is noted that the horse, with six placental membranes, passes little or no antibodies transplacentally and relies on colostrum for protection of the foal. Humans and monkeys, having three placental membranes, receive all the antibodies via the placenta and little, if any, from the colostrum. The transfer of IgG in the human is accomplished, according to Bellanti and Hurtado,[3] by means of active transport mechanism of the immunoglobulin across the placenta. Bellanti and Hurtado do point out, however, that secretory IgA immunoglobulins are found in human milk and provide local protection on the mucous membranes of the gastrointestinal tract. The lowered incidence of enteric and respiratory infections seen in breast-fed infants has been recognized. It has been established by other investigations that the mammary glands and their secretion of milk are of importance in protecting the infant, not only through the colostrum but through mature milk from birth through the early months of life. Some information has been available for decades to support the acknowledgment of the protective role of human milk. Many recent discoveries have broadened knowledge. All the mysteries of the protective value of human milk, however, have not been unraveled. Cells do constitute an important postpartum component of maternal immunological endowment.

The protective properties of human milk can be divided into cellular factors and humoral factors for facility of discussion, although they are closely related in vivo.

CELLULAR COMPONENTS OF HUMAN COLOSTRUM AND MILK

Over 100 years ago cell bodies were described in the colostrum of animals. As with much lactation research, further study of colostrol corpuscles was undertaken by the dairy industry for commercial reasons in the early 1900s. This research afforded an opportunity to make major progress in the understanding of cells in milk. Initially it was believed that these cells represented a reaction to infection in the mammary gland and were even described as "pus cells."

It has become clear that the cells of milk are normal constituents of that solution in all species. Cells include macrophages, lymphocytes, neutrophils, and epithelial cells and total 4000/mm³. Living leukocytes are normally present in human milk.

The overall concentration of these leukocytes is of the same order of magnitude as that seen in peripheral blood, although the predominant cell in milk is the macrophage rather than the neutrophil. Macrophages comprise about 90% of the leukocytes, and 2000 to 3000/mm³ are present. Lymphocytes make up about 10% of the cells (200 to 300/mm³), which is much lower than in human blood. There are large and small lymphocytes. By indirect immunofluorescence with anti-T anti-

Table 5-1. Distinguishing characteristics of T-lymphocytes, B-lymphocytes, and macrophages*

Membrane markers	T-lympho-cytes	B-lympho-cytes	Macro-phages
IgG	−	+	−
Receptor for C3 (erythrocyte-antibody-complement [EAC] rosettes)	−	+	+
Receptor for immunoglobulin or antibody-antigen complexes (Fc)	−	+	+
Thymus-specific antigens (θ, mouse thymocyte leukemia antigen, and so on)	+	−	−
Receptors for sheep red blood cells (erythrocyte [E] rosettes)	+	−	−
In vitro stimulation of DNA synthesis by mitogens			
Phytohemagglutinin (PHA)	+	−†	−
Concanavallin A (Con A)	+	−	−
Lipopolysaccharide (bacterial endotoxin)	−	+	−
Anti-immunoglobulin	−	+	−
Specific binding to antigen-coated beads	−	+	−
Mixed lymphocyte culture reactivity	+	−	−
Graft-versus-host (GVH) reaction-inducing capacity	+	−	−
Adherence to surfaces (glass, plastic)	−‡	−§	+
Phagocytic	−	−	+

*From Bellanti, J. A., and Hurtado, R. C.: Immunology and resistance to infection. In Remington, J. S., and Klein, J. O., editors: Infectious diseases of the fetus and newborn infant, Philadelphia, 1976, W. B. Saunders Co.
†Some B-lymphocytes may be recruited to divide secondarily because of factors elaborated by activated T-lymphocytes. B cells may also be stimulated when the mitogen is attached to solid support.
‡Except for blast cells.
§Except for mature plasma cells or when immune complexes are attached to B cells.

body to identify thymus-derived lymphocytes, it has been shown that 50% of human colostrol lymphocytes are T cells. By immunofluorescence procedures to detect surface immunoglobulins characteristic of B-lymphocytes, 34% were identified as B-lymphocytes (Table 5-1).

Macrophages

Macrophages are large complex phagocytes, which contain lysosomes, mito-chondria, pinosomes, ribosomes, and a Golgi apparatus. The monocytic phago-cytes are lipid laden and were previously called the colostrol bodies of Donne. They have the same functional and morphological features as those in other human tissue sources. These functions are (1) to be motile due to amoeboid movement, (2) to adhere to and spread on glass surfaces, (3) to phagocytose microorganisms (fungi and bacteria) and kill bacteria, (4) to phagocytose vital dyes, (5) to produce complement components C_3 and C_4, and (6) to produce lysosome and lactoferrin.

The mobility of macrophages is inhibited by the lymphokine migration inhibitor factor (MIF), which is produced by antigen-stimulated sensitized lymphocytes. The activities of macrophages have been demonstrated in both fresh colostrum and in colostrol cell cultures.

Lymphocytes

It has been established that both T- and B-lymphocytes are present in human milk and colostrum. They synthesize IgA antibody. Human milk lymphocytes respond to mitogens by proliferation, with increased macrophage-lymphocyte interaction and the release of soluble mediators, including MIF. Cells destined to become lymphopoietic cells are derived from two separate influences, the thymus (T) and the bursa (B) or bursal equivalent tissues. The population of cells called B cells comprise the smaller part of the total. The term B cell is derived from its origination in a different anatomical site from the thymus; in birds it has been identified as the bursa of Fabricius. The B cells can be identified by the presence of surface immunoglobulin markers. The B cells in human milk include cells with IgA, IgM, and IgG surface immunoglobulins.

T cell system. More rapid mitotic activity occurs in the thymus gland than in any other lymphatic organ, yet 70% of the cells die within the cell substance. Thymosin has recently been identified as a hormone produced by thymic epithelial cells to expand the peripheral lymphocyte population. After emergence from the thymus gland, T cells acquire new surface antigen markers. The T cells circulate through the lymphatic and vascular systems as long-lived lymphocytes, which are called the recirculating pool. They then populate restricted regions of lymph nodes, forming thymic-dependent areas.

The significance of the leukocytes in human milk in affording immunological benefits to the breast-fed infant continues to be investigated. It is suggested that the lymphocytes can sensitize, induce immunological tolerance, or incite graft-versus-host reactions. According to Head and Beer, lymphocytes may be incor-porated into the suckling's tissues, achieving short-term adoptive immunization of the neonate.[16]

Studies of the activities of lymphocytes have been carried out by a number of investigators who collected samples of milk from lactating women at various times postpartum, examined the number of cell types present, and then studied the

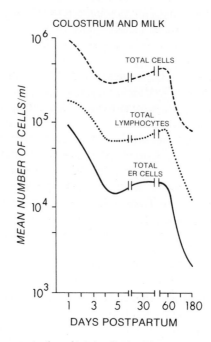

Fig. 5-1. Geometric mean concentration of total cells, lymphocytes, and E rosette-forming cells *(ER)* in the colostrum and milk of 200 lactating women. (Modified from Ogra, S. S., and Ogra, P. L.: J. Pediatr. **92:**546, 1978.)

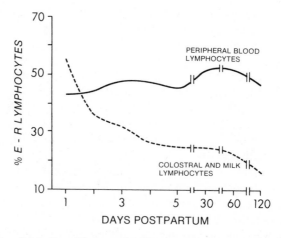

Fig. 5-2. Comparative distribution of E rosette-forming cells *(ER)* in peripheral blood and in colostrum and milk of 200 lactating women. (Modified from Ogra, S. S., and Ogra, P. L.: J. Pediatr. **92:**546, 1978.)

activities of these cells in vitro. Ogra and Ogra[29] collected samples from 200 women and measured the cell content from 1 through 180 days (Fig. 5-1). They then compared the response of T-lymphocytes in colostrum and milk with that of the T cells in the peripheral blood (Fig. 5-2).

The greatest number of cells appeared on the first day, with the counts ranging from 10,000 to 100,000/mm³ for total cells. By the fifth day, the count had dropped to 20% of the first day's count. In addition, the number of E rosette–forming cells was determined by using sheep erythrocyte–rosetting technique. The E rosette formation (ERF) lymphocytes constituted a mean 100/mm³ on the first day and a tenth of that by the fifth day.

At 180 days, total cells were 100,000/mm³, lymphocytes, 10,000/mm³, and ERF lymphocytes, 2000/mm³. The investigators compared the values to those in the peripheral blood of each mother (Fig. 5-2).

Ogra and Ogra[29] also studied the lymphocyte proliferation responses of colostrum and milk to antigens. Their data show response to stimulation from the viral antigens of rubella, cytomegalovirus, and mumps. Analysis of cell-mediated immunity to microbial antigens shows milk lymphocytes are limited in their potential for recognizing or responding to certain infectious agents, compared to cells from the peripheral circulation. To date human milk lymphocytes have not been shown to respond to *Candida albicans,* tetanus toxoid, or streptokinase. This is believed to be an intercellular action and not due to lack of external factors. On the other

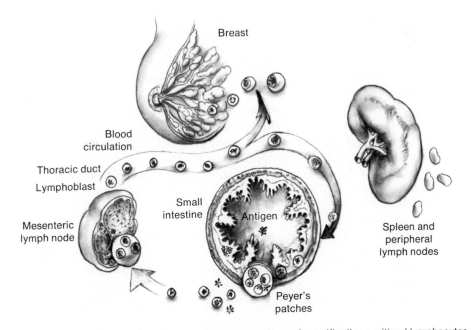

Fig. 5-3. Schematic diagram of mechanism by which progeny of specifically sensitized lymphocytes originating from gut-associated lymphoid tissue may migrate to and infiltrate mammary gland and its secretions, supplying breast with immune cells. (Modified from Head, J. R., and Beer, A. E.: The immunologic role of viable leukocytic cells in mammary exosecretions. In Larson, B. L., editor: Lactation, vol. IV. Mammary gland/human lactation/milk synthesis, New York, 1978, Academic Press, Inc.)

hand, the T cells and B cells have been shown to have unique reactivities not seen in peripheral blood. Goldblum and co-workers[11] were able to show a response in human colostrum to *E. coli* given orally, which was not accompanied by a systemic response in the mother. This suggests that milk provides a site for local humoral or cell-mediated immunity induced at a distant site such as the gut with the reactive lymphoid cells migrating to the breast. This concept has been further refined to suggest that IgA and IgM immunoglobulin in colostrum may represent migration of specific antibody-producing cells from the gut lymphoid tissue, specifically Peyer's patches, to the mammary gland. Ogra and Ogra[29] suggest that the cells may be selectively accumulated in the breast during pregnancy. The responses of milk cells and their antibodies are not representative of the total immunity of the individual. Parmely and co-workers[31] have provided a scheme to describe this mechanism (Fig. 5-3). The diagram depicts the progeny of specifically sensitized lymphocytes that originated in the lymphoid tissue of the gut as they migrate to the mammary gland. As they infiltrate the mammary gland and its secretion, they supply the breast with immune cells capable of selected immune responses.

Parmely and associates[31] partially purified and propagated milk lymphocytes in vitro to study their immunological function. Milk lymphocytes responded in a unique manner to stimuli known to activate T-lymphocytes from the serum. Milk lymphocytes are hyporesponsive to nonspecific mitogens and histocompatible antigens on allogenic cells in their laboratory. They, too, found them unresponsive to *Candida albicans*. Significant proliferation of lymphocytes occurred in response to K_1 capsular antigen of *E. coli*. Lymphocytes from blood failed to respond. This supports the concept of local mammary tissue immunity at the T-lymphocyte level.

More recent experiments in rodents have provided evidence the T-lymphocytes reactive to transplantation alloantigens can adoptively immunize the suckling newborn. Foster nursing experiments performed in rodents have shown that newborn rats exposed to allogenic milk manifested alterations in their reactivity to skin allografts of the foster mother's strain. In animals, mothers may give their suckling newborn immunoreactive lymphocytes. The influence of maternal milk cells on the development of neonatal immunocompetence has been demonstrated in several different immunological contexts. Congenitally, athymic nude mice nursed by their phenotypically normal mothers or normal foster mothers had increased survival. The mothers contributed their T cell–helper activity to the suckling newborn.

The accumulated research data support the concept that lymphocytes from colostrum and milk provide the human infant with immunological benefits. Both T- and B-lymphocytes are reactive against organisms invading the intestinal tract. Investigations on allergy, necrotizing enterocolitis, tuberculosis, and neonatal meningitis support the concept that milk fulfills a protective function.

SURVIVAL OF MATERNAL MILK CELLS

Although it is clear that cells are provided in the colostrum and milk, the effectiveness or impact of these cells on the neonate depend on their ability to survive in the gastrointestinal tract. It has been demonstrated in several species, including the human, that the pH of the stomach is as low as 0.5, but the output of HCl is minimal for the first few months, as is the peptic activity. Immediately after a feeding begins, the pH rises to 6.0 and returns to normal in 3 hr. The cells from milk tolerate this. Studies have also shown that intact nucleated lymphoid cells are found in the stomach and intestines. These cells, when removed from rat stomachs, are capable of phagocytosis. Lymphoid cells in milk have been shown to traverse the mucosal wall.

When human milk is stored, however, it has been shown that the cellular components do not tolerate heating to 63° C or cooling to −23° C or lyophilization. Although a few cells may be identified, they are not viable, according to Liebhaber and colleagues.[23]

HUMORAL FACTORS
Immunoglobulins

All classes of immunoglobulins are found in human milk. Immunological techniques developed in the past decade have enhanced the study of immunoglobulins through electrophoresis, chromatographics, and radioimmune assays. More than thirty components have been identified, and of these eighteen are associated with proteins in the maternal serum and the others are found exclusively in milk. Table 5-2 shows the relationship of antibody type with transplacental transfer.

The concentrations are highest in the colostrum of all species, demonstrated by the following figures developed by Michael and associates,[27] expressed in milligrams per 100 ml of colostrum:

> First day   600 IgA, 80 IgG, and 125 IgM
> Second day 260 IgA, 45 IgG, and 65 IgM
> Third day   200 IgA, 30 IgG, and 58 IgM
> Fourth day   80 IgA, 16 IgG, and 30 IgM

The main immunoglobulin in human serum is IgG; IgA is only a fifth the level of IgG. In milk, however, the reverse is true. IgA is the most important immunoglobulin in milk not only in concentration but also in biological activity. Of the IgA

Table 5-2. Relationship of antibody type with transplacental transfer*

Good passive transfer	Poor passive transfer	No passive transfer
Diphtheria antitoxin	*Haemophilus influenzae*	Enteric somatic (0)
Tetanus antitoxin	*Bordetella pertussis*	antibodies (Salmonella,
Antierythrogenic toxin	*Shigella flexneri*	Shigella, *E. coli*)
Antistaphylococcal antibody	Streptococcus MG	Skin-sensitizing antibody
Salmonella flagella (H) antibody		Heterophile antibody
Antistreptolysin		Wassermann antibody
All the antiviral antibodies		
present in maternal circulation		
(rubeola, rubella, mumps,		
poliovirus)		
VDRL antibodies		

*From Bellanti, J. A., and Hurtado, R. C.: Immunology and resistance to infection. In Remington, J. S., and Klein, J. O., editors: Infectious diseases of the fetus and newborn infant, Philadelphia, 1976, W. B. Saunders Co.

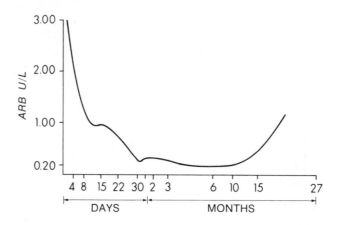

Fig. 5-4. IgA content during period of lactation. Concentration of IgA is given in arbitrary units based on mass concentration values (g/L). (Modified from Peitersen, B., et al.: Acta Paediatr. Scand. **64:**709, 1975.)

immunoglobulins, secretory IgA is the most significant and is likely synthesized in the mammary alveolar cells.

Quantitative determinations of immunoglobulins in human milk were made from milk collected at birth up to as long as 27 months postpartum by Peitersen and co-workers.[32] The IgA content was high immediately after birth, averaging 2.7 units, dropped to 0.3 units in 2 to 3 weeks, and then remained constant (Fig. 5-4). The researchers used an arbitrary unit of expression based on the mass concentration values (g/l) developed by Behring Werke for the quantitative result. Similar observations were made on IgG levels and IgM levels, demonstrated by Figs. 5-5 and 5-6. Simultaneously, they also compared milk and serum values in nineteen mothers and found the serum levels to be comparable to standard adult levels. Ogra and Ogra[29] have compared serum and milk levels at various times postpartum (Fig. 5-7). Samples obtained separately from the left and right breast showed similar values. The levels remained constant during a given feeding and for a 24 hr period as a whole. In all quantitative determinations, IgA is the predominant immunoglobulin in breast milk, constituting 90% of all the immunoglobulins in colostrum and milk.

Ogra and Ogra[29] studied the serum of postpartum lactating mothers and nonpregnant matched controls and noted that the individual and mean concentrations of all classes of immunoglobulin were lower in the postpartum subjects. The levels were statistically significant in IgG, being 50 to 70 mg higher in the nonpregnant women.

It is important to note as one records the fact that immunoglobulin levels, particularly IgA and IgM, are very high in colostrum and drop precipitously in the first 4 to 6 days, that the volume of mammary secretion also increases dramatically in this same period of time, thus the absolute number is more nearly constant than it would first appear. IgG does not show this decline. Local production and concentration of IgA and probably IgM may take place in the mammary gland at the time of delivery.

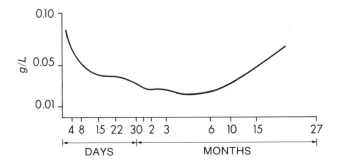

Fig. 5-5. IgG content during period of lactation recorded in arbitrary units. (Modified from Peitersen, B., et al.: Acta Paediatr. Scand. **64:**709, 1975.)

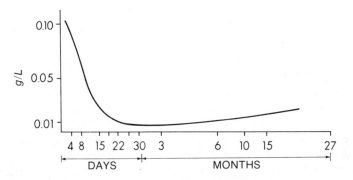

Fig. 5-6. IgM content during period of lactation. (Modified from Peitersen, B., et al.: Acta Paediatr. Scand. **64:**709, 1975.)

Stability of immunoglobulins. A study by Ford and associates[8] showed no change at 56° C but a 20% reduction in IgA with heating to 62.5° C for 30 min. IgM was totally destroyed by heat at 62.5° C. Freezing to −23° C for 4 weeks caused no alteration in IgA.

Secretory IgA differs antigenically from serum IgA. Secretory IgA can by synthesized in the nonlactating as well as the lactating breast. It is a compact molecule and resistant to proteolytic enzymes of the intestinal tract and the low pH of the stomach. It is manufactured by the mammary gland and by the cellular lymphocytes in milk. Levels in milk are 10 to 100 times higher than in serum. Levels in cow's milk are very low, that is, a tenth the level in mature milk (0.03 mg/100 ml). Later in life the intestinal tract subepithelial plasma cells secrete IgA, but not in the neonatal period.

Discussion continues as to whether or not antibodies are absorbed from the intestinal tract. There is, however, a wealth of evidence to demonstrate the activity of the immunoglobulins, especially sIgA, at the mucosal levels. These antibodies provide local intestinal protection against viruses such as poliovirus and bacteria such as *E. coli*, which may infect the mucosa or enter the body via the gut.

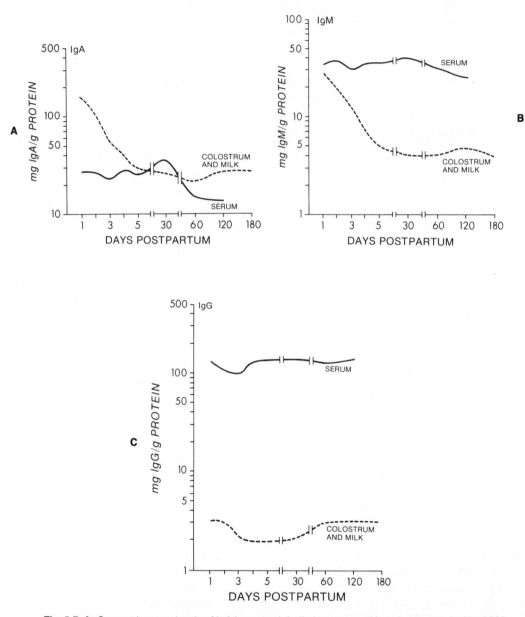

Fig. 5-7. A, Geometric mean levels of IgA immunoglobulin in serum and in colostrum and milk of 200 lactating women. **B,** Geometric mean levels of IgM immunoglobulin in serum and in colostrum and milk of 200 lactating women. **C,** Mean levels of IgG immunoglobulin in serum and in colostrum and milk of 200 lactating women at various times postpartum. (Modified from Ogra, S. S., and Ogra, P. L.: J. Pediatr. **92:**546, 1978.)

Bifidus factor

It has been established since the work of Tissier in 1908 on the intestinal flora of the newborn infant that the predominant bacteria of the breast-fed infant is bifid bacteria. This is a gram-positive, nonmotile anaerobic bacillus. Many observers have shown the striking difference between the flora of the gut of breast- and bottle-fed infants. György[14] demonstrated the presence of a specific factor in colostrum and milk that supported the growth of *Lactobacillus bifidus*. Bifidus factor has been characterized as a dialyzable nitrogen-containing carbohydrate that contains no amino acid.

In a prospective study of breast-fed Mayan Indian infants from birth to 3 years of age, bifid bacteria predominated and constituted 95% to 99% of the flora. Other culturable microorganisms were streptococci, bacteroides, clostridia, micrococci, enterococci, and *E. coli*. A change occurred when large amounts of solid foods were added at about a year of life. The solids were notably protein poor. *E. coli* progressively increased in numbers. *L. bifidus* metabolizes milk saccharides, producing large amounts of acetic acid, lactic acid, and some formic and succinic acids, which create the low pH of the stool of breast-fed infants. The intestinal flora of bottle-fed infants is gram-negative bacteria, especially coliform organisms and bacteroides.

The flora of bifid bacteria is inhibitory to certain pathogenic bacteria. Substantial clinical evidence is available to demonstrate that there is a resistance mechanism against intestinal infections from *Staphylococcus aureus,* Shigella, and Protozoa.

Resistance factor

The fact that human milk protects the human infant against staphylococcal infection was well known in the preantibiotic era. The protection continued

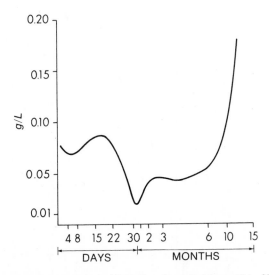

Fig. 5-8. Lysozyme content during period of lactation. In period from 15 to 27 months of lactation, lysozyme was found in only three samples, values varying considerably. (Modified from Peitersen, B., et al.: Acta Paediatr. Scand. **64:**709, 1975.)

Table 5-3. Antibacterial factors in colostrum and mature milk*

Group	Hemo-globin (g/100 ml)	Serum albumin (g/100 ml)	Immunoglobulins (mg/100 ml)			Lysozyme (mg/100 ml)	Lactoferrin (mg/100 ml)
			IgA	IgG	IgM		
Colostrum (1 to 5 days)							
Well-nourished women	11.5 ± 0.37	2.49 ± 0.065	335.9 ± 37.39 (17)†	5.9 ± 1.58 (17)	17.1 ± 4.29 (17)	14.2 ± 2.11 (15)	420 ± 49.0 (28)
Under-nour-ished women	11.3 ± 0.60	2.10 ± 0.081	374.3 ± 42.13 (10)	5.3 ± 2.30 (10)	15.3 ± 2.50 (10)	16.4 ± 2.39 (21)	520 ± 69.0 (19)
Mature milk (1 to 6 months)							
Well-nourished women	12.8 ± 0.43	3.39 ± 0.120	119.6 ± 7.85 (12)	2.9 ± 0.92 (12)	2.9 ± 0.92 (12)	24.8 ± 3.41 (10)	250 ± 65.0 (17)
Under-nour-ished women	12.6 ± 0.56	3.47 ± 0.130	118.1 ± 16.2 (10)	5.8 ± 3.41 (10)	5.8 ± 3.41 (10)	23.3 ± 3.53 (23)	270 ± 92.0 (13)

*From Reddy, V., et al.: Acta Paediatr. Scand. **66:**229, 1977.
†Figures in parentheses indicate number of samples analyzed.

throughout the lactation period. György[14] identified the presence of an ''antistaph-ylococcal factor'' in experiments with young mice who had been stressed with staphylococci. It has no demonstrable direct antibiotic properties. It was termed a ''resistance factor'' and described as nondialyzable, thermostable, and part of the free fatty acid part of the phosphide fraction, probably $C_{18:2}$, distinct from linoleic acid.

Lysozyme

Human milk contains a nonspecific antimicrobial factor, lysozyme, which is a thermostable, acid-stable enzyme. It is found in large concentrations in the stools of breast-fed infants and not in stools of formula-fed infants and thus is thought to influence the flora of the intestinal tract. Lysozyme levels show an increase over time during lactation (Fig. 5-8); this finding is more apparent in Indian women than in those of the Western world. Reddy and colleagues[32] studied the levels of lyso-zyme in well-nourished and poorly nourished women in India and found no differ-ence between them (Table 5-3). As shown in this study, lysozyme levels increase during lactation. Levels in human milk are 14 to 39 mg/100 ml, which is 300 times the level in cow's milk (13 μg/100 ml). Lysozyme is bacteriostatic against Entero-bacteriaceae and gram-positive bacteria.

Lactoferrin

Lactoferrin is an iron-binding protein that has a strong bacteriostatic effect on staphylococci and *E. coli,* apparently by depriving the organism of iron. Lactofer-rin is normally unsaturated with iron. It has been suggested that oral iron therapy can interfere with the bacteriostatic function of lactoferrin, which depends on its unsaturated state. Reddy and associates[32] showed that giving iron to the mother did not interfere with the saturation of lactoferrin in the milk and therefore its potential microbicidal effect (Table 5-4). Lactoferrin is less than 50% saturated with iron in human milk.

The concentration of lactoferrin is high in colostrum, 600 mg/100 ml, and then progressively declines over the next 5 months of lactation, leveling off at about 180 mg/100 ml (Table 5-3). It also contains small amounts of transferrin (10 to 15 μg/ml).

Unsaturated lactoferrin has been demonstrated by Kirkpatrick and co-workers[20] to inhibit the growth of *Candida albicans.* A combination of lactoferrin and specific antibody had a powerful bacteriostatic effect on *E. coli.* Inhibited *E. coli* appears to be markedly iron deficient. A significant factor that has been clearly demonstrated in preserving the bacteriostatic properties of human milk is the fact that milk proteins, including lysozyme and lactoferrin, reach the duodenum with-out any digestion taking place. They are stable in the acid pH of the stomach.

Table 5-4. Effect of iron therapy on lactoferrin in milk*†

	Total lactoferrin (mg/100 ml)	Saturated lactoferrin (% of total)
Before iron therapy	240 ± 29.0	9.0 ± 7.15
After iron therapy	260 ± 80.0	8.6 ± 3.32

*From Reddy, V., et al.: Acta Paediatr. Scand. **66:**229, 1977.
†Values are mean ±SE of eleven subjects.

Trypsin inhibitor has been identified in human milk, which temporarily delays the hydrolysis of protein.

Interferon

Colostrum cells in culture have been shown by Lawton and Shortridge[21] to be stimulated to secrete an interferon-like substance with strong antiviral activity up to 150 NIH units/ml. They did not find this property in the supernatant of colostrum or milk.

Complement

The C_3 and C_4 components of complement, known for their ability to fuse bacteria bound to a specific antibody, are present in colostrum in low concentrations compared to the levels in serum. IgG and IgM activate complement. C_3 proactivator has been described, and IgA and IgE have been identified as stimulating the system. Activated C_3 has opsonic, anaphylactic, and chemotactic properties and is important for the lysis of bacteria bound to a specific antibody.

B_{12}-binding protein

Unsaturated B_{12}-binding protein of high molecular weight has been found in very high levels in human milk and in the meconium and stools of breast-fed infants, compared to infant formulas and the infants who are formula-fed. The protein binding renders the B_{12} unavailable for bacterial growth of *E. coli* and bacteroides.

FLORA OF THE INTESTINAL TRACT

As has been pointed out, the normal flora of the intestinal tract of the breast-fed infant is *L. bifidus*. The gram-negative population in the gut is kept small. Two actions are apparent. The first encourages the growth of *L. bifidus* and thus crowds out the growth of other bacteria. Second, the number of pathogens is further kept low by the direct action of lysozyme and lactoferrin. When the number of pathogenic bacteria are kept low, the immune antibodies can keep the growth under control and prevent the absorption of bacteria through the gut wall into the bloodstream.

EVIDENCE OF EFFECTIVENESS OF HUMAN MILK IN CONTROLLING INFECTION

The properties of human milk do appear to control infection. There are specific disease entities that have shown a clear differential in the incidence between infants fed cow's milk and those fed human milk.

Bacterial infection

Breast milk IgA has antitoxin activity against enterotoxins of *E. coli* and *Vibrio cholerae*, which may be significant in preventing infantile diarrhea. Gindrat and colleagues[9a] found antibodies against 0 antigen of some of the most common serotypes of *E. coli* in high titer in breast milk samples collected from healthy mothers in Sweden. The infants who had consumed reasonable amounts of breast milk with high titers of *E. coli* antibodies had antibodies in their stool.

In studies by Gothefors and co-workers[12], it was shown that *E. coli* isolated from stools of breast-fed infants differed from those strains found in formula-fed infants in two respects. They were more sensitive to the bactericidal effect of human serum. More often, spontaneously agglutinated bacteria from other sites, such as the prepuce or periurethral area, were less sensitive in breast-fed infants. These findings support the theory that breast milk favors proliferation of mutant strains, which have decreased virulence. This mutation of bacterial strains is another way breast-feeding may protect against infection.

It has been suggested that milk immunization is a dynamic process because a mother's milk has been found to contain antibody to virtually all her infant's strains of intestinal bacteria. The mother exposed to the infant's microorganisms either via the breast or the gut responds immunologically to those microorganisms and thus protects her immunologically immature infant automatically.

The orderly review of data regarding the presence of antibodies in human milk has produced a substantial list of affected organisms. In addition to *E. coli*, there have been identified antibodies to *Bacteroides fragilis, Clostridium tetani, Haemophilus pertussis, Diplococcus pneumoniae, Corynebacterium diphtheriae, Salmonella, Shigella, Vibrio cholerae, Staphylococcus aureus,* and several strains of *Streptococcus.*

A study in Oslo by Hansen[15] of an outbreak of severe diarrhea due to *E. coli* strain 0111 showed six severely ill children were formula-fed. Two infants who were breast-fed had *E. coli* strain 0111 in their stools but showed few symptoms. Their mothers had no detectable antibodies for strain 0111 in their milk, which would suggest that other factors in human milk protect the infant from serious illness when there are no antibodies in the milk. Hansen[15] also showed in another study that after colonization with a specific strain of *E. coli*, mothers had large numbers of lymphoid cells in their milk with antibodies to that *E. coli*. Their serum produced no such response. This supports the concept that antigen-triggered lymphoid cells from Peyer's patches seek out lymphoid-rich tissue, producing IgA in the mammary gland. The mother is immunized in the gut at the same time her milk is. It has also been shown that *E. coli* enteritis can be cured by feeding human milk.

Infants with septicemia, meningitis, and urinary tract infections who were also breast-fed were studied by Winberg and Wessner.[36] The infants were compared to matched controls as to the amount of breast milk consumed. The sick infants consumed significantly less breast milk. The infants who received little at the breast were given supplementary formula feeding.

A study of possible cell-mediated immunity in breast-fed infants was undertaken by Schlesinger and Covelli.[34] They showed that tuberculin-positive nursing mothers had reactive T cells in their colostrum and early milk. Furthermore, eight of thirteen infants nursed by tuberculin-positive mothers had tuberculin-reactive peripheral blood T cells after four weeks. Cord blood had no such activity.

Viral infection

Protection against viruses has been the subject of similar studies. Breast milk contains antibodies against poliovirus, coxsackievirus, echovirus, influenza virus, reovirus, and rhinovirus. It has been confirmed that human milk inhibits the growth of these viruses in tissue culture. Nonspecific substances in human milk are active against arbovirus and murine leukemia virus, according to work by Fieldsteel.[7]

A high degree of antiviral activity against Japanese B encephalitis virus as well as the two leukemia viruses has been found in human milk. The factor was found in the fat fraction and was not destroyed by extended heating, which distinguishes it from antibodies.

Specimens of human colostrum have been found to contain neutralizing activity against respiratory syncytial virus. Respiratory syncytial virus (RSV) has become a major threat in infancy and is the most common reason for hospitalization in infancy in some developed countries. It has a high mortality. Epidemics have occurred in special-care nurseries. Statistically significant data collected by Downham[6] showed that few breast-fed babies (8 out of 115) were among the infants hospitalized for RSV infection, compared to controls who were breast-fed (46 of 167).

Necrotizing enterocolitis has been a serious threat to premature infants in acute care newborn nurseries in recent years. Animal studies have demonstrated a protective quality to breast milk. Efforts to confirm a similar relationship in human infants have been encouraging but not conclusive. Leukocytes in milk fulfill a protective function, possibly as a consequence of their natural transplantation, according to Beer and Billingham.[2]

The relationship of sudden infant death to formula-feeding is supported by circumstantial evidence and retrospective studies. The fact remains that in all series reported, sudden infant death is rare in breast-fed infants. Whether this is related to protection against infection is not clear.

The apparent predisposition of bottle-fed infants to purulent otitis media as compared to breast-fed infants may be due to IgA-conferred immunity in human milk. It may also be due to the mechanics of bottle-feeding. Of a group of infants with otitis media, 85% had had their bottles propped up, whereas only 8% of a matched bottle-feeding control group who did not have otitis media had had their bottles propped up. When one swallows fluid lying flat on the back, it is possible to regurgitate it into the eustachian tube.[1]

ALLERGIC PROTECTIVE PROPERTIES

In discussing the antiallergic properties of human milk, it is more difficult to identify specific protective properties.

During the neonatal period, the small intestine has increased permeability to macromolecules. Infants have more serum and secretory antibodies against dietary proteins than children or adults. Production of secretory IgA in the intestinal tract is delayed until 6 weeks to 3 months of age. Secretory IgA in colostrum and breast milk prevents the absorption of foreign macromolecules when the infant's immune system is immature. Protein of breast milk is species specific and therefore nonallergic for the human infant. No antibody response has been demonstrated to occur with human milk in human infants. It has also been shown that macromolecules in breast milk are not absorbed.

Indirect evidence can be inferred from a demonstration of the response to cow's milk protein. Within 18 days of taking cow's milk, the infant will begin to develop antibodies. Since the advent of prepared formulas, in which the protein has been denatured by heating and drying, the incidence of cow's milk allergy has been considered to be 1%. The most reliable means of diagnosing it is by challenging with isolated cow's milk protein. Although circulating antibodies and co-proantibodies have been identified, these are not reliable techniques for the clinician involved in patient care.

The allergic syndromes that have been associated with cow's milk allergy include gastroenteropathy, atopic dermatitis, rhinitis, chronic pulmonary disease, eosinophilia, failure to thrive, and sudden death, or cot death, which has been attributed to anaphylaxis to cow's milk. The gastrointestinal symptoms have received the greatest attention and include spitting, colic, diarrhea, blood in the stools, frank vomiting, weight loss, malabsorption, colitis, and failure to thrive. It has been associated in the gastrointestinal protein and blood loss. The diagnosis is best made by elimination diet and, when appropriate, challenge tests. Cutaneous testing is of little help.

The association of nasal-secretion eosinophilia with feeding cow's milk and/or solid foods as compared to eosinophilia in strictly breast-fed infants was shown by Murray.[28] Of free-fed infants 32% had high eosinophilic secretions and only 11% of breast-fed infants had eosinophils in nasal secretions.

It is not surprising that many different antigenic specificities are recognized when the colostrum or milk of one species is fed to or is injected into another species. Cow's milk is high on the list of food allergens, particularly in children; sensitivity to cow's milk is responsible for at least 20% of all pediatric allergic conditions, according to Gerrard.[9] Evidence exists that IgA antibodies play an important role in confining food antigens to the gut. Food antigens given to a bottle-fed infant before he can make his own IgA and when he is deprived of that in human milk and the plasma cells may be expected to be more readily absorbed.

The association of the drop in breast-feeding and the rise in allergy was first made by Glaser.[10] He pioneered the theory of prophylactic management of allergy. The management of the potentially allergic infant will be discussed in Chapter 15.

REFERENCES

1. Beauregard, W. G.: Positional otitis media, J. Pediatr. **79:**294, 1971.
2. Beer, A. E., and Billingham, R. E.: Immunologic benefits and hazards of milk in maternal-perinatal relationships, Ann. Intern. Med. **83:**865, 1975.
3. Bellanti, J. A., and Hurtado, R. C.: Immunology and resistance to infection. In Remington, J. S., and Klein, J. O., editors: Infectious diseases of the fetus and newborn infant, Philadelphia, 1976, W. B. Saunders Co.
4. Bullen, J. J.: Iron-binding proteins and other factors in milk responsible for resistance to E. coli. In Ciba Foundation Symposium no. 42, New York, 1976, Elsevier North Holland, Inc.
5. Chandon, R. C., Shahani, K. M., and Holly, R. G.: Lysozyme content of human milk, Nature **204:**76, 1964.
6. Downham, M. A. P. S., et al.: Breast feeding protects against respiratory syncytial virus infections, Br. Med. J. **2:**274, 1976.
7. Fieldsteel, A. H.: Nonspecific antiviral substance in human milk active against arbovirus and murine leukemia virus, Cancer Res. **34:**712, 1974.
8. Ford, J. E., et al.: Influences of the heat treatment of human milk on some of its protective constituents, J. Pediatr. **90:**29, 1977.
9. Gerrard, J. W.: Allergy in infancy, Allerg. Pediatr. Ann. **3:**9, Oct. 1974.

9a. Gindrat, J. J., et al.: Antibodies in human milk against *E. coli* of the serogroups most commonly found in neonatal infection, Acta Paediatr. Scand. **61:**587, 1972.

10. Glaser, J.: The dietary prophylaxis of allergic disease in infancy, J. Asthma Res. **3:**199, 1966.

11. Goldblum, R. M., et al.: Antibody-forming cells in human colostrum after oral immunization, Nature **257:**797, 1975.

12. Gothefors, L., Olling, S., and Winberg, J.: Breast feeding and biological properties of faecal E. coli strains, Acta Paediatr. Scand. **64:**807, 1975.

13. Gullberg, R.: Possible influence of vitamin B_{12} binding protein in milk on the intestinal flora in breast-fed infants. II. Contents of unsaturated B_{12}-binding protein in meconium and faeces from breast-fed and bottle-fed infants, Scand. J. Gastroenterol. **9:**287, 1974.

14. György, P.: A hitherto unrecognized biochemical difference between human milk and cow's milk, Pediatrics **11:**98, 1953.

15. Hanson, L. A.: Escherichia coli infections in childhood: significance of bacterial virulence and immune defense, Arch. Dis. Child. **51:**737, 1976.

16. Head, J. R., and Beer, A. E.: The immunologic role of viable leukocytic cells in mammary exosecretions. In Larson, B. L., editor: Lactation, vol. IV. Mammary gland/human lactation/milk synthesis, New York, 1978, Academic Press, Inc.

16a. Ho, P. C., and Lawton, J. W. M.: Human colostral cells: phagocytosis and killing of *E. coli* and *C. albicans,* J. Pediatr. **93:**910, 1978.

17. Iyengar, L., and Selvaraj, R. J.: Intestinal absorption of immunoglobulins by newborn infants, Arch. Dis. Child. **47:**411, 1972.

18. Jelliffe, D. B., and Jelliffe, E. F. P.: Human milk in the modern world, Oxford, 1978, Oxford University Press.

19. Johnstone, D. E., and Dutton, A. M.: Dietary prophylaxis of allergic disease in children, N. Engl. J. Med. **274:**715, 1966.

20. Kirkpatrick, C. H., et al.: Inhibition of growth of Candida albicans by iron-unsaturated lactoferrin: relation to host-defense mechanisms in chronic mucocutaneous candidiasis, J. Infect. Dis. **124:**539, 1971.

21. Lawton, J. W. M., and Shortridge, K. F.: Protective factors in human breast milk and colostrum, Lancet **1:**253, 1977.

22. Lebenthal, E.: Symposium on gastrointestinal and liver disease, cow's milk protein allergy, Pediatr. Clin. North Am. **22:**827, 1975.

23. Liebhaber, M., et al.: Alterations of lymphocytes and of antibody content of human milk after processing, J. Pediatr. **91:**897, 1977.

24. Mata, L. J., and Urrutia, J. J.: Intestinal colonization of breast-fed children in a rural area of low socioeconomic level, Ann. N.Y. Acad. Sci. **176:**93, 1971.

25. Mata, L. J., and Wyatt, R. G.: Host resistance to infection. In Jelliffe, D. B., and Jelliffe, E. F. P., editors: The uniqueness of human milk, Am. J. Clin. Nutr. **24:**976, 1971.

26. Matthews, T. H. J., et al.: Antiviral activity in milk of possible clinical importance, Lancet **2:**1387, 1976.

27. Michael, J. G., Ringenback, R., and Hottenstein, S.: The antimicrobial activity of human colostral antibody in the newborn, J. Infect. Dis. **124:**445, 1971.

28. Murray, A. B.: Infant feeding and respiratory allergy, Lancet **1:**497, 1971.

29. Ogra, S. S., and Ogra, P. L.: Immunologic aspects of human colostrum and milk, I. Distribution characteristics and concentrations of immunoglobulins at different times after the onset of lactation, J. Pediatr. **92:**546, 1978.

30. Ogra, S. S., and Ogra, P. L.: Immunologic aspects of human colostrum and milk, II. Characteristics of lymphocyte reactivity and distribution of E-rosette forming cells at different times after the onset of lactation, J. Pediatr. **92:**550, 1978.

31. Parmely, M. J., Beer, A. E., and Billingham, R. E.: In vitro studies of the T-lymphocyte population of human milk, J. Exp. Med. **144:**358, 1976.

32. Peitersen, B., Bohn, L., and Andersen, H.: Quantitative determination of immunoglobulins, lysozyme, and certain electrolytes in breast milk during the entire period of lactation, during a 24-hour period, and in milk from the individual mammary gland, Acta Paediatr. Scand. **64:**709, 1975.

32a. Pittard, W. B., III: Breast milk immunology, a frontier in infant nutrition, Am. J. Dis. Child. **133:**83, 1979.

33. Reddy, V., et al.: Antimicrobial factors in human milk, Acta Paediatr. Scand. **66:**229, 1977.
34. Schlesinger, J. J., and Covelli, H. D.: Evidence for transmission of lymphocyte responses to tuberculin by breast-feeding, Lancet **2:**529, 1977.
35. Stoliar, O. A., et al.: Secretory IgA against enterotoxins in breast milk, Lancet **1:**1258, 1976.
36. Winberg, J., and Wessner, G.: Does breast milk protect against septicaemia in the newborn? Lancet **1:**1091, 1971.

CHAPTER 6

Psychological bonding

Although the previous chapters provide more than adequate information to support the urgency of breast-feeding in almost every case, the critical impact in the return to breast-feeding in modern cultures rests with the issue of the mother's role and her perception of breast-feeding as a biological act. The maternal influences include psychophysiological reactions during nursing, long-term psychophysiological effects, maternal behavior, sexual behavior, and attitudes toward men. All professionals providing support care in the perinatal period will also need to have a clear view not only of the biological benefits but also their own psychological hang-ups regarding the breast itself. The breast has been a sex object in the Western world in this century and its biological benefits have been downplayed. This is clearly demonstrated by the conflicting mores that permit pornographic pictures in newspapers and movies and nude theater but arrest a mother, discretely nursing her baby in public, for indecent exposure.

It has been generally accepted by proponents of breast-feeding, even prior to the upsurge of interest and research in bonding, that the major reason to breast-feed is to provide that special relationship and closeness that accompanies nursing. Conversely, the major contraindication to breast-feeding was lack of desire to do so. This was evidenced by the fact that it was considered more appropriate to present breast-feeding as a matter of personal choice with no compelling reasons to urge a mother to consider nursing. The concern over creating guilt in the mother who chose not to nurse has been significant to the clinician.

MOTHER-INFANT INTERACTION

The studies done in recent years to understand bonding have largely been done without reference to breast-feeding. It has been pointed out that a comprehensive book, *Attachment and Loss* by Bowlby,[4] which reviews early mother-infant interactions extensively, never mentions breast-feeding. In addition, sucking is given extensive treatment without making a distinction between bottle and breast or implying there is an alternative to the bottle. Work by Spitz[22] and others has identified the devastating effects on the infant when he is deprived of long-term maternal contact. These investigators demonstrated major deficits in development, both mental and motor, as well as general failure to thrive. What had yet to be described was the impact on the mother. Klaus and Kennell[15] have provided those data in their many writings on mother-infant interaction, which are summarized in their book, *Maternal-Infant Bonding*. There is reason to believe that the maternal-infant bond is the strongest human bond, when two major facts are considered, that is, the infant's early growth is within the mother's body and after birth his survival depends on her care. Although the process had not been meticulously described, it had been noted by Budin[6] that when a mother was separated from her infant and was unable to provide the early care of her sick child, she lost interest and even abandoned the infant.

Klaus and Kennell[15] point out that there is probably a critical period in which ideal bonding takes place in the human. This critical period has been described for many animal species, in which the mother rejects or even destroys her offspring if they are taken from her at a critical early postpartum time. For the goat this time is the first 5 min. For the human, Kennell and co-workers[14] described this critical period as within the first 12 hr. Further, they noted that mothers in the United States showed different attachment behavior when permitted early contact with their premature infants compared to mothers who have first contact at 3 weeks of age. Mothers of full-term infants who were allowed contact within the first 2 hr and subsequently extra contact behaved differently at 1 month and 1 year with their babies, compared with controls. Klaus and Kennell's[15] further work in Guatemala confirmed these findings. Actually, Jackson and associates[13] made similar observations in the Yale Rooming-In Unit in 1945 to 1955, but failed to provide control observations.

Kennell and colleagues[14] conclude, "These and other studies in the human suggest that shortly after birth there is a sensitive period which appears to have long-lasting effects on maternal attachments and which may ultimately affect the development of the child."

The impact of early mother-infant interaction and breast-feeding on the duration of breast-feeding has been reported; no data appear to be available as to whether or not mothering is different in breast-feeding and bottle-feeding mothers. Sosa and co-workers[21] reported the effect of early mother-infant contact on breast-feeding, infection, and growth. Breast-feeding mothers who were permitted early contact but not early breast-feeding were compared with mothers without early contact who also breast-fed. The mothers with early contact were observed to nurse 50% longer than the controls. The early-contact infants were heavier and had fewer infections. Sosa and associates[21] conducted a similar study in Brazil, in which study mother nursed immediately on delivery and the infant was kept beside mother's bed until they went home. At home they had a special nurse make continual contacts to help in the breast-feeding. The control had traditional therapy, that is, contact at feeding times after an early glimpse. Infants were housed in a separate nursery. At two months, 77% of the early-contact mothers were successfully nursing and only 27% of the controls.

An additional study by DeChateau[9] in Sweden investigated a group of twenty-one mothers with early contact and nineteen control mothers, all of whom were breast-feeding to begin with. The only difference in management was the first 30 min of early contact, since 24 hr rooming-in was provided for all mothers after 2 hr postpartum. The length of breast-feeding differed: early contact, 175 days, and control, 105 days. Follow-up observations at 3 months of age showed different mothering behavior. The study group had more attachment behavior, fondling, caressing, and kissing than the controls.

On the basis of several such studies, Klaus and Kennell[15] ". . . strongly believe that an essential principle of attachment is that there is a sensitive period in the first

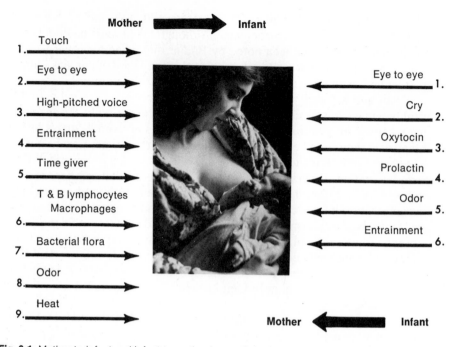

Fig. 6-1. Mother-to-infant and infant-to-mother interactions that can occur simultaneously in first days of life. (From Klaus, M. H., and Kennell, J. H.: Maternal-infant bonding, the impact of early separation or loss on family development, St. Louis, 1976, The C. V. Mosby Co.)

minutes and hours after an infant's birth which is optimal for parent-infant attachment." This sensitive period seems to coincide with the period of quiet alert in the first hour of life. Unless heavy medication or difficult delivery intervene, an infant experiences a period when his eyes are wide open, he can see, has visual preferences, turns to the spoken word, and responds to his environment. Such a period in the state of consciousness of the infant may last only seconds or minutes at a time over the next few days.

When Klaus and Kennell[15] diagramed the reciprocal interaction in the first few hours of life, they chose a nursing mother-infant couple. They included in their scheme the factors that are limited to breast-feeding, such as the transfer of lymphocytes and macrophages from mother to infant and the stimulation of oxytocin and prolactin by suckling of the infant as part of the reciprocal interaction (Fig. 6-1).

PSYCHOLOGICAL DIFFERENCE BETWEEN BREAST- AND BOTTLE-FEEDING

Professionals have spent decades reassuring mothers that they can capture the same emotional and behavioral experience feeding their infant a bottle as they can feeding at the breast. The same warmth and love is there. Technically speaking, the same warmth is not there, as the lactating breast has been shown to be warmer than the nonlactating. It can be demonstrated by infrared pictures as well.

Newton and Newton[17] suggest that special caution should be used in evaluating statistical associative studies that purport to study the hypothesis that breast- and bottle-feeding are psychological equivalents. "Because breast-feeding involves a large measure of personal choice and because it is related to attitudinal and personality factors, no groups of breast- and bottle-feeders are likely to be equal in other respects. Therefore the relation of breast-feeding to any particular psychosocial measure may not be cause and effect, but simply the differences due to other uncontrolled covariables."[17] A human mother's care of her infant is derived from a complex mixture of her genetic endowment, the response of the infant, a long history of interpersonal relationships with others, her family constellation, this and previous pregnancies, and the community and culture.

Before reviewing specific psychological attributes relating to breast-feeding, it might be well to deal with the distinction between styles of nursing. Newton[16] has described two distinct groups: unrestricted breast-feeding and token breast-feeding.

Unrestricted breast-feeding

Unrestricted breast-feeding means the infant is put to the breast whenever he cries or fusses. Feeding is ad lib and not by the clock, usually leading to ten or more feedings a day. The infant receives no bottles, and solids are not introduced until the second half of the first year. Breast milk continues to be a major source of nourishment beyond the first year of life. It is interesting to note that this was routine practice in the United States in the beginning of this century as attested by writings on the subject of child rearing.

Token breast-feeding

Token breast-feeding is characterized by rules and regulations. Feeding is done by the clock both in frequency and duration. It is deemed unnecessary to permit unlimited suckling. Weaning usually occurs by the third month, if not before. Supplementary bottles and solids are not uncommon. As a result, the let-down reflex is never well established. Engorgement is not uncommon. The infant is frequently too frantic from crying or too sleepy to feed well at the appointed times.

A study at the University of Rochester of urban physicians revealed that many of the pediatricians prescribed solids by three months or earlier and suggested supplementary bottles. Most of the physicians in the family medicine program in the same community, however, provided no supplements and no solids until 6 months. Over 50% of mothers in that community who planned to breast-feed had made contact with some childbirth or breast-feeding program and chose their physician according to his practice style.

PERSONALITY DIFFERENCES BETWEEN BREAST- AND BOTTLE-FEEDING MOTHERS

There are clear differences between mothers who practice unrestricted breast-feeding and those who bottle-feed. There are actually some distinctions between token-feeders and bottle-feeders. It has been said that maternal personality is more important to the development of the infant's personality than either breast- or bottle-feeding per se. Experimenters looking at these questions have provided a wealth of somewhat conflicting information. Chamberlain[8] undertook to decipher the differences between mothers who bottle-fed and those who practiced unrestricted breast-feeding with their second child. The groups were similar in age, education, parity, intelligence, and socioeconomic status. The breast-feeding mothers were less defensive about their method of feeding, were more oriented toward home life, and had higher radicalism scores. The bottle-feeding mothers confirmed the hypothesis that they had problems in trying to breast-feed their first child due to inadequate lactation, possibly a psychosomatic reaction. They also had a greater incidence of sexual anomalies, as indicated from a higher surgency score. The breast-feeding mothers wanted their children to do things typical of children; the bottle-feeding mothers preferred their children to be conservative and other-person oriented.

Call[7] had studied the emotional factors favoring successful breast-feeding and noted that of 104 consecutive mothers delivering at an Air Force hospital, 42.6% of the multiparas and 50% of the primiparas chose bottle-feeding. Of the breast-feeding mothers, 48% of those multiparas and 40% of the primiparas were successful beyond 3 weeks. Failure was associated with engorgement, lack of let-down reflex, and psychological conflict. The two conflicts seen in those who did not nurse and those who failed were as follows:

1. They had a conflict in accepting the biological maternal role in relation to the infant versus other roles society holds for women. The maternal role is considered a general class attitude in middle-class American society.
2. They had a conflict regarding the functioning of the breast itself, that is, as an organ for nourishment of the young versus a sexual organ affording the breast the same psychological value as the penis in the male. Nursing thus becomes a castration threat.

PSYCHOPHYSIOLOGICAL REACTIONS DURING NURSING

Newton and Newton[17] have equated psychophysiological reactions during nursing to the degree of successful lactation. During unrestricted suckling the gentle stroking of the nipple occurs 3000 to 4000 times. This should result in an increase in temperature of the mammary skin and rhythmical contraction of the uterus. Failure to experience these signs is related to failure to produce adequate milk.

The long-term psychophysiological reaction of unrestricted nursing is a more even mood cycle compared to the mood swings associated with ovulation and menstruation. Unrestricted nursing is associated with secondary amenorrhea for at least sixteen months, if nursing continues that long.

From studies in animals, Thoman and co-workers[23] have stated "The present experiments do indicate that there is a unique buffering system which appears to protect the lactating female from large variations in responsiveness during the process of lactating. Inasmuch as there exists considerable information that indicates that maternal factors have profound and long-lasting effects on the psychophysiological function of offspring in adulthood, the existence of such buffering systems in the lactating females would appear to be of importance in the mother-young interaction."

When the rate of success in breast-feeding is related to experiences at birth, Jackson and associates[13] reported that the more difficult the labor, the less successful the breast-feeding. A direct correlation has also been made with the amount of medication and anesthetic given during labor and delivery and subsequently the sleepiness of the infant and, ultimately, the inadequacy of the suckling.

Newton observed that mothers who talked to their babies on the second day nursed their babies longer, that is, beyond the second month.

IMPACT OF SOCIETY, MEDICAL PROFESSION, AND FAMILY
Society

Newton[16] has pointed out that a woman's joy in and acceptance of the female biological role in life may be an important factor in her psychosexual behavior, which includes lactation. She found that women who wished to bottle-feed also believed that the male role was the more satisfying role. Nulliparous women who planned to breast-feed their children more often stated their satisfaction with the female role, according to Adams.[1] Breast-feeding behavior has been related to a woman's role in life as influenced by her cultural locale, education, social class, and work. Breast-feeding rates and weaning times vary in the United States by geographical area, as pointed out by Robertson.[20] The smaller the community, the longer the duration of breast-feeding. Cross-cultural studies in large cities show variation in rates of nursing. These rates are influenced by education and, in this generation, the higher the education, the higher the incidence of breast-feeding.

The attitudes of the husband, close family, and friends have an influence on the mother's attitude toward breast-feeding. More important, their attitudes influence the rate of success and the age at weaning more negatively than positively. One study showed that a grandmother's interest did not influence the mother's decision to nurse as frequently as a friend's (peer) decision to bottle-feed.

The unrestricted breast-fed infant cries and his mother has the urge to suckle him because the cry has triggered her let-down reflex. The breast is turgescent and ready for the infant. Unrestricted crying is rarely seen in these infants. With token breast-feeding, such a response does not occur on schedule and from feeding to feeding the milk supply may be little or, conversely, gushing. The infant is unable to cope with the unpredictability.

Medical profession

The enthusiastic physician can influence the number of breast-feeding mothers in his practice; this has been demonstrated. If the physician provides knowledgeable medical and psychological support, the success rate of the patients who intended to breast-feed will increase. Some patients who had not formed an opinion or given it any thought in their preparation for motherhood will be persuaded to try. In addition, this physician will attract patients to the practice who are already successfully breast-feeding but find their own physician unable or unwilling to support their efforts.

A study was done at the University of Rochester in a small city where over fifty pediatricians practiced. The pediatricians described their own practices according to the number of breast-feeding mothers there were (high, 75%; moderate, 50%; low, 25%). They were also asked when they started solid foods and general practice "regulations" and, finally, how their own children were fed. The physicians with a high incidence of breast-feeding in their practices started solids after 4 months, had few rules and regulations about the office, and usually their own children had been breast-fed. The physician with a high number of bottle-feeders started solids by 6 weeks, had many rules and regulations about the practice, and their own children had been bottle-fed. When asked about using lay groups to help their patients breast-feed, the female physicians were more apt than the male physicians to discredit what these mothers could do to help other mothers.

The family

Impact on the infant. For the infant, there are differences in the alleviation of hunger, the mother-infant interaction, oral gratification, activity, development, personality, and adaption to the environment.

DEVELOPMENT. Early assessment of newborns in the first or second week of life shows more body activity with breast-fed than bottle-fed infants. They are more alert and have stronger arousal reaction. Statistics reported by Douglas[10] on age of learning to walk in Great Britain showed a distinct difference, with breast-fed infants starting 2 months earlier than bottle-fed. The longer the infant was nursed, the more striking the differences. Thus prolonged breast-feeding does not impede development, as has been implied by advocates of early weaning. A study in Illinois[12] in 1929 compared children exclusively breast-fed for 4 months, 9 months, and over a year to bottle-fed infants. The children who were exclusively breast-fed 4 and 9 months scored significantly higher on achievement tests, but the difference was reversed beyond a year. Exclusively breast-feeding beyond a year increased morbidity as well, which is in keeping with the concept that solids should be added in the second half of the first year.

Animal work has also shown a relationship of weaning time to learning skills. Since it has become evident that there are species-specific proteins and amino acids, it is possible that the brain develops more physiologically with the precise basic nutrients. Comparisons with animal species show that the more intelligent and skillful groups within a species are nursed longer.

PERSONALITY. The personality and adjustment of infants as related to their early feeding experiences have been the subject of much discussion. It must be acknowledged that the personality of the mother and the temperament of the child need to be considered. Some conflicting information is reported in studies analyzing retrospectively the effects of breast-feeding on outcome in terms of security and behavior. The emphasis has been on the duration of the breast-feeding rather than the quality of the relationship. When abrupt weaning takes place, it may be psychologically very traumatic for the infant and the mother. In animals, when the mother is stressed while lactating, the nursling's plasma cortisone levels are elevated. The psychologically depressed mother may not experience postpartum depression until the infant is weaned from the breast. It has been accepted that early experience, including feeding experience, does influence later behavior in the long run, but much more study must be done before the impact of nursing at the breast is truly understood in this complex culture today.

Impact on the father. Since the birthing process moved into the hospital setting, the father has been moved further and further from the nucleus of his new family. Fortunately, in recent years this trend has been reversed. Research on interaction with the infant had focused on the mother until Parke and associates[18] observed all three together. In the triadic situation, the father tends to hold the baby twice as much as mother, touches the baby slightly more, but smiles significantly less than the mother. The father plays the more active role when both are present. The study was conducted with middle-class participants who had been to childbirth classes, but the same results were obtained among low-income families without preparation or the presence of the father in the labor and delivery room. The infant had to be relatively active and responsive to capture the father's attention. The investigators felt fathers were far more involved in and responsive toward their infants than our culture had acknowledged. Other studies have shown that when fathers were asked to undress their babies and establish eye-to-eye contact with them in the first few days of life, they showed more care giving behavior than the controls 3 months later.

Newton describes the early attachments of the new family as follows:

Father	interacts with baby	engrossment
Mother	interacts with baby	bonding
Baby	interacts with mother	attachment

The father has been brought back into the childbirth scene as a coach, which has been described as the father's role in shared childbirth. The idea of coaching has negative connotations, since a coach is one who develops the players to work and try harder but always to win. The father should be a partner and supporter in labor, delivery, and breast-feeding. Raphael[19] has suggested that the father may well play the role of the doula. The doula is one who provides psychological encouragement and physical assistance to the newly delivered mother. Raphael further indicates that it is the lack of a doula to support the mother that predisposes her to failure with breast-feeding.

There is more to nurturing the infant than feeding. The father therefore should play a very significant role with the infant. For instance, when the infant is fussy and does not need to be fed, comforting is often best done by the father.

Fathers who object to their wives breast-feeding may do so because they do not want to share this part of their lover with an infant. Some fathers express concern that the breasts will leak and destroy any sexual mystique. On the other hand, many men take great pride in the knowledge that their infants will be breast-fed and support their wives in this effort. The decision to breast-feed should be made with the full involvement of the father in most cases.

Impact on siblings. Although there is some information about siblings and breast-feeding with regard to behavior patterns, there are no known studies comparing siblings of bottle- and breast-fed infants. Just as siblings frequently wish to try the infant's bottle, they may wish to nurse at the breast. The child will reflect the mother's attitude toward the breast and nursing. If the mother nurses secretly or in private and isolates herself from the family, it may cause concern in the sibling and produce feelings of shame or guilt regarding the breasts.

WHY WOMEN DO NOT BREAST-FEED

Before the trend to bottle-feeding can be reversed, one has to understand why some women do not breast-feed. It cannot be blamed on society or the medical profession when a woman cannot accept this as part of the biological role of a mother. A physician who does not understand the complexities of rejecting breast-feeding cannot hope to assist a mother to succeed in breast-feeding.

Bentovim[3] has taken a systems approach, pointing out that a range of physical, psychological, and sociological factors are involved. A general systems-theory approach provides an explanatory model in which the elements are envisioned as interacting dynamically (Fig. 6-2). ''Breast-feeding is a systemic product of many

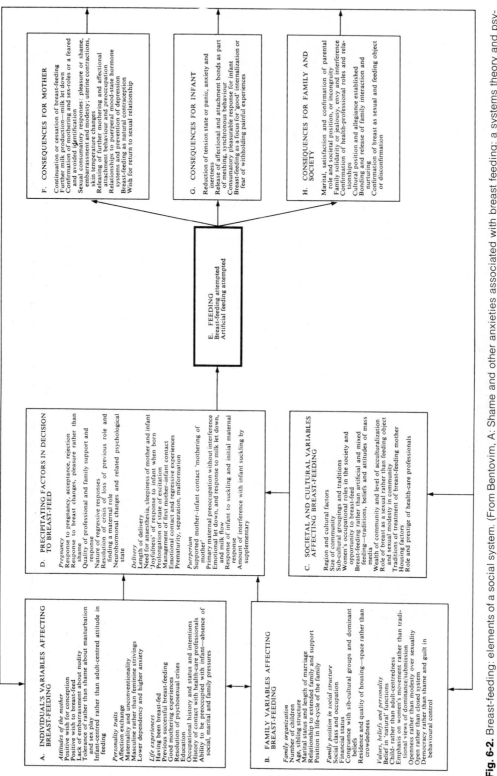

Fig. 6-2. Breast-feeding: elements of a social system. (From Bentovim, A: Shame and other anxieties associated with breast feeding: a systems theory and psychodynamic approach. In Ciba Foundation Symposium no. 45, breast feeding and the mother, Amsterdam, 1976, Elsevier Scientific Publ. Co., p. 159.)

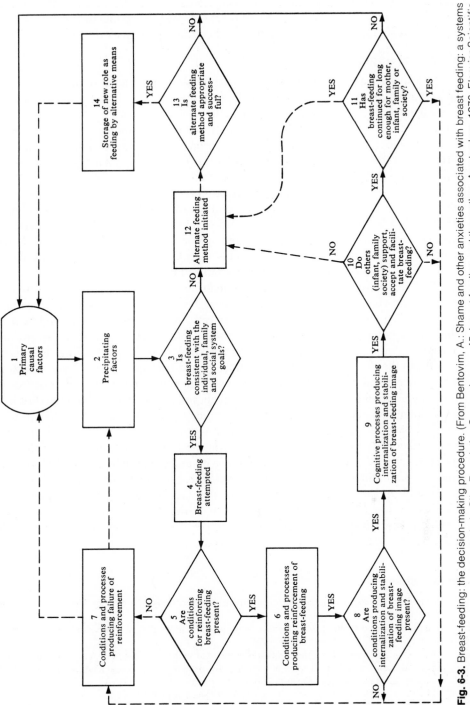
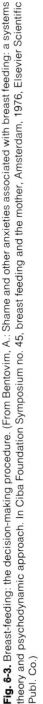

Fig. 6-3. Breast-feeding: the decision-making procedure. (From Bentovim, A.: Shame and other anxieties associated with breast feeding: a systems theory and psychodynamic approach. In Ciba Foundation Symposium no. 45, breast feeding and the mother, Amsterdam, 1976, Elsevier Scientific Publ. Co.)

interacting factors rather than a product of individual behavior only,"[3] according to Bentovim. A good experience with breast-feeding can ensure an intense interaction and synchronous response of giving and taking. According to Brazelton,[5] this is the essence of the infant's beginning to create a secure world for himself.

Block diagram approach

Bentovim[3] has created a block diagram (Fig. 6-2) as the first step, describing quantitative and conceptual relationships. Following the diagram, block A contains the variables relating to the mother and her characteristics that convinced her to breast-feed. Block B includes the characteristics of the family relating to breast-feeding. Block C contains variables in society that influenced the decision to breast-feed. Block D is the precipitating factors (such as pregnancy!) that are acted on by A, B, and C to make the decision to breast-feed this particular infant. Block E represents the attempt to feed, which has consequences for the mother as listed in block F, for the child as in block G, and for the family and society as in block H. Through neurohormonal response and sexual response, suckling can produce secondary pleasure or displeasure, shame, and anxiety. The infant responds to the mothering and attachment behavior. This interacts with the family and society, which feed back to and influence the variables in blocks A, B, and C.

This diagram (Fig. 6-2) cannot demonstrate negative and positive feedback. The same variables, however, are used to illustrate the decision-making procedure and are diagramed in Fig. 6-3. Solid lines refer to positive feedback and broken lines to negative feedback. From this it is clear that beliefs and attitudes toward breast-feeding influence the choice and the success of breast-feeding. Bentovim points out that it may be possible to restore breast-feeding to be the natural choice. This would depend on society finding a system in which the breast can be accepted not only as good for the infant and his development, but also as the object of less ambivalent and secret pleasure. Bentovim suggests, "The role of the health professionals in this area is important in that only through the right relationship with the mother will a new source of mothering be found that can act as a form of extended family for the woman to identify with and to counteract personal, family, and cultural influences."[3] Hendricks[11] confirms this view and states that the biggest block in the minds of women relates to feelings of shame associated with breast-feeding. More than half the women in the Newcastle[2] survey were prevented from breast-feeding because of a sense of shame. The shame is a result of relating the breast to concepts of sexuality.

REFERENCES

1. Adams, A. B.: Choice of infant feeding technique as a function of maternal personality, J. Consult. Clin. Psychol. **23:**143, 1959.
2. Bacon, C. J., and Wylie, J. M.: Mothers' attitudes to infant feeding at Newcastle General Hospital in summer 1975, Br. Med. J. **1:**308, 1976.
3. Bentovim, A.: Shame and other anxieties associated with breast feeding: A systems theory and psychodynamic approach. In Ciba Foundation Symposium no. 45, breast feeding and the mother, Amsterdam, 1976, Elsevier Scientific Publ. Co., p. 159.
4. Bowlby, J.: Attachment and loss. London, 1969, The Hogarth Press Ltd.
5. Brazelton, T. B.: The early mother-infant adjustment, Pediatrics **32:**931, 1963.
6. Budin, P.: The nursling, London, 1907, The Caxton Publishing Co.
7. Call, J. D.: Emotional factors favoring successful breast feeding of infants, J. Pediatr. **55:**485, 1959.

8. Chamberlain, R. E.: Some personality differences between breast and bottle feeding mothers, Birth Fam. J. **3:**31, 1976.
9. deChâteau, P., et al.: A study of factors promoting and inhibiting lactation, Dev. Med. Child. Neurol. **19:**575, 1977.
10. Douglas, J. W. B.: Extent of breast feeding in Great Britain in 1946 with special reference to health and survival of children, J. Obstet. Gynaecol. Br. Empire **57:**335, 1950.
11. Hendrickse, R. G.: Discussion from Ciba Foundation Symposium no. 45, breast feeding and the mother, Amsterdam, 1976, Elsevier Scientific Publ. Co.
12. Hoeffer, C., and Hardy, M. C.: Later development of breast fed and artificially fed infants, J.A.M.A. **92:**615, 1929.
13. Jackson, E. B., Wilkin, L. C., and Auerbach, H.: Statistical report on incidence and duration of breast feeding in relation to personal, social and hospital maternity factors, Pediatrics **17:**700, 1956.
14. Kennell, J. H., Trause, M. A., and Klaus, M. H.: Evidence for a sensitive period in the human mother. In Ciba Foundation Symposium no. 33, Parent-infant interaction, Princeton, N.J., 1975, Excerpta Medica, Associated Scientific Publishers.
15. Klaus, M. H., and Kennell, J. H.: Maternal-infant bonding, the impact of early separation or loss on family development, St. Louis, 1976, The C. V. Mosby Co.
16. Newton, N.: Psychologic differences between breast and bottle feeding. In Jelliffe, D. B., and Jelliffe, E. F. R., editors: Symposium, the uniqueness of human milk, Am. J. Clin. Nutr. **24:**993, 1971.
17. Newton, N., and Newton, M.: Psychologic aspects of lactation, N. Engl. J. Med. **277:**1179, 1967.
18. Parke, R. D., O'Leary, S., and West, S.: Mother-father-newborn interaction: effects of maternal medication, labor, and sex of infant, Am. Psychol. Assoc. Proc. 85, 1972.
19. Raphael, D.: The tender gift: breastfeeding. New York, 1976, Schocken Books, Inc.
20. Robertson, W. O.: Breast feeding practices: some implications of regional variations, Am. J. Public Health **51:**1035, 1961.
21. Sosa, R., et al.: The effect of early mother-infant contact on breast feeding, infection and growth. In Ciba Foundation Symposium no. 45, breast feeding and the mother, Amsterdam, 1976, Elsevier Scientific Publ. Co., p. 179.
22. Spitz, R. A.: An inquiry into the psychiatric conditions in early childhood, Psychoanal. Study Child **1:**53, 1945.
23. Thoman, E. B., Wetzel, A., and Levine, S.: Lactation prevents disruption of temperature regulation and suppresses adrenocortical activity in rats, part A, Community Behav. Biol. **2:**165, 1968.

CHAPTER 7

Contraindications to and disadvantages of breast-feeding

In reviewing the contraindications to breast-feeding, it is important to look at the entities that put the mother or infant at significant risk and are not remedial. Contraindications are medical; the disadvantages of breast-feeding are a second group of factors to be considered.

CONTRAINDICATIONS
Breast cancer

A mother with a diagnosis of breast cancer should not nurse her infant in the interest of having definitive treatment immediately. All lumps in the lactating breast are not cancer and are not even benign tumors. The lactating breast is lumpy and the "lumps" shift day by day. If a mass is located, and the physician thinks it should be biopsied, it can be done under local anesthesia without weaning the infant. A Rochester surgeon[8] has performed ten such procedures following my referral in the past 15 years without postoperative complications. The diagnosis of benign masses was made in all cases. The performance of immediate surgery relieved tremendous anxiety without unnecessarily sacrificing breast-feeding.

Is cancer more or less common in women who breast-feed? The answer is not easy to find, but in countries where breast-feeding is common, breast cancer is uncommon. In the United States, the incidence of breast cancer has steadily risen while the frequency of breast-feeding declined. At one time it had been suggested that nursing protected a woman against breast cancer. This concept was investigated in an international study and shown to be invalid.[10] Breast-feeding, however, does not predispose a woman to cancer.[5]

The critical question remains—does breast-feeding increase any child's risk of breast cancer, especially in female offspring? This haunting question, first posed by an experimental scientist, created tremendous publicity and genuine concern among physicians asked this question by patients. One needs to explore the available data.

Virus in breast milk. In the laboratory, it has been reported that particles physically identical to mouse mammary tumor virus have been found in human milk. Other investigators have attempted to duplicate this work. Chopra and co-workers[3] reported that the particles they located in human milk resembled virus from monkey breast tumor, which had been shown to possess biophysical, biochemical, and in vitro transforming properties of known oncogenic RNA viruses. They reserved judgment on the exact identity of the particles until they could be cultured or shown to produce tumor, since they may well not be viruses. Roy-Burman and colleagues[14] reported their efforts to detect RNA tumor virus in human milk using milks taken from women with varied histories of viruses. They found no correlation between RNA-directed DNA polymerase activity and family history of breast cancer. They suggest, as have others, that the RNA-directed DNA polymerase activity is a normal feature of lactating breast tissue.

Epidemiological study. Epidemiological data conflict with the suggestion that the tumor agent is transmitted via the breast milk. The incidence of breast cancer is low among groups that had nursed their infants, including lower economic groups, foreign-born groups, and those in sparsely populated areas.[10] The frequency of breast cancer in mothers and sisters of a woman with breast cancer is two to three times that expected by chance. This could be genetic or environmental. Cancer actually is equally common on both sides of the family of an affected woman. If breast milk were the cause, it should be transmitted from mother to daughter. When mother-daughter incidence of cancer was looked at, there was no relationship to breast-feeding.

Sarkar and associates[16] reported that human milk, when incubated with mouse mammary tumor virus, caused degradation of the particle morphology and decreased infectivity and reverse transcriptase activity of the virions. They suggest that the significance of this destructive effect of human milk on mouse mammary tumor virus may account for the difficulty in isolating the putative human mammary tumor agent. Sanner[15] has provided data to show that the inhibitory enzymes in milk can be removed by special sedimentation technique. He ascribes the discrepancies in isolating virus particles in human milk to these factors, which inhibit RNA-directed DNA polymerase.

Current position. Miller and Fraumeni[11] from the Epidemiology Branch of the National Cancer Institute reviewed the information and concluded that it did not support the belief that breast cancer is related to breast-feeding and further suggested that the fear of cancer in the breast-fed female offspring does not justify avoiding breast-feeding.

Morgan and co-workers[12] did a retrospective study by interviewing women over 60 years of age about their history of cancer and the feeding history of their daughters, as well as the incidence of cancer in their daughters. This study showed that the younger the interviewed woman was, the younger her daughters were, and the less breast cancer in the daughters. However, this could be attributable to their young age. Since the incidence of breast-feeding has declined, fewer daughters have been breast-fed. This factor could have skewed the results. They found breast-fed women have the same breast cancer experience as nonbreast-fed. There was no increase in benign tumors, either. Daughters of breast cancer patients have an increased risk of developing benign and malignant tumors by merit of their heredity, not their breast-feeding history.

Unilateral breast-feeding (limited to the right breast) is a custom of women of the fishing villages in Hong Kong. Ing and associates[7] investigated the question, ''Does the unsuckled breast have an altered risk of cancer?'' They studied breast cancer data from 1958 to 1975. Breast cancer occurred equally on the left and the right breast. Comparison of patients who had nursed unilaterally with nulliparous patients and with patients who had borne children but not breast-fed indicated a highly significantly increased risk of cancer in the unsuckled breast. The authors conclude that in postmenopausal women who have breast-fed unilaterally, the risk of cancer is significantly higher in the unsuckled breast. They believed that breast-feeding may help protect the suckled breast against cancer.

Papaionnou,[13] in a collective review of the etiological factors in cancer of the breast in humans, concludes, "Genetic factors, viruses, hormones, psychogenic stress, diet and other possible factors, probably in that order of importance, contribute to some extent to the development of cancer of the breast."

Wing[20] concludes in her update on human milk and health that "in view of the complete absence of any studies showing a relationship between breast-feeding and increased risk of breast cancer, the presence of virus-like particles in breast milk should not be a contraindication to breast-feeding."

Hepatitis B virus

The transmission of hepatitis B from mothers whose blood contains hepatitis B antigen to their infants has been described in several parts of the world.[9] Such transmission of an infectious agent from mother to infant is termed vertical transmission. The mode of transmission is transplacentally in utero, at delivery, or shortly after delivery. Horizontal transmission occurs between two individuals in close contact. Taiwan and Japan report a high incidence of transmission from carrier mothers to their infants, in contrast to reports from the rest of the world.[19] Follow-up from 4 to 12 months of age indicated the infants of carrier mothers in most studies remained serum negative. In the United States, the rate of transmission to infants from carrier mothers is very low.

Transmission from mothers with acute hepatitis B in pregnancy is very different. It was shown that with mothers in active disease just before, during, or after pregnancy, the infants had up to a 50% chance of being hepatitis B antigen positive. Hepatitis was acquired transplacentally or at birth, but not by breast milk because they were not breast-fed. There is a 50% risk of hepatitis if a mother has the disease at the end of pregnancy.[4]

In addition to transplacental infection there is the risk of fecal-oral transmission at delivery and transcolostrolly. Hepatitis B antigen has been found in saliva, stool, urine, prostatic fluid, and seminal fluid. Some infants do pick up the virus at birth. Hepatitis B antigen is found in breast milk.[18] Transmission by this route has not been well documented. The mothers of some infants who did become infected did not have the virus in the colostrum.[1]

Beasley and co-workers[2] write that although breast milk transmission is possible, their work showed no difference in frequency of antigenemia among breast-fed and nonbreast-fed babies in a long-term follow-up study of 147 mothers who were carriers of hepatitis B antigen. The time of transfer of the antigen from mother to infant may be during labor and delivery, when microscopic blood leaks may occur across the placenta, rather than via the breast milk.

Cytomegalovirus infection

Cytomegalovirus (CMV) has been identified in human milk of women with CMV-CF (complement fixation) antibody. Hayes and associates[6] showed 10.8% incidence at one to six days and 50% incidence at one to thirteen weeks. There is no correlation between the presence of viruria and the finding of CMV in the milk.

Breast milk ranks with cervical secretions as a potential source of CMV infection in infants according to these researchers.

β-streptococcal disease

A case of recurrent β-streptococcal disease in an infant who was breast-fed has been reported. The infant was infected at birth and treated with antibiotics. Six weeks later the mother developed bilateral mastitis, and the infant became moribund 2 days later. The infant and the milk grew out β-streptococcus. In the same journal two other cases of β-streptococcal infection in breast-fed infants are reported. The same type of β-streptococcus was found in mother and infant. It is highly likely that the mother was infected by the infant. It is rare to see bilateral mastitis in humans, but in all three cases of streptococcal mastitis, it was bilateral. Any time there is streptococcal disease in the newborn, recurrence should be watched for.[17] Bilateral mastitis should be considered a suspicious sign.

DISADVANTAGES

Disadvantages to breast-feeding are those factors perceived by the mother as being an inconvenience to the mother, since there are no known disadvantages for the infant. Our society has created the milieu for the mother to develop concerns. In cultures in which nursing in public is commonplace, nursing is not considered inconvenient, since the infant and the feeding are always available.

The fact that the mother is committed to the infant for six to twelve feedings a day for months is overwhelming to a woman who has been free and independent. Motherhood itself, however, changes one's life-style.

Guilt from failure, shame, and other anxieties are of considerable concern. Surveys evaluating the decline of breast-feeding have revealed that feelings of shame, modesty, embarrassment, and distaste have been described. These feelings are more common in lower social groups. Research on wider sociological and psychological factors regarding the feelings and attitudes toward breast-feeding can have a considerable influence on the choice to breast-feed and will be helpful in dealing with these issues.

REFERENCES

1. Beasley, R. P.: Transmission of hepatitis by breast feeding (letter to the editor), N. Engl. J. Med. **292:**1354, 1975.
2. Beasley, R. P., et al.: Evidence against breast feeding as a mechanism for vertical transmission of hepatitis B, Lancet **2:**740, 1975.
3. Chopra, H., et al.: Electron microscopic detection of Simian-type virus particles in human milk, Nature New Biol. **243:**159, 1973.
4. Crumpacker, C. S.: Hepatitis. In Remington, J. S., and Klein, J. O., editors: Infectious diseases of the fetus and newborn infant, Philadelphia, 1971, W. B. Saunders Co.
5. Fraumeni, J. F., and Miller, R. W.: Breast cancer from breast feeding, Lancet **2:**1196, 1971.
6. Hayes, K., et al.: Cytomegalovirus in human milk, N. Engl. J. Med. **287:**177, 1972.
7. Ing, R., Ho, J. H. C., and Petrakis, N. L.: Unilateral breast feeding and breast cancer, Lancet **2:**124, 1977.
8. Kingsley, H. S.: Personal communication, 1975.
9. Linnemann, C. C., and Goldberg, S.: HBAg in breast milk, Lancet, **2:**155, 1974.
10. MacMahon, B., et al.: Lactation and cancer of the breast. A summary of an international study, Bull. W.H.O. **42:**185, 1970.

11. Miller, R. W., and Fraumeni, J. F.: Does breast feeding increase the child's risk of breast cancer? Pediatrics **49**:645, 1972.
12. Morgan, R. W., Vakil, D. V., and Chipman, M. L.: Breast feeding, family history, and breast disease, Am. J. Epidemiol. **99**:117, 1974.
13. Papaioannou, A, N.: Etiologic factors in cancer of the breast in humans: collective review, Surg. Gynecol. Obstet. **138**:257, 1974.
14. Roy-Burman, P., et al.: Attempts to detect RNA tumour virus in human milk, Nature New Biol. **244**:146, 1973.
15. Sanner, T.: Removal of inhibitors against RNA-directed DNA polymerase activity in human milk, Cancer Res. **36**:405, 1976.
16. Sarkar, N. H., et al.: Effect of human milk on mouse mammary tumor virus, Cancer Res. **33**:626, 1973.
17. Schreiner, R. L., Coates, T., and Shackelford, P. G.: Possible breast milk transmission of group B streptococcal infection (letter to the editor), J. Pediatr. **91**:159, 1977.
18. Smith, J. L., and Hindman, S. H.: Transmission of hepatitis by breast-feeding (letter to the editor), N. Engl. J. Med. **292**:1354, 1975.
19. Stevens, C. E., et al.: Vertical transmission of hepatitis B antigen in Taiwan, N. Engl. J. Med. **292**:771, 1975.
20. Wing, J. P.: Human versus cow's milk in infant nutrition and health: update 1977, Curr. Prob. Pediatr. **8**(1):entire issue, Nov., 1977.

CHAPTER 8

Management of the mother-infant nursing couple

Successful nursing depends on the successful association of mother and infant with appropriate support from the father and available medical resources. Since both mothers and infants vary, a simple set of rules cannot be outlined to guarantee success for everyone. In fact, one of the difficulties has been that a rigid system was established in hospitals for initiating lactation that did not fit all mother-infant couples. Furthermore, physicians do not receive formal education on breast-feeding; thus they resort to gaining information from nonmedical sources and assume that this is the only way to approach the situation.

Nowhere in medicine does one's personal interests or prejudices become more evident than in the area of counseling about childbirth and breast-feeding. Having a child does not make one an expert on the subject. As pointed out previously, the University of Rochester study of physicians revealed that there is direct correlation with the way a physician's child was fed and how the physician counsels patients. Nowhere else does personal experience influence medical management so greatly. There is a distinct difference in hospital care among nurses who have breast-fed and those who have not. In addition, having had this personal experience it is common for the professional to then assume his experience is the model to recommend for everyone. One must be especially careful in one's enthusiasm for the process not to overlook the view of a patient less inspired or actually repelled by the thought of nursing.

The key to the management of the nursing couple is establishing a sense of confidence in the mother and supporting her with simple answers to questions when they arise.

Management is best discussed in terms of the three stages: (1) the prenatal period, (2) the immediate postpartum, or hospital, management, and (3) the postnatal, or posthospital, period.

PRENATAL PERIOD

It is most effective to prepare for breast-feeding well in advance of delivery. Prospective parents should consider feeding plans for the infant during the prenatal period, after the pregnancy is well established. Once quickening has occurred the infant becomes more of a reality for the mother and she can relate to planning. Except in sophisticated cultures, the parents will not initiate this decision-making discussion, and it is appropriately introduced by the obstetrician in the second trimester. This then gives the parents plenty of time to begin planning

109

more realistically for the infant. Particularly with first children, it is appropriate to suggest to the parents that they select a pediatrician early. They should request a prenatal conference with the pediatrician to discuss not only feeding but other points of management and child rearing that they might have questions about. If the mother is receiving prenatal care from a family practice physician, this step is an automatic one because the parents are being groomed psychologically as well as medically for the birth.

In a University of Rochester study of feeding practices in the Rochester community, mothers were asked who and what had influenced them to feed their infants in the manner they had chosen. None of 104 consecutive mothers from two local hospitals refused to respond to some questions on how they fed their infants. Fifty-four were breast-feeding and fifty were bottle-feeding. The same questionnaire was given to all mothers. Mothers who had elected to bottle-feed discussed feeding with their husbands before deciding in 32% of the cases and with their obstetrician in 10% of the cases; 37% discussed feeding with neither. Only one mother consulted her pediatrician. She was told there was no medical evidence that breast-feeding was advantageous. Mothers who had chosen to breast-feed discussed their choice with their husbands in 80% of the cases, with their obstetrician in 38% of the cases, and with their pediatrician in 20% of the cases. Only two multiparas did not discuss feeding with any of these persons. Because some breast-feeding mothers consulted more than one person, the figures total more than 100% (Table 8-1). This clearly demonstrates the role of the obstetrician or provider of prenatal care in a mother's decision making and also points out the need to involve both husband and wife in the discussion. These results indicate that it is necessary for the physician to initiate a discussion regarding feeding plans, since in most cases in which no discussion was held with the physician the mother chose bottle-feeding.

The mothers were also asked why they had made the choice they did. The reasons available to them were simple, leaving opportunity for the mother to add her own (Table 8-2). Bottle-feeding mothers were influenced by their mothers and friends, and fewer had attended childbirth classes. Breast-feeding mothers were less influenced by their mothers and friends, and 80% attended childbirth classes. The significant difference was in the "other" reasons for the choice of feeding (Table 8-3). Bottle-feeding mothers gave more negative reasons, and not one included the infant's welfare as the reason. Breast-feeding mothers all had positive reasons for nursing, and all did it because it was better for the infant in some way. A few had a second reason that involved their personal gain from nursing.

The medical profession as a group has been hesitant to take anything but a neutral position in such discussions for fear of pressuring the mother. Today the evidence is strong that there are distinct advantages to the infant as well as the mother to breast-feed. Parents do have the right to hear the data. They can make

Table 8-1. Prenatal decision making

Persons mothers consulted	Bottle-feeding	Breast-feeding
Husband	32%	80%
Obstetrician	10%	38%
Pediatrician	2%	20%

their own choice and need not be pressured. Newton and Newton[12] have shown that parents who had negative feelings about breast-feeding were successful at breast-feeding 26% of the time. Those who were ambivalent were 35% successful. Those patients who were positive about breast-feeding had a 74% success rate under the same management in the hospital.

The prenatal discussion should also include any questions the parents may have about the lactation process and mother's ability to provide adequately for the infant. An examination of the breasts is part of good prenatal care but the emphasis has been on ruling out cancer and not on the functional capacity of the gland. The breast tissue should be checked for lumps and cysts that might need treatment, of course. The size of the mass of mammary tissue is not correlated with the ability to produce milk. The more generous gland is usually due to a more generous fat pad. During pregnancy the fat is replaced by proliferating acini. A mother should not be discouraged from nursing because of small breasts. This may be the mother who needs most to prove herself.

Breast texture should be assessed by palpation. The inelastic breast gives the impression it is firmly knit together and the overlying skin is taut and firm so it cannot be picked up. The elastic breast is looser and the overlying skin free, and

Table 8-2. Factors that influenced decision to breast- or bottle-feed

Factors	Bottle-feeding	Breast-feeding
Childbirth classes	44%	80%
"That's how my mother fed her babies"	40%	16%
"That's how my friends fed their babies"	30%	16%
"That's how I fed my other baby"	96% of all bottle-feeding multiparas*	94% of all breast-feeding multiparas†
Other reasons	34%	68%

*60% of bottle-feeding mothers were multiparas.
†53% of breast-feeding mothers were multiparas.

Table 8-3. Reasons volunteered for the choice made

Bottle-feeding		Breast-feeding	
Breast-feeding:		Best for baby	8
Did not appeal to me	3	More natural	8
Too annoying	1	More nutritional	2
Makes breasts big	1	More beneficial	2
Ties me down	2	Special immunities	2
More convenient for me	3	More satisfying	2
No medical proof for breast milk	2	Prevent allergies	3
Infant won't sleep through night if breast-fed	2	Health reasons for infant	4
		Wanted to	2
Best for me	3	Satisfying	3
Want to take birth control pills	1	More convenient	2
Want to go to work	1		
Too nervous to breast-feed	2		
TOTAL	21		38

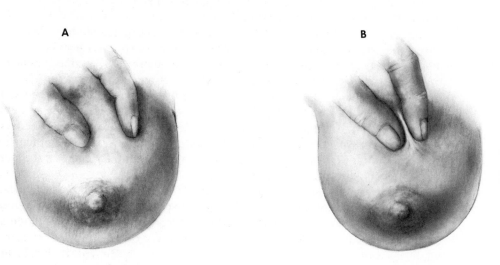

Fig. 8-1. Texture of breast tissue can be assessed by picking up skin of breast. **A,** Inelastic breast tissue; **B,** elastic breast tissue.

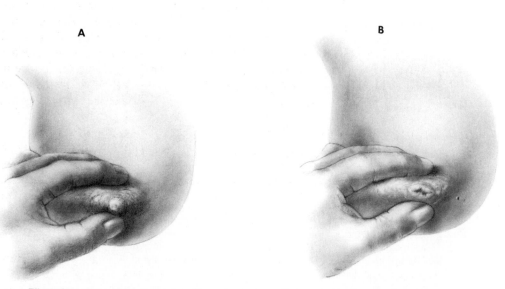

Fig. 8-2. A, Normal nipple everts with gentle pressure. **B,** Inverted or tied nipple inverts with gentle pressure.

the tissue is more easily picked up. Inelastic breasts are more prone to engorgement and seem improved by prepartum massaging and close attention to preventing of engorgement (Fig. 8-1).

Examination of the areola and nipple is equally important to identify any anatomical problems that may need some preparation prior to delivery. Gross malformations and inversion of the nipple will be easily detected, but lesser problems may go unnoticed. One must test for freedom of protrusion. When the areola is squeezed and it retracts, it indicates a "tied nipple" or inverted nipple due to the persistence of the original invagination of the mammary dimple (Fig. 8-2).

The physician may provide literature regarding breast-feeding or suggest reading sources for the patient. (See Appendix J for available reading materials for parents.) One should avoid dismissing the parents' questions by merely suggesting appropriate readings, since their personal decision making will be enhanced by open discussion with a knowledgeable professional. Although parents may have access to childbirth preparation programs in the community, the parents should not be put off to seek all their information from such sources. It often causes tremendous disappointment and misunderstanding when the parents have no opportunity to discuss with their care provider such issues as early infant contact, nursing the infant in the delivery room, and family-centered maternity care. Although the most vocal groups on the subject of childbirth and the family in our society today lump all these options together, including breast-feeding, as a package, there are many mothers who want to breast-feed but do not wish to have rooming-in, for instance. Therefore, all patients should be provided with adequate information to make a choice in each matter separately.

The concerns most frequently expressed by mothers considering breast-feeding are related to the mother, not the infant. Mothers who are more concerned about their own well-being have more trouble adjusting to motherhood and should be provided with more support in adapting to the role. They may be helped by selecting a doula to support them, since our modern culture tends to isolate the young couple. Raphael[14] describes a doula as one of "those individuals who surround, interact with, and aid the mother at any time within the perinatal period, which includes pregnancy, birth and lactation."

Concerns most frequently expressed prenatally include the following:

1. What is the effect on the figure? Data indicate that the breast is affected by heredity, age, and pregnancy in that order and only minimally by lactation. Women who have never borne children may "lose their figures" long before a grand multipara who nurses her infants. Pregnancy enlarges breasts temporarily, as does early lactation, but the effect is temporary. Poor diet and lack of exercise will destroy a figure in both male and female long before any other influence.

2. What is the effect on the mother's freedom? Obviously only a mother can breast-feed the infant; however, there are ample data to support the fact that it is possible to maintain a career, keep a job, or just get away from the house and still nurse one's infant in today's world. Actually, mothers in primitive cultures have returned to the fields or some form of productivity outside the home out of sheer necessity for generations. Mothers concerned about this often are best reassured by their peers, that is, mothers who are nursing. In communities with nursing mother groups, it is a simple referral.

3. Many women are concerned with exposing the breasts. Despite the constant barrage of publicity about the breast in the modern press, many women are embarrassed to consider their breasts being bared. As pointed out in Chapter 5, shame is an important consideration when helping a mother accept breast-feeding. Bentovim[4] suggests that shame and anxieties arise from the influence of one's life history and current events; thus intervention is necessary at many levels. Bacon and Wylie[2] found in their study that the most common reason for giving up breast-feeding was embarrassment. They suggest that, since their study showed a higher percentage of the high social class are breast-feeding, ". . . the higher social classes will lead the swing back to breast-feeding, just as they led the fashion to the bottle 40 years ago." The lower social classes expressed more modesty and shame for nudity.

Preparation of the breasts

In addition to affording the couple an opportunity to discuss options and learn about breast-feeding and the mechanisms of lactation, the prenatal period is a time to prepare the breast for its new role as a source of nourishment for the newborn infant. Many mothers do no special preparation and are very successful. Fair-skinned women, especially redheads, are more prone to developing cracked, sore nipples than others. Mothers who have had trouble with tender, cracked nipples when nursing a previous infant would do well to do some preparation. The activity has a good psychological effect as well as getting the process off on a positive note.

Bathing should be as usual with minimal or no soap directly on the nipples and thorough rinsing. Buffing the nipple with a soft towel is recommended by some. Montgomery glands in the areola secrete a sebaceous material for the cleansing and lubrication of the areola and nipple. This should not be removed by soaps or chemicals. Tincture of benzoin, alcohol, and other drying agents are contraindicated because they predispose the nipples to cracking during early lactation. Wearing a protective brassiere, modern women do not get the friction to the nipples that looser clothing provides, which may be why cracked nipples are such a common problem. In Scandinavia, it is suggested that the pregnant woman get as much air and sunshine as possible directly on the breasts prior to delivery. In countries where this is not possible, a cautiously used sunlamp can provide the same effect.

The use of lanolin or A and D ointment around the nipple, but not over the ducts and areola, twice a day, accompanied by gentle traction on the nipple to the point of discomfort but not pain, has been shown to prepare the delicate tissue for a vigorous suckling infant. The incidence of tender nipples in the early period of lactation was reduced to zero in some studies by this simple procedure (Fig. 8-3).

Preparation of the nipples

Flat nipples or inverted nipples do not preclude breast-feeding, but it is important to prescribe some form of treatment prior to delivery rather than waiting until the infant is frustrated and the breast engorged. Flat nipples need a consistent program of stretching, described in general breast preparation, but it should be done at least twice daily during the last 6 weeks of pregnancy.

Inverted nipples (Fig. 8-2) can be diagnosed by pressing the areola between the thumb and the forefinger. A flat or normal nipple will protrude; a truly inverted

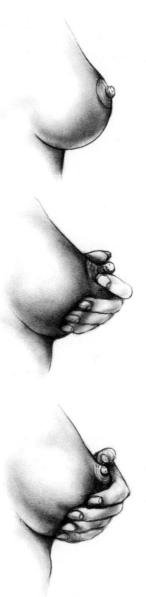

Fig. 8-3. To prepare nipple for breast-feeding during pregnancy, support breast gently with fingers while grasping nipple with thumb and index finger. Draw nipple out to point of discomfort, then release. Repeat exercise five or six times, several times a day.

nipple will retract. True inverted nipples are actually rare. Inverted nipples can be treated with massage as just described, but will respond more effectively if a nipple shield is also used when a brassiere is worn. The physician can recommend a pair of nipple shields available in any drugstore and intended for use in shielding the human nipple when the infant is nursing. The rubber nipple tip of the shield should be removed and only the plastic base with the hole in the center applied over the

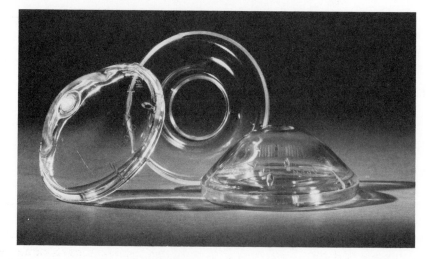

Fig. 8-4. Eschmann.shields are designed for use in pregnancy and early lactation to correct flat or inverted nipples. They may also be used to correct retraction during engorgement. Shield is slipped into cup cf well-fitting bra. When in position nipple is at center of opening in bottom piece. Outer convex piece fits over it and provides protection for nipple. It should not be used to collect milk or while nursing infant. Shields should be worn during pregnancy, at first for a few hours at a time, increasing the time as pregnancy progresses. (Manufactured by Eschmann Brothers & Walsh Limited, West Sussex, England; courtesy Eschmann-Canada Ltd., Toronto, Ontario.)

areola inside a well-fitting brassiere. The constant, even pressure will cause the nipple to evert through the hole. Shields can be worn daily for the last weeks or months of pregnancy. Only the plastic or glass ones should be used because the all-rubber shields pull on the skin, holding the moisture in. A special shield, either the Woolrich or Eschmann Shield, which forms a plastic tent over the areola, is very effective in everting nipples. Because it holds the moisture in over the nipple and areola, it should only be worn a few hours at a time (Fig. 8-4). Many women who find nipple manipulation unappealing find the shields work well. It is appropriate to exercise and also use the shield.

Hand expression

Some breast-feeding instructions suggest hand expressing the breast to produce a few drops of colostrum every day for the last few weeks of pregnancy. Fortunately, the instructions usually suggest the patient consult her physician first. Manual or any kind of pumping of the breasts may, indeed, stimulate the uterus to contract. It has been the cause of premature labor. It has no particular benefit and means the early sequestered cells are expressed away in the drops of colostrum prior to delivery and are lost to the infant. Occasionally, prepartum mastitis has developed from this treatment. Any seeming benefit is far outweighed by the risks.

•   •   •

Following is a summary of prenatal preparation:
1. During the first trimester, make the initial breast examination. Suggestions to consider how the infant is to be fed can be initiated.

2. Once the mother has experienced quickening in the second trimester, suggest that definite plans be made regarding feeding.
3. During the third trimester, discuss any preparations that may be appropriate, such as nipple care. Also discuss nursing immediately after delivery.

IMMEDIATE POSTPARTUM, OR HOSPITAL, PERIOD

Immediately after the placenta has separated the establishment of lactation begins. This is a critical period because many mothers who do not receive the proper support in the hospital are driven to failure by inept management.

Nursing in the delivery room

The mother will probably want to nurse her infant immediately after birth, if she has read the current literature. If she does not ask, the obstetrician should suggest it.

Disease-oriented physicians who have been trained to give trials of water first, hours after delivery, are always concerned that the infant may aspirate. Actually, all infants born elsewhere in the world go straight to the breast on delivery. It has a physiological effect on the uterus as well, causing it to contract. Because sugar water and cow's milk formulas are very irritating if aspirated, delay in feeding has been the rule in the United States, where most infants are bottle-fed. Colostrum is not irritating, however, and is readily absorbed. There are a few contraindications to immediate nursing: (1) a heavily medicated mother, (2) an infant with a 5 min Apgar score under 6, or (3) a premature infant under 36 weeks of gestation. The concern for the infant with a tracheoesophageal (TE) fistula is important, but a few precautions should suffice. If there is hydramnios or excess secretions at birth, a tube should be passed to the stomach to make sure the esophagus is patent. If all is well, the infant may nurse. If there is a TE fistula, it is a surgical emergency. Choanal atresia is another anomaly that would be of concern, but an infant cannot suck on the breast or anything if he cannot breathe through his nose. Usually an infant with choanal atresia has a low Apgar score or needs some assistance in establishing respirations.

For this first breast-feeding, it may be best to have the mother on a stretcher or bed wide enough to have the infant lay beside her (not the delivery table). The infant should not be dangled in midair over the breast. Both mother and infant will do better if there is an atmosphere of tranquility in the room. The only other risk to the infant is thermal stress. If the room is air-conditioned, it may be necessary to provide a warmer over the infant, especially if the infant is naked for skin-to-skin contact. Some mothers have shaking chills following the strenuous athletic event of labor and cannot provide adequate warmth for the infant without some external source of heat.

Chilling an infant may set off a chain of events from hypothermia to hypoglycemia to tachypnea to mild acidosis to the extent of requiring a septic work-up. Hypothermia, therefore, is more easily prevented than treated.

If possible, mother, father, and infant should remain together for the next hour. The first hour for the infant is usually one of quiet alertness, a state that will usually recur only briefly for the next few days. It is important to delay the instillation of silver nitrate drops until after this time together with the mother. If the drops are put in the eyes, blepharospasm will prevent the infant from opening his eyes and mar the eye-to-eye contact. Only if there is a known risk of gonorrhea should the drops be put in immediately. If the mother has delivered in a birthing center, early contact and nursing should be part of the routine.

Days in the hospital

The physician should see that his patients are permitted to have their infants with them as much as they wish, within the guidelines of reasonable medical care. Only the few patients with difficult deliveries, C sections with medication, postpartum complications, or toxemia need be excluded, but the physician should make that judgment. An experienced nursing staff is critical to the management of the nursing mother at this point. Advice should be reasonable and consistent, and nurses should be cautioned against interjecting their own personal opinion or experience. Key points in management should include the following:

1. Help the mother find a comfortable position. There should be no rules about sitting up or lying down.
2. Help the infant to the breast.
3. Help the mother reposition the infant on the second breast, since moving may be hard at first.
4. If the infant falls asleep after the first breast, wait a little, wake him, and then move to the second side.
5. Allow the infant to nurse 5 min on a side at first. This will usually assure that the infant takes both sides and will help the breasts adapt gradually. Frequent small feedings will provide good stimulation to the breast without stressing the mother. The milk supply is stimulated best by suckling.

Many physicians believe that until the milk is in, the 2 AM feeding can be replaced by water in the nursery, if the infant wakes up, so that the mother gets a full night's sleep. A mother should be given the infant if she requests to have him. On the other hand, modern hospitals are a hubbub of activity, and with liberalized visiting hours there is no time for the mother to rest unless naps are scheduled. In the early days of the Rooming-In Unit at the Yale–New Haven Hospital, Jackson insisted that all postpartum mothers have a nap after lunch. Every day the shades were drawn and traffic decreased on the unit for an hour. This is part of mothering the mother. In primitive cultures, mothers are groomed, fed, and protected after delivery, often for weeks. Furthermore, adequate rest is essential to successful lactation. In 1953, Jackson, with her colleagues Barnes and co-workers,[3] prepared a classic description of the management of breast-feeding, which still remains the single most valuable source of information.

Diagnosing problems with nursing

To solve the problem of unsuccessful nursing one should observe the mother feeding the infant. Often the problem is a simple one such as a mother so uncomfortable and tense the let-down reflex will not trigger or perhaps an infant with a poor suck. In these cases and others the diagnosis will be made most easily by direct observation.

Understanding the mechanism of suckling in the neonate, however, is essential to recognize ineffective sucking on the part of the infant (Fig. 8-5). As the breast is offered to the infant, the lips gently clamp the areola to hold it in place as the tongue thrusts forward to grasp the nipple and areola. In a rhythmical motion the

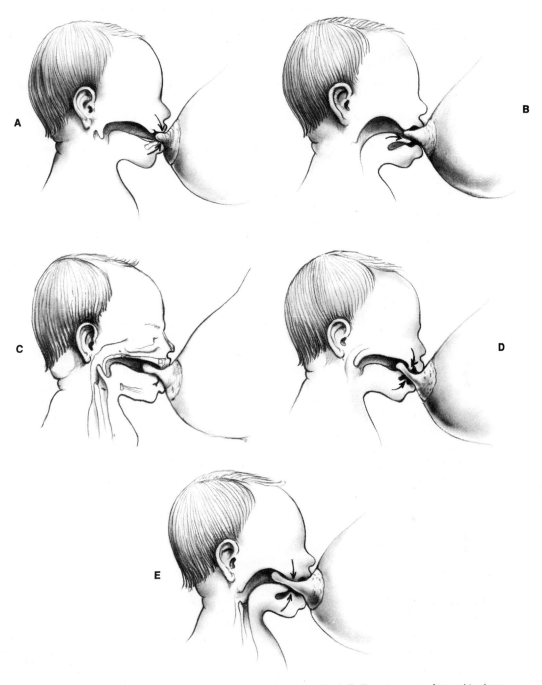

Fig. 8-5. A, Infant grasps breast (note *arrows* showing jaw action). **B,** Tongue moves forward to draw nipple in. **C,** Nipple and areola move toward palate as glottis still permits breathing. **D,** Tongue moves along nipple, pressing it against hard palate and creating pressure. **E,** Ductules under areola are milked and flow begins. Glottis closes.

tongue moves up against the hard palate drawing the nipple and areola into the mouth. The cheeks fill the mouth because of the sucking fat pads and provide further negative pressure. The tongue returns to the gum and lips and draws back along the areola, compressing the collecting ductules in the areola and "milking" them as the tongue moves along the nipple, which is compressed against the hard palate, sustaining the relative negative pressure. Milk flows from the nipple and is swallowed as a response of the swallowing reflex. If the infant has a fluttering tongue, it may not be as productive in stimulating ejection. If the infant cannot coordinate suck and swallow, choking occurs. Sometimes if ejection is strong, the first rush of milk will cause choking. Stopping and starting again should solve the problem. If the infant's jaw is slightly receding, the nipple may not stay in place. Gentle support at the angle of the jaw will help.

An infant who is given a bottle or rubber nipple to suck becomes confused because the sucking action is different (Fig. 8-6). The relatively inflexible rubber nipple may keep the tongue from its usual rhythmical action. In addition, the flow may be so rapid, even without sucking, that the infant learns to put the tongue against the rubber nipple holes to slow down the flow. Some infants who have been breast-fed gag when the relatively large rubber nipple is put in their mouths. When an infant uses the same tongue action he has needed for a rubber nipple at the breast, he may even push the human nipple out of the mouth. Sometimes, when he can not grasp an engorged areola properly, he will clamp down on the nipple with his jaws, causing pain in the nipple and disrupting the ejection reflex.

Engorgement. The best management of engorgement is prevention. The degree of engorgement lessens with each infant because the time at which the milk comes in seems to shorten in multiparas. The primipara suffers most from engorgement. Engorgement involves two elements: one is congestion and increased vascularity; the second is accumulation of milk. Engorgement may involve only the areola, only the body of the breast (so-called peripheral engorgement), or both.

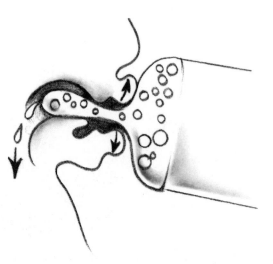

Fig. 8-6. Infant sucking on rubber nipple, which fills mouth and thus prevents tongue action and provides flow without stroking. Flow occurs even if lips not tight around rubber hub.

AREOLAR ENGORGEMENT. When the areola is engorged, it obliterates the nipple and makes grasping the areola properly impossible for the infant. If he sucks only the nipple, it is exquisitely painful, since that is the only area of the breast where there are pain fibers. In addition, the collecting ductules are not "milked" and therefore do not empty, and the infant is frustrated by lack of milk.

The treatment is directed at reducing the engorgement so that the infant can nurse effectively, which will further reduce the overdistended ducts. Gentle manual expression by the mother herself will usually produce a small amount of flow and soften the areola. The presence of milk on the nipple will further encourage the infant's sucking. A mother should be taught how to manually express (Fig. 8-7). By placing the thumb and forefinger at the margins of the areola and pressing back in toward the chest, and then bringing the fingers together, rhythmically simulating the action of the infant's jaw, the flow will start and the tense tissue soften. When the infant is put to the breast, the mother should compress the areola between two fingers to make it easier for the infant to grasp. Offering the breast this way makes it easier for any infant to grasp, especially when he needs encouragement to nurse (Fig. 8-8).

PERIPHERAL ENGORGEMENT. Initially, the breasts increase in vascularity and begin to swell. This usually starts in the second 24 hr period after delivery. Initially, engorgement is vascular; thus pumping mechanically is not productive and may be traumatic. The mother should be advised to wear a well-fitting but adjustable nursing brassiere that does not have thin straps or permanent plastic lining. She should wear it 24 hr a day. With moderately severe engorgement, the breasts become full, hard, and tender. The swelling starts at the clavicle and goes to the lower rib cage and from the midaxillary line to the midsternum. The breasts may even become hard, tense, and warm. The mother complains of throbbing and aching pain and can find no comfortable position except flat on her back and very still.

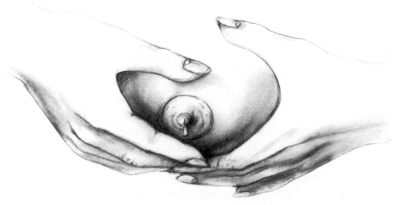

Fig. 8-7. Position for manual expression of breast. Thumbs are brought toward areola, compressing areola between thumb and supporting fingers. With areola grasped, pressure is applied toward chest wall, and then pressure is released. This compression and pressure stimulates milking action.

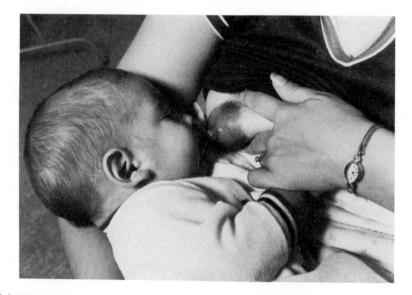

Fig. 8-8. When breast is offered to infant, areola is gently compressed between two fingers and breast supported to assure that infant is able to grasp areola adequately.

Management is centered on making the mother comfortable so that she can continue to nurse and stimulate milk production as well as nourish the infant. Proper support to elevate the breasts is important. The axilla are particularly painful, probably due to the tension on Cooper's ligament. Cold packs may help initially to reduce vascularity. Warm packs may help other patients. Standing in a warm shower and having the mother manually express some milk at the same time may be the best preparation to feed the infant. Some find comfort in alternating hot and cold water. Aspirin may give the mother some relief and should not bother the infant An aspirin-codeine preparation has been recommended as well. It may be necessary to provide the mother with some sleep medication.

It is important to maintain drainage during this period of engorgement to prevent back pressure from developing and eventually depressing milk production. Manual expression of the breasts is extremely helpful. The mother should support the breast with her fingers and place her thumbs distally and massage gently toward the areola, rotating gradually around the breast to include all quadrants. Then, once the peripheral lobules have been softened, areolar expression as previously described should be used to encourage complete emptying of the collecting ducts in the areola. This is a procedure best done by the mother, but it takes a skilled and experienced nurse to teach this technique. We have in recent years used the Egnell pump (Fig. 18-5) in cases of engorgement; it is very effective. The traditional electric pump is an instrument of unphysiological torture.

Hand pumps can be used but only exert negative pressure on the areola. Unless accompanied by manual expression of the distal segments they are only temporizing. The Egnell pump does simulate the infant's stroking tongue.

Currently maternity patients are going home in 2 to 3 days or less, which is certainly before lactation is well established, but it may also be before engorgement is full blown. At the time maternity floors were run so rigidly that ad lib breast-feeding was an impossible feat, it was often suggested a mother go home and get away from the negative hospital atmosphere to a place where she could relax and concentrate on feeding the infant and resting. This is a point at which the doula, so well described by Raphael,[14] could make the difference between success and failure. It may be appropriate for the obstetrician to order the mother to have some assistance at home, whether it is the husband, mother, or friend. "The common denominator for success in breast-feeding is the assurance of some degree of help from some specific person for a definite period of time after childbirth," according to Raphael.[14] She studied mothers in the cycle of anxiety while she became the doula for the individuals she studied at about 6 to 10 days postpartum. The remarkable calm that can be experienced in the presence of a confident caring person will relax the mother. The infant senses the calm and confidence and sleeps. When he feeds again he nurses well. Breaking the cycle of panic that seizes a new mother when she finds herself home alone with a new infant who needs frequent feeding requires an ability to instill confidence.

Although the physician cannot provide the doula role, he can be sure the family understands the need and can suggest community resources if no personal ones are available. Successful breast-feeding is not automatic, as is demonstrated by the failure rate. Some of the problems have been generated by the disturbance of the synchronization of interaction between mother and infant by rigid hospital protocol. This is continued at home when feeding is by the clock rather than by instinct.

Nipples

PAINFUL NIPPLES. Presumably the nipples will adapt to the nursing experience naturally; however, often there are discomforts. It is common for the initial grasp of the nipple and sucks to cause discomfort in the first few days of lactation. It is not cause for alarm, only reassurance. This sensation is created by the negative pressure on the ductules, which are not yet filled with milk. Later, when lactation is well established and the let-down reflex is experienced, mothers will describe a turgescence, which is the increased fluid pressure being relieved by suckling. Occasionally the pain persists throughout the nursing. This is the time to observe the feeding, looking for malpositioning or other abnormalities.

Finding none, it may be due to a "barracuda baby" with a vigorous suck. The breast will gradually adapt to it, and it will not last indefinitely. Sometimes the maternal tissues are unusually tender and delicate. Dry heat may help between feedings. The mother should remove the waterproofing from her brassiere and expose her breasts to air or an electric lamp with a 60-watt bulb for 20 min two to three times per day. A lamp similar to the perineal lamp can be used in the hospital.

Nipple shields should not be used unless all else has failed, since it often becomes hard to wean the infant back. The infant becomes confused in learning his sucking routine. Shields made entirely of rubber should never be used because they draw and pull the skin. Glass or plastic with a rubber nursing nipple work well and have the advantage that the mother can see the milk through the glass or plastic.

SMALL OR FLAT NIPPLES. When the nipples are small or flat, care to flatten the breast and areola between two fingers to provide as much nipple as possible to the infant will assist him in getting a hold. Sometimes a shield is necessary to draw the nipple out, but the shield should be removed and the infant placed directly on the breast for the rest of the feeding. Once engorgement is diminished and nursing is well established, small and/or flat nipples are no longer a problem.

LARGE NIPPLES. Large nipples are occasionally a problem with a small infant or an infant with an indecisive suck. A shield may help the infant cope at first, but it is best to just work patiently with the infant. Manual expression, which softens the areola to make it more pliable, prior to putting the infant to the breast, often helps.

CRACKED NIPPLES. Whenever the mother complains of nipple pain on nursing, the nipple should be examined in good light to look for cracks or subepithelial pete-chiae, which may be the precursor to cracking. Watching the nursing process may identify abnormal positioning at the breast. If there are true cracks, however, therapy is indicated. In the precracked stage, dry heat between nursings will be most effective. When true fissures have developed Barnes and associates[3] recommend that the infant be taken off the affected breast for 24 to 48 hr, nursing only on the other side. That is drastic treatment, and in our experience, opening both sides of the nursing brassiere at feedings and beginning to nurse on the opposite side first will permit the initial let-down to occur "atraumatically," then the infant can be put carefully to the affected breast. The heat treatments will assist in the therapy. When nursing has to be stopped on a given breast it sets up a chain reaction of engorgement, reduced flow, and plugging of the ducts. A nipple shield should be tried before stopping the nursing on a breast.

A very successful treatment described by Young,[15] which has now been adopted as a hospital routine in New Zealand, is the use of the mother's milk on the cracked nipple. A small amount is expressed and applied gently to the nipple and areola and allowed to dry on. Healing is rapid, and the success rate is excellent.* The application of any ointment that must be removed prior to nursing has disadvantages, since the removal is traumatic. A and D ointment and hydrous lanolin, which do not have to be removed, are the most effective of the ointments.

Following is a summary of management of sore, painful, or cracked nipples:

1. Examine the breast, nipple, and nursing scene.
2. Conduct prefeeding manual expression.
3. Carefully position infant on breast.
4. Nurse on unaffected breast first with affected side exposed to air.
5. Apply expressed breast milk to nipples and let dry on between feedings.
6. Apply dry heat 20 min, four times a day with a 60-watt bulb, 18 inches (45 cm) away.
7. If necessary, use nipple shield while nursing.
8. Rarely, temporarily stopping the nursing on affected side, replacing it with manual expressing or pumping, may be indicated.
9. If necessary, give aspirin or codeine in short-acting preparation just after nursing (Chapter 11).

The infant in the hospital

Infants have been aptly classified by their feeding characteristics by Barnes and colleagues[3] as "barracudas," excited ineffectives, procrastinators, gourmets or mouthers, and resters.

BARRACUDAS. When put to the breast, barracudas vigorously and promptly grasp the nipple and suck energetically for from 10 to 20 min. There is no dallying.

---

*Human milk has also been used in some cultures very successfully as eye drops in cases of bacterial ophthalitis.

Occasionally this type of infant puts too much vigor into his nursing and hurts the nipple.

EXCITED INEFFECTIVES. Excited ineffective infants become so excited and active at the breast that they alternately grasp and lose the breast. They then start screaming. It is often necessary for the nurse or mother to pick up the infant and quiet him first, and then put him back to the breast. After a few days the mother and infant usually become adjusted.

PROCRASTINATORS. Procrastinators often seem to put off until the fourth or fifth postpartum day what they could just as well have done from the start. They wait till the milk comes in. They show no particular interest or ability in sucking in the first few days. It is important not to prod or force these infants when they seem disinclined. They do well once they start.

GOURMETS OR MOUTHERS. Gourmets insist on mouthing the nipple, tasting a little milk and then smacking their lips before starting to nurse. If the infant is hurried or prodded, he will become furious and start to scream. Otherwise, after a few minutes of mouthing he settles down and nurses very well.

RESTERS. Resters prefer to nurse a few minutes and then rest a few minutes. If left alone, they often nurse well, although the entire procedure will take much longer. They cannot be hurried.

• • •

These descriptions serve to demonstrate the facts that infants are different and the management of the nursing experience will vary accordingly. Therein lies the secret to appropriate counseling—recognizing the differences between infants and responding to them.

Weight loss. Newborns usually lose some weight, and it tends to be a function of whether they are appropriate, large, or small for gestational age as well as how many kilocalories are ingested in the first few days. The infants of multiparas who are breast-feeding often lose little weight because the milk comes in so quickly. On the other hand, the normal primipara may not have a full supply for 72 to 96 hr. If the weight loss is over 5% (150 g in a 3 kg infant) one should evaluate the process to identify any problems before they become serious. A 10% weight loss is acceptable if all else is going well and the physical examination is negative, but it should be justified in the record, and the infant should be seen shortly after discharge from the hospital to assure resolution of the problem. Weighing before and after feedings is successful only in producing tremendous anxiety in the mother and affords little information because it is so inaccurate. It is therefore almost never indicated.

Vomiting blood. A breast-fed baby who vomits blood should have the blood evaluated for fetal or adult hemoglobin by the alum-precipitated toxoid (APT) test. (Suspend blood in a small amount of saline solution, and add an equal amount of 10% NaOH. Adult hemoglobin turns brown; fetal hemoglobin stays pink.) If it is adult hemoglobin, the nipple may be bleeding. Sometimes this bleeding is unknown to the mother, and sometimes she is afraid to report it.

Let-down reflex. The most important single function that affects the success of breast-feeding is the let-down reflex. Any mother can produce the milk, but if she does not excrete it, further production is suppressed. Much has been written on this single reflex by physiologists, endocrinologists, biochemists, pathologists, anatomists, psychologists, psychiatrists, obstetricians, and pediatricians. Indeed, it is a complex function that depends on hormones, nerves, and glands, which can be inhibited most easily by psychological block.

The hormonal mechanism of milk ejection is described in Chapter 3. The reflex stimulation of milk ejection has been meticulously studied by Caldeyro-Barcia[5] while he studied intramammary pressures. The more efficient stimulus for the milk-ejection reflex is suckling of the nipple. The frequency of suckling is 70 to 120 strokes/min, and the mean pressure is between -50 and -150 mm Hg. The maximum recorded was -220 mm Hg. Within 1 min of the onset of suckling, the first contraction of the mammary myoepithelium is recorded. Uterine contractions are also stimulated by suckling. Amplitude and frequency may increase over time during nursing. Mechanical stimulation of the nipple can produce the same effect on the breast and uterus. The milk-ejection reflex is inhibited centrally by cold, pain, and emotional stress. Ejection response can be elicited by seeing the infant or hearing him cry.

The milk-ejection reflex can be at least partially blocked by alcohol, which seems to be a central effect preventing the release of oxytocin, since the mammary gland and uterine response to injected oxytocin are not changed by alcohol. Studies on mothers with diabetes insipidus suggest that the patient retains the ability to synthesize and release oxytocin despite the fact that she is unable to

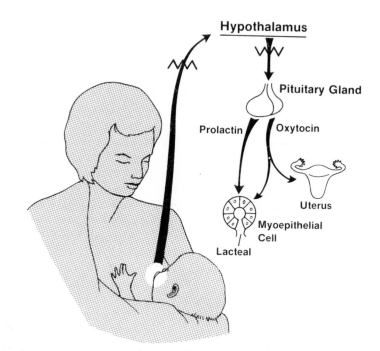

Fig. 8-9. Diagrammatical outline of ejection reflex arc. When infant suckles breast, he stimulates mechanoreceptors in nipple and areola that send stimulus along nerve pathways to hypothalamus, which stimulates the posterior pituitary to release oxytocin. It is carried via bloodstream to breast and uterus. Oxytocin stimulates myoepithelial cell in breast to contract and eject milk from alveolus. Prolactin is responsible for milk production in alveolus. It is secreted by anterior pituitary gland in response to suckling. Stress such as pain and anxiety can inhibit let-down reflex. The sight or cry of infant can stimulate it.

produce ADH (vasopressin) in response to stimuli. Artificial cervical dilation postpartum will also cause milk ejection.

Injection of oxytocin reproduces the effect of suckling. A rapid series of injections of 1 to 10 mU intravenously will simulate suckling. A continuous drip is less effective. Use of pitocin as a snuff or nasal spray is the best method for home use of oxytocin to initiate let-down.

The oxytocin concentration in the blood rises with suckling, which supports the hypothesis that suckling elicits the release of oxytocin.

The data on the question of ADH release during suckling are confused but it would seem there is independent release of oxytocin and ADH.

The mammary myoepithelium is stimulated to contraction by oxytocin, and the milk-ejection reflex results in the contraction of the myoepithelium and the release, or let-down, of milk (Fig. 8-9). In the first weeks of lactation, the threshold dose of oxytocin is very low, averaging 0.65 mU from the fifth day. Thirty days after weaning it is 100 mU. Vasopressin is not as effective and requires 100 times the dosage of oxytocin to produce the same effect during lactation. Deamino-oxytocin is 1.5 times as potent as oxytocin on the third postpartum day, but the difference disappears over time, probably due to the rapid breakdown of natural oxytocin by oxytocinase early in the postpartum period.

Practical aspects of the milk-ejection reflex. When the nipple is stimulated, the receptors at the nipple and areola are stimulated and nervous impulses are transmitted to the hypothalamus via the somatic afferent nerves. The hypothalamus stimulates the pituitary gland to secrete prolactin, which induces the alveoli in the breast to secrete milk. The cell membranes release fat globules and protein into the lumen. This produces the hind milk, which has a higher protein and fat content. Foremilk has been present since the previous nursing and is released first. It is a more dilute, less fatty solution that empties into the lacriferous sinuses awaiting the next suckling. The ejection reflex induces the holocrine excretion of milk from the cells. The posterior pituitary gland secretes oxytocin, which stimulates the myoepithelial cells to contract and eject the milk from the ducts.

Newton and Newton[11] have studied the ejection reflex and clearly show the effect of distraction to the let-down effect. Distractions included immersing feet in ice water (reported to be the worst), being asked mathematical questions in rapid series, which resulted in electric shock if wrong answer was given, or having painful traction on the big toe (Table 8-4). In practice, for some mothers pain, stress, and mental anguish interfere with let-down. When simple adjustments such as making the mother more comfortable, playing soft music, or leaving the mother in a quiet room do not work, other techniques should be tried.

Table 8-4. Ejection reflex* †

Maternal disturbance	Mean amount of milk obtained by infant
No distractions (no injection)	168 g
Distraction (saline injection)	99 g
Distraction (oxytocin injection)	153 g

*Interrupted milk flow can be restarted with hormone injection.
†Modified from Newton, M., and Newton, N.: J. Pediatr. **91**:1, 1977.

The most direct therapy is oxytocin. When simple supportive measures fail, this can be prescribed at home as a nasal spray, most readily available as synthetic oxytocin (Syntocinon). It is packaged in 2 and 5 ml spray bottles. A mother almost never needs a second bottle. It contains 40 USP units (IU) of synthetic oxytocin, a polypeptide hormone of the posterior pituitary gland, per milliliter of spray. (A prescription is required.) It is destroyed in the gastrointestinal tract, therefore it must be sprayed nasally, where it is rapidly absorbed. One spray into one or both nostrils 2 to 3 min before putting the infant to breast (or pumping in the case of collecting for a infant unable to nurse at the breast) is sufficient.

POSTNATAL, OR POSTHOSPITAL, PERIOD

When the family makes the transition from hospital to home it can be stressful. The infant who has been passive and content wakes up and cries for the first time. Because of all the procedures necessary to discharge an infant from the hospital (discharge physicals, blood tests, etc.) the well-planned discharge is often delayed and everyone is frantic, including the infant. The mother should be reassured about this and not be alarmed if she has to feed the infant frequently, the first day at home.

Feeding frequency

Hospital schedules are on a 4 hr feeding program, based on the feedings of bottle infants whose slow emptying time of the stomach with cow's milk formulas requires 4 hr. The emptying time for breast milk is about 1½ hr, thus frequent feedings are not unusual. Pediatric textbooks at the turn of the century described ten to twelve feedings a day as normal. Comparison of mammalian care patterns and composition of their milk shows an inverse relationship with protein content and frequency of feedings. From this it might be deduced that the human infant might well need to be fed more frequently than every 4 hr (Table 8-5).[10] Infants who sleep 5 to 6 hr at a stretch at night may make up for skipped feedings during the day.

Table 8-5. Mammalian care patterns and breast milk composition*†

	Example of species (number of species studied)			
	Deer (n = 13)	Dogs (n = 18)	Goats (n = 22)	Human beings
Infant care pattern	Nest or cache	Nest or cache	Carry, follow, hibernate	???
Feeding interval	5-15 hr	2-4 hr	Continuous	???
Mean % breast milk component				
Protein	10.5	9.6	3.9	1.2
Fat	16.5	9.4	4.5	3.8
Carbohydrate	3.0	3.3	5.1	7.0
Water	67.0	76.3	86.9	87.6

*From Lozoff, B., et al.: J. Pediatr. **91**:1, 1977.
†The mean percent of each breast milk component in species that hibernate, carry, or follow is significantly different (p < 0.01) from the corresponding value in species that nest or cache their young, even those which feed as frequently as every 2 to 4 hours. Calculations derived from Ben Shaul.

New mothers are often most insecure and most concerned about lack of sched-uling, especially if an ad lib program of feeding has been suggested. Other mothers seem to thrive on random scheduling. When a mother expressed concerns about frequent feedings and worries about the adequacy of her milk (she is often disturbed that it looks so thin and blue after the luxurious color of colostrum), Jackson would suggest she keep a record of feeding times and duration, as well as sleep and wakeful times. A chart was provided (Appendix B). The mother was usually surprised to find how quickly her infant developed a schedule. Often the infant was sleeping longer than she thought. The chart is also reassuring to the physician, especially if weight gain is marginal. In some cases it will highlight a problem not previously identified such as a poor gainer who sleeps all night, missing several feedings.

Adequate rest

If nursing is not going well, the most likely cause of problems is fatigue on the part of the mother. She may need to be ordered by her physician to nap and rest. She will have to learn to nap when the infant is napping. This becomes more difficult when there are other young children, but a simultaneous nap for all the little ones and mother may have to be engineered. Otherwise she may have to go to bed with the children at night and just concentrate on resting and feeding the infant. When the need for rest is acute, the father should be assigned the infant care with the possible inclusion of a bottle-feeding, while the mother sleeps undis-turbed.

Sore breasts—caked breasts

Tender lumps in the breasts in a mother who is otherwise well are probably due to plugging of a collecting duct. The best treatment is to continue nursing. Manual-ly massaging the area to initiate and assure complete drainage should be recom-mended. Hot packs prior to feedings may help. If the breast is especially tender, initiating nursing on the opposite breast first permits the affected breast to "let-down" without the pressure of suckling. The affected breast should be completely emptied by nursing or manual expression. One should be sure the brassiere is not cutting off an alveolus with the undue pressure of a narrow strap.

Repeated "caking". When this condition is recurrent, one needs to look for a major cause such as exhaustion and fatigue. Several women have come to my attention who have had repeated lumps in their breasts with poor flow of milk, often as if the ducts were plugged. The condition responded fairly well to manual expression prior to each feeding, often with the expulsion of small plugs. The condition dramatically improved by limiting the mother to polyunsaturated fats and adding lecithin to the diet. It was also necessary but effective for subsequent pregnancies as well in all three cases.

Galactocele

Milk-retention cysts are uncommon and when found are almost exclusively in lactating women. The contents at first are pure milk. Owing to absorption of the fluid they later contain thick creamy, cheesy, or oily material. The swelling is smooth and rounded, and compression of it may cause milky fluid to exude from the nipple. Galactoceles are believed to be caused by the blockage of a milk duct.

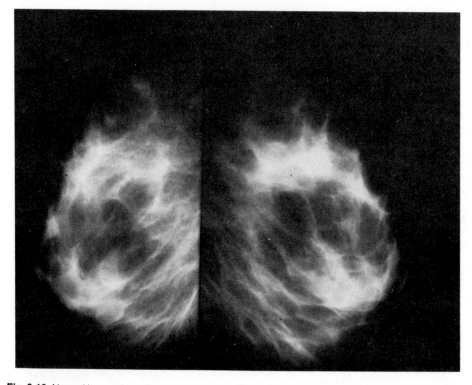

Fig. 8-10. Normal breast tissue by mammography. Tissue is one-third fat and appears cystic in nature. (Courtesy Dr. Wende Logan.)

The cyst may be aspirated to avoid surgery but will fill up again. It can be removed surgically under local anesthesia without stopping the breast-feeding. Its presence does not require cessation of the lactation. A firm diagnosis can be made by ultrasound; a cyst and milk will appear the same and a tumor will be distinguishable (Figs. 8-10 and 8-11).

Breast rejection

Infants have been observed to reject the breast intermittently, most often at 3 to 4 months and then go back after several feedings or a day or so. A bottle can be substituted. Total rejection of both breasts may be due to the return of menstruation. A mother will notice the infant will reject the breast for a day or so with each period. Other infants seem unaffected. Strong foods in the diet may cause rejection of milk. It usually occurs 8 to 12 hr after ingestion and disappears by 24 hr after ingestion.

Unilateral breast rejection. Some infants prefer one breast and even refuse the other. When this occurs manual expression or softening the nipple for easier grasp may help, thus enticing the infant to suckle. Holding the infant in the same position (i.e., on same side in same direction, so-called football hold) for the other breast may lead the infant to take the second breast. Sometimes applying honey to the rejected nipple or using a breast shield will help. Unilateral breast feeding is a custom in some parts of China.

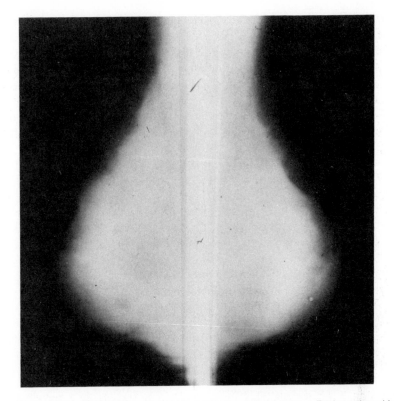

Fig. 8-11. Breast tissue during pregnancy and lactation by mammography. Fat is replaced by lactation tissue and presents solid appearance. Tumor would be easily distinguished by this procedure in lactating breast. It is safe, noninvasive technique that does not interfere with nursing. (Courtesy Dr. Wende Logan.)

Goldsmith[9] reported five cases of lactating women whose infants suddenly rejected a single breast. Weeks or months later a mass was noted by the mother and biopsy revealed malignancy. It would be wise to examine any patient who complains of unilateral breast rejection that does not respond to simple measures while lactating to rule out a tumor. Ultrasound followed by a mammogram, if necessary, can be performed without discontinuing lactation.

Mastitis

Mastitis is an infectious process in the breast, producing localized tenderness, redness, and heat, together with systemic reactions of fever, malaise, and sometimes nausea and vomiting. Mastitis is rarely seen in the hospital because it does not usually occur until several weeks postpartum. It no longer occurs in epidemics as seen in hospitals at one time, prior to the common use of antibiotics and when hospital stays were prolonged for normal childbirth. The infection may be hospital acquired if the mother or infant is colonized with a virulent bacteria before leaving the hospital. Devereux[8] describes 20 years of experience with fifty-three lactating patients who experienced seventy-one acute attacks of mastitis. The highest incidence was in the second and third weeks postpartum. No infant was weaned because of the mastitis. No infants were sick in association with the mastitis.

All but five mothers nursed subsequent infants. Six patients had mastitis with other pregnancies. Eight of seventy-one patients (11.1%) developed abscesses, six requiring incision and drainage. The bacterial cause was not stated. When treatment was delayed beyond 24 hr, the abscess rate increased.

The management regimen that has been most successful at the University of Rochester is as follows:

1. Continue to nurse on both breasts, but start the infant on the unaffected side while the affected side "lets down." Be sure to empty affected side by feeding or pumping.
2. Insist on bed rest (mandatory). The mother can take the infant to bed and obtain assistance for the care of the rest of the family.
3. Choose an antibiotic that can be tolerated by the infant as well as the mother, such as ampicillin (avoid sulfa drugs when the infant is under 1 month) or erythromycin. Regardless of the course of the disease, the antibiotic should be given for 10 days. Shorter courses are associated with relapses.
4. Apply ice packs or warm packs to the breast, whichever provides the most comfort. Experience indicates heat is better.
5. Provide plenty of fluids for the mother.
6. Give an analgesic such as aspirin.
7. The mother should wear a supporting brassiere that does not cause painful pressure.

Supplementary feedings

Many physicians suggest to mothers that a supplementary bottle can be added any time. Actually, when lactation is going well it is not needed, and when it is not going well, a bottle may aggravate the problem. During hospitalization, giving a substitute bottle may confuse a new infant, who may be having trouble sucking at first. Complementary bottles, that is, ones given after a breast-feeding to top off the feeding, are the beginning of a downhill course that may doom lactation to failure. It would be better to take the infant to breast more often. If it is necessary for the mother to be away at feeding time, she can pump a feeding ahead of time and save it in the refrigerator or freezer for someone else to give by bottle. If this is not practical, a bottle of formula can be given. It can be made up from a formula powder more economically one feeding at a time, and there is no waste. Powder preparations have a long shelf life even when open and are better tolerated by the infant because lower temperatures are required to manufacture powders, thus there is no carmelizing of the sugars or denaturing of the proteins. A powder goes quickly into solution if the water is warm when mixing is attempted. (Prepare formula powder as follows: one scoop of powder to 2 oz of water gives 20 kcal/oz.)

Solid foods

Successfully nursing mothers are never impatient to start solid foods like bottle-feeding mothers frequently are. Milk, and especially human milk, supplies the appropriate nutrients. (Some physicians, however, prescribe additional fluorine, 0.5 mg, and vitamin D, 200 units [Chapter 9].) At about 6 months a normal infant begins to use his iron stores and that is probably an appropriate time to start solid foods, especially iron-containing ones. This permits the entire process of weaning to cup and solid foods to be a gradual one. An infant does not need teeth to eat baby food and conversely he does not have to be weaned from the breast because teeth have erupted. By 6 months the number of feedings usually has decreased, and the timing and volume are beginning to cycle to a schedule that resembles three meals a day and some snacks. A breast-fed infant should have started some solids by 6 months of age.

Colic

Colic by definition is spasmodic contractions of smooth muscle, causing pain and discomfort. It can be experienced in many organs, such as the gastrointestinal or genitourinary tract, and at all ages. When the term colic is used in reference to infants it usually means a syndrome in which the young infant cries for a prolonged period of time, often the same time of day, in the early months of life. The infant usually draws his legs up as if in pain. There are a myriad of remedies directed at various possible causes, including allergy, hypertonicity, and hormone withdrawal.

Although colic is less common in the breast-fed infant, it does occur. Characteristically, the infant will cry and scream as if in pain from 3 to 4 hr at a stretch, usually between 6 and 10 PM at night. The infant will nurse frequently, then scream and pull away from the breast as if in pain, only to cry out a few minutes later. Sometimes the infant can be comforted by another adult such as his father or grandmother. The infant will respond to gentle rocking when held against a warm shoulder. If the infant is put down, the screaming starts up again. If the nursing mother holds the infant, he is frantic unless nursed and yet does not need to be fed. This may disturb a new mother who wonders why she cannot console her infant (Is her milk weak? Does it disagree with her infant? Is she an inadequate mother?). None of these options is true, but the fact that the infant smells her milk makes him behave as if he needs to nurse. Anyone who is not nursing can quickly quiet the infant. Picking the infant up does not spoil him, and rocking and cuddling are appropriate.

If true colic is diagnosed because of the consistency of the screaming for several hours each day at the same time, treatment is in order. Elixir of diphenhydramine (Benadryl) or pyribenzamine (1 to 2 tsp immediately and every 4 hr as necessary) is usually very effective. If the medication is given 30 min before the anticipated colic begins, it works best. The elixir is sedating as well as having an "antiallergic" component. Spiritus fermenti or other forms of alcohol, such as 5 drops of whiskey in 1 tsp of warm water, may help the colic. When wine or beer is suggested to the mother as an aperitif before dinner, it may serve to relax the frantic mother as well as the colicky infant. It is recognized that excessive alcohol while nursing can produce failure to thrive and hypoglycemia in the neonate, but when used in moderate dosage it may be very effective.

Acute 24 hr colic in a breast-fed infant may be due to something in the maternal diet. When a strong vegetable like beans, onions, garlic, or rhubarb is taken for the first time and the infant starts to cry within a few hours and continues for 20 to 24 hr it may be transient colic. This colic is self-limited and does not need any treatment. The colic foods are different for different infants. Some infants have no trouble. During the period of colic the infant may need frequent small feedings and much cuddling. Sometimes they overfeed, then vomit and settle down postvomiting and go quietly to sleep, just as an overfed bottle infant does.

The distress or discomfort may be due to tension, and "colic" has been noted to be more common in infants of high-strung mothers with their first infants. Colic has been associated with hormone withdrawal and has been treated with progesterone. In the breast-fed baby this is a less likely cause because of the presence of hormones in breast milk. Allergy to cow's milk can be manifest by bouts of pain and crying and switching to hypoallergenic milk may help the bottle-fed infant. The breast-fed infant may be reacting to something in the mother's diet, which can be easily eliminated after it is identified by association. Colicky breast-fed infants who are weaned to formula are usually much worse. Weaning is not an appropriate treatment for the colicky breast-fed infant in most cases. Colic usually diminishes in the third month of life, when the infant's gastrointestinal tract matures.

REFERENCES

1. Applebaum, R. M.: The modern management of successful breast feeding, Ped. Clin. North Am. **17:**203, 1970.
2. Bacon, C. J., and Wylie, J. M.: Mothers' attitudes to infant feeding at Newcastle General Hospital in summer 1975, Br. Med. J. **1:**308, 1976.
3. Barnes, G. R., et al: Management of breast feeding, J.A.M.A. **151:**192, 1953.
4. Bentovim, A.: Shame and other anxieties associated with breast feeding: A systems theory and psychodynamic approach. In Ciba Foundation Symposium no. 45, breast feeding and the mother, Amsterdam, 1976, Elsevier Scientific Publ. Co.
5. Caldeyro-Barcia, R.: Milk ejection in women. In Reynolds, M., and Folley, S.J., editors: Lactogenesis, Philadelphia, 1969, University of Pennsylvania Press.
6. Countryman, B. A.: Breast care in the early puerperium, J. Obstet. Gynecol. Nurs. **2:**36, 1973.
7. Deem, H., and McGeorge, M.: Breastfeeding, N.Z. Med. J. **57:**539, 1958.
8. Devereux, W. P.: Acute puerperal mastitis, Am. J. Obstet. Gynecol. **108:**78, 1970.
9. Goldsmith, H. S.: Milk-rejection sign of breast cancer, Am. J. Surg. **127:**280, 1974.
10. Lozoff, B., et al.: The mother-newborn relationship: limits of adaptability, J. Pediatr. **91:**1, 1977.
11. Newton, M., and Newton, N.: The let-down reflex in human lactation, J. Pediatr. **33:**698, 1948.
12. Newton, N., and Newton, M.: Relationship of ability to breast feed and maternal attitudes toward breast feeding, Pediatrics **5:**869, 1950.
13. Newton, M., and Newton, N.: The normal course and management of lactation, Clin. Obstet. Gynecol. **5:**44, 1962.
14. Raphael, D.: The tender gift: breast feeding, New York, 1976, Schocken Books, Inc.
15. Young, D.: Personal communication, 1978.

CHAPTER 9

Diet and dietary supplements for the mother and infant

The Committee on Recommended Dietary Allowances of the Food and Nutrition Board considers the question of diet for the lactating mother fully answered by saying the diet should supply somewhat more of each nutrient, except vitamin D, than that recommended for the nonpregnant female. Most writings for the nursing mother make the sweeping statement that maternal diet during lactation should be simple and well balanced with several glasses of milk and extra calories. All over the world women produce adequate and even abundant milk on very inadequate diets. Women in primitive cultures with modest but adequate diets produce milk without any obvious detriment to themselves and none of the fatigue and loss of well-being that some well-fed Western mothers seem to experience.

IMPACT OF MATERNAL DIET ON MILK PRODUCTION

Much can be learned from the study of the diets of lactating women of different cultures[15] about critical dietary differences. Accepting the limitations imposed by the methods of sampling and the variations inherent in pumping samples, (associated with time of day and length of lactation), there are some important observations.

Volume

The volume of milk produced by mothers has been measured in many studies and in many countries. Malnutrition does seem to have an effect on the total volume of milk produced. In the extreme, when famine occurs the milk supply dwindles and ceases, with ultimate starvation of the infant. In countries where food supplies vary with the season, milk supplies drop 100 ml/day during the periods of food shortage. Conversely, when food is supplemented, the volume output and protein content increase (Table 9-1). Edozien and co-workers[5] showed in a Nigerian village that the ultimate result of supplementing maternal diet with protein and kilocalories was an increased rate of weight gain in the infant. Sosa and associates[20] have shown a dramatic increase in milk volume by supplementing maternal diets in Guatemala (Fig. 9-1, *A*). The weight gain in these infants is shown in Fig. 9-1, *B* . Thus an inadequate diet seems to affect volume and not the composition because the breast depletes the maternal stores of nutrients to maintain the proper composition of milk.

135

Table 9-1. Effect of maternal dietary supplementation with protein on the volume and protein content of breast milk and weight gained by baby (Nigeria)*†

	Daily protein intake					
	50 g (initially, mean ± SD)	100 g (mean ± SD)	P	25 g (initially, mean ± SD)	100 g (mean ± SD)	P
Number of subjects	7	7		3	3	
Total milk solids (g/100 ml)	13.8 ± 1.3	13.4 ± 0.9		12.0 ± 0.6	11.9 ± 0.5	
Milk protein (g/100 ml)	1.61 ± 0.15	1.57 ± 0.19		1.20 ± 0.21	1.25 ± 0.23	
Milk lactose (g/100 ml)	8.1 ± 0.9	7.9 ± 1.0		7.3 ± 1.4	8.0 ± 1.8	
Milk produced (ml/day)	742 ± 16	872 ± 32	<0.05	817 ± 59	1059 ± 63	<0.05
Milk consumed (ml/day)	617 ± 15	719 ± 10	<0.05	777 ± 38	996 ± 74	<0.05
Weight gained by infant (g/day)	30.4 ± 3.6	45.7 ± 2.0	<0.05	10.5 ± 3.6	32.2 ± 10.1	<0.05

*From Edozien, J. C., Rahim-Khan, M. A., and Waslien, C. I.: J. Nutr. **106:**312, 1976, copyright © American Institute of Nutrition.

†Subjects were fed the initial diets for the first 14 days and then a diet providing 100 g protein/day for the next 14 days. Results for each subject represent the mean values for milk samples collected during days 8 to 14 (for initial diet) and days 21 to 28 (for diet providing 100 g protein/day). Duration of lactation for all subjects was between 30 and 90 days.

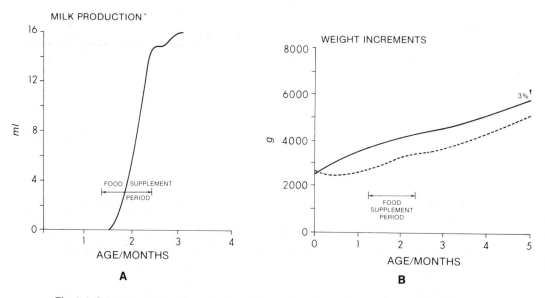

Fig. 9-1. A, Increments in milk production during maternal supplementation period. *Milliliters of milk obtained 1 hr after milk production. **B,** Weight increments of infants during maternal supplementation and follow-up period. †Boston growth curves. (From Sosa, R., Klaus, M., and Urrutia, J. J.: J. Pediatr. **88:**668, 1976.)

Protein content

Since the recent work of Hambraeus and colleagues[10] has reestablished the norms for protein in human milk to be 0.8 to 0.9 g/100 ml in well-nourished mothers, figures from previous studies will have to be recalculated to consider the fact that all nitrogen in human milk is not protein (25% of the nitrogen is nonprotein nitrogen [NPN] in human milk, and 5% of the nitrogen is NPN in bovine milk). The protein content of milk from poorly nourished mothers is surprisingly high.[17] An increase in dietary protein increases volume but not overall protein content, given the normal variations seen in healthy well-nourished women.

Observations made over a 20-month period of continued lactation showed that milk quality did not change although the quantity decreased slightly, which Von Muralt[21] attributed to the decreasing demand of a child who is receiving other nourishment. Therefore the total protein available with the decreased volume of milk and increased weight of the child decreased from 2.2 g/kg of body weight to 0.45 g/kg. The need for additional protein sources for the child after 1 year of age becomes obvious (Table 9-2).

A very painstaking study by Hanafy and co-workers[11] comparing maternal nutrition and lactation performance demonstrates what most clinicians have believed must be true: the well-fed lactating mother is more likely to produce a healthy infant. The investigators compared two groups of urban mothers of a moderate to poor socioeconomic standard in Egypt. The groups were similar except for the state of nutrition that was assessed (Table 9-3). The comparison of

Table 9-2. Constituents of maternal milk in areas of socioeconomic deprivation compared to average figures from the Western world*

Constituent	Western world	India, New Guinea, and Pakistan
Protein (g/100 ml of milk)	1.16	0.9
Total lipids (g/100 ml of milk)	4.78	2.5
Lactose (g/100 ml of milk)	6.95	6.20
Phospholipids (mg/100 ml of milk)	2.3	1.11
Cholesterol (mg/100 ml of milk)	18.8	21.1
Calcium (mg/100 ml of milk)	30.9	28.4

*Modified from Jelliffe, D. B., and Jelliffe, E. F. P.: Human milk in the modern world, New York, 1978, Oxford University Press.

Table 9-3. The nutritional state of healthy and malnourished mothers*

Factors	Apparently healthy		Clinically malnourished	
	Range	Mean	Range	Mean
Arm circumference (cm)	20-40	32.9	16-22	19.3
Weight (% of predicted)	80-168	121.4	76-96	85.1
Serum albumin (g/100 ml)	2.8-5.9	3.81	1.6-3.2	2.53
Urea N/Creatine N	6-44	22.1	2-26	11.3
NSIM†	82.5-152.5	116.3	50-95	71.5

*Modified from Hanafy, M. M., et al.: J. Trop. Pediatr. **18:**188, 1972.
†Nutritional state index of mothers.

Table 9-4. Comparison of the milks of healthy and malnourished mothers*

Factors	Apparently healthy		Clinically malnourished	
	Range	Mean	Range	Mean
Protein (g/100 ml)	0.95-1.36	1.09	0.76-1.32	0.93
Lactose (g/100 ml)	5.58-7.95	6.65	4.08-8.29	6.48
Fat (g/100 ml)	2.8-6.8	4.43	2.8-6.2	4.01
Calories (kcal/100 ml)	61-92	70.8	48-78	65.8
Amount (ml/day)	450-1290	922	180-1770	723
Protein (g/day)	4.3-15.0	10.02	1.6-14.9	6.65
Calories (kcal/day)	310-900	648	100-1080	475

*Modified from Hanafy, M. M., et al.: J. Trop. Pediatr. **18**:188, 1972.

Table 9-5. Comparison of the infants of healthy and malnourished mothers*

Factors	Apparently healthy		Clinically malnourished	
	Range	Mean	Range	Mean
Age (mo)	1-10	5.0	1-12	4.7
Arm circumference (% of predicted)†	43-133	72	43-102	70
Weight (% of predicted)†	60-139	102	43-120	86
Height (% of predicted)†	87-106	94	76-106	93
Serum albumin (g/100 ml)	1.8-4.6	3.11	1.2-3.7	2.50
NSII‡	55-119	83	45-101	70

*Modified from Hanafy, M. M., et al.: J. Trop. Pediatr. **18**:189, 1972.
†Percent of predicted value.
‡Nutritional state index of infants.

their milks is presented in Table 9-4. The ultimate goal of lactation is a healthy, growing infant. One must recognize that the foundation for good nutrition in any infant is established in utero. Nonetheless, significant differences in growth were shown by the two groups (Table 9-5).

Fat and cholesterol

Considerable interest has been focused on the impact of dietary fat and cholesterol on the composition of human milk. Fat is the main source of kilocalories in human milk for the infant. The concern about fat compostion in terms of the polyunsaturated to saturated fatty acid (PUFA) ratio and the high level of cholesterol normally found in breast milk has led to monitoring of mothers on altered lipid intakes. Potter and Nestel[18] studied lactating women who were placed on one of two experimental diets after a period of a study of their normal Australian diet, which includes 400 to 600 mg of cholesterol/day and fat that is rich in saturated fatty acids. Following this baseline study, the mothers were either given diet A, with 580 mg cholesterol and a high level of saturated fats, or diet B, with 110 mg cholesterol and a higher level of polyunsaturated fats from vegetable oils. A second study was carried out with the two diets high in either saturated or unsaturated fats, but the cholesterol remained the same, 345 to 380 mg/day.

The low-cholesterol diets lowered the maternal blood cholesterol but not the

Table 9-6. Lipid concentrations of mature human milk*

		Diet		Lipid concentration in milk		
Study	Plan	Saturation of fat†	Cholesterol (mg/day)	Cholesterol (mg/100 ml)	Triglyceride (g/100 ml)	Phospholipid (mg P/100 ml)
I (n = 7)	A	S	580	18.1 ± 2.7‡	3.42 ± 0.61	4.04 ± 0.71
	B	P	110	19.3 ± 3.6	3.57 ± 0.82	4.18 ± 0.91
II (n = 3)	C	S	380	23.3 ± 2.3	4.11 ± 0.42	
	D	P	345	21.3 ± 2.4	4.12 ± 0.56	

*From Potter, J. M., and Nestel, P. J.: Am. J. Clin. Nutr. **29**:54, 1976.
†S, rich in saturated fatty acids (P/S ~ 0.07); P, rich in polyunsaturated fatty acids (P/S ~ 1.3).
‡Mean ± SEM.

triglyceride levels. The cholesterol level of the milk, however, was unaffected in any diet combination. The increase in PUFA in the diet rapidly increased the levels of linoleate in the milk to twice the previous level at the expense of myristate and palmitate. Protein levels remained the same in the milk throughout the study. Infant plasma cholesterol levels decreased in response to an increase in the concentration of linoleate in the milk. The significant dietary change seemed to depend on the consumption of high PUFA and low cholesterol to alter the levels in the milk and thus in the infant's plasma (Table 9-6).

Guthrie and associates[9] have provided data on the fatty acid patterns of human milk in correlation with the current American diet, which has a high PUFA ratio. Compared with previous studies in 1953, 1958, and 1967, there was a shift toward higher levels of $C_{18:2}$ fatty acids, linoleic acid, and $C_{18:3}$, linolenic acid. Depot fat reflects dietary fatty acid patterns and thus the pool for mammary gland synthesis of milk fats. The mammary gland can dehydrogenate saturated and monosaturated fatty acids.

A word of caution on the lowering of fats in the diet inordinately—evaluation of the effects of a low-fat maternal diet on neonatal rats by Sinclair and Crawford[19] is pertinent. They made the distinction between two types of lipid in animals—storage and structural. This is correlated with histological findings of visible and invisible fats. Visible fats are triglycerides found in body depots. Invisible or structrual fats include phosphoglycerides, sphingolipids, and some neutral lipids, including cholesterol. The structural fats are key constituents of cellular membranes, certain enzymes, and myelin. The brain contains more structural lipids than protein.

Sinclair and Crawford[19] found that neonatal rats born to mothers raised on low-fat diets had a higher mortality, and survivors had smaller body, brain, and liver weights than controls. The lipid content of the body, brain, and liver was significantly less than controls. During life, the rat pups had depended entirely on their mother's milk for nutrition.

Lactose

The lactose level is recognized as being reasonably stable in human milk, which may be a function of the fact that lactose is a determinant of volume. Changes in the carbohydrate levels in the diet have been studied by Morrison[16] and reported by Hytten and Thomson.[13] Comparison of mothers on diets with three different levels of carbohydrate shows that the amounts of protein, fat, and carbohydrate in their milk are similar (Table 9-7).

Water

There are no data to support the assumption that increasing fluid intake will increase milk volume. Conversely, restricting fluids has not been shown to decrease milk volume, according to Hytten and Thomson.[13] From a practical standpoint, mothers have an increased thirst, which usually maintains a need for added fluid intake. When restricted, mothers will experience a decrease in urine output, not in milk. From a management standpoint, sharply decreasing fluids to prevent engorgement in the mother who is not lactating is ineffectual and only adds another inconvenience and discomfort.

Kilocalories

The caloric content, sample by sample, of milk from well-nourished mothers does vary somewhat but averages about 75 kcal/100 ml. Since fat is the chief

Table 9-7. Effect of various carbohydrate diets on milk composition*

Milk components	Carbohydrate level in diet (g/kg of body weight)		
	5 to 6	6 to 7	7 to 8
Protein (g/100 ml)	1.168	1.146	1.177
Fat (g/100 ml)	4.09	4.40	4.67
Lactose (g/100 ml)	7.30	7.38	7.38

*Modified from Hytten, F. E., and Thomson, A. M.: Nutrition of the lactating woman. In Kon, S. K., and Cowie, A. T., editors: Milk: the mammary gland and its secretion, vol. II, New York, 1961, Academic Press, Inc.; and Morrison, S. D.: Technical communication bulletin no. 18, London, 1952, Commonwealth Bureau of Animal Nutrition.

Table 9-8. Average daily intake of nutrients by twenty Australian women during the second and third trimesters of pregnancy* †

	Second trimester	Third trimester
Weight (kg)	58.7 ± 1.53	63.5 ± 1.42
Height (cm)	163.1 ± 1.38	163.1 ± 1.38
Age (yr)	25 ± 1.0	25 ± 1.0
Protein (g)	75.5 ± 2.98	70.7 ± 2.63
Fat (g)	95.0 ± 3.41	85.8 ± 4.40
Calories (kcal)	2150 ± 64	2030 ± 80
Calcium (mg)	1097 ± 90	1072 ± 70
Iron (mg)	11.3 ± 0.28	10.1 ± 0.36
Vitamin A value (IU)	8467 ± 940	8750 ± 857
Thiamin (mg)	1.1 ± 0.05	1.0 ± 0.05
Riboflavin (mg)	2.1 ± 0.14	2.0 ± 0.13
Nicotinic acid equivalent (mg)	24 ± 0.7	22 ± 0.8
Ascorbic acid (mg)	101 ± 9.1	97 ± 7.0
Calories (kcal/kg of body weight)	36.6	32.0

*From English, R. M., and Hitchcock, N. E.: Br. J. Nutr. **22**:15, 1968.
†Mean values with their standard errors.

Table 9-9. Weight changes of Australian women related to physical activity, calorie intake, appetite and dietary advice*

Group	Weight (kg)†	Physical activity	Calorie intake (kcal)†	Appetite	Dietary advice
Breast-feeders					
Nonpregnant	54.5 ± 1.92 (recall)	Grade 1‡	—	Normal	None
Third trimester of pregnancy	62.3 ± 2.11	Between grade 0‡ and grade 1‡	2090 ± 78	Decrease noted by 10 subjects (62%)	Restrict calorie intake
6-8 weeks postpartum	55.4 ± 1.77	Grade 1‡	2460 ± 111	Increase noted by 6 subjects (38%)	None
6 months postpartum or after cessation of breast-feeding	54.1 ± 2.06	Grade 1‡	2260 ± 95	Normal	None
Nonbreast-feeders					
Nonpregnant	52.6 ± 1.89 (recall)	Grade 1‡	—	Normal	None
Third trimester of pregnancy	62.3 ± 1.44	Between grade 0‡ and grade 1‡	1910 ± 110	Decrease noted by 6 subjects (60%)	Restrict calorie intake
6-8 weeks postpartum	54.5 ± 1.98	Grade 1‡	1880 ± 161	Normal	None
6 months postpartum	53.0 ± 2.06	Grade 1‡	1980 ± 193	Normal	None

*From English, R. M., and Hitchcock, N. E.: Br. J. Nutr. **22:**16, 1968.
†Mean values with their standard errors; ± SE.
‡National Health and Medical Research Council: Nutrition Committee (1965).

source of kilocalories, the fat content has the greatest impact on total kilocalories, with lactose and protein also contributing to the total. Thus in malnourished mothers the caloric content may be reduced.

How does this correlate with the caloric needs of the mother to produce the milk? The calculations for energy requirement have been made by comparing the energy intakes of nursing mothers and nonnursing mothers who were matched for other variables. English and Hitchcock[6] found nursing mothers consumed 2460 kcal and nonnursing mothers comsumed 1880 kcal, a net difference of 580 kcal (Tables 9-8 and 9-9).

Lactation will not produce a net drain on the mother if the amount of energy available and the requirement of any given nutrient is replaced in the diet. There is an energy cost to milk production because the breast does not work at 100% efficiency. During pregnancy, fat and other nutrients are stored for the fetus and in preparation for lactation. Lactation is subsidized, as is fetal growth, by maternal stores, even though the diet on any given day may be relatively deficient in a specific nutrient. This can be clarified by Fig. 9-2, which shows that diet and stores are available for milk as well as for maintenance of the mother.

The energy requirement can be calculated by determining the caloric content of the milk itself, plus an allowance for the energy cost of production. Using this formula, if there is 850 ml of milk with 600 kcal and the production efficiency is estimated at 60%, then the additional caloric need each day will be 1000 kcal. English and Hitchcock[6] collected their data between days 6 and 8 postpartum, when milk production is adequate for a newborn and the mother may be less active. If one assumes a production efficiency of 90%, as stated by Worthington,[23] then, indeed, the added caloric requirement to produce 850 ml of milk is less (945 kcal).

ENERGY UTILIZATION
IN LACTATION

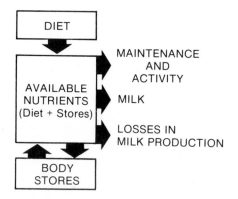

Fig. 9-2. Energy utilization in lactation, showing availability of body stores and dietary sources.

Vitamins

Water-soluble vitamins. Water-soluble vitamins move with ease from serum to milk, thus dietary fluctuation is more apparent. Levels of water-soluble vitamins in milk are raised or lowered by change in the maternal diet. Vitamin C levels reflect ingestion of vitamin C–laden beverages within 30 min. It has been pointed out by Anderson and colleagues[1] that the body's requirement for vitamin C increases under stress, including lactation. Furthermore, the vitamin C content of human organs at autopsy is much higher in the neonate than at any other time of life. This is true of all the major organs, including the brain.

The level of B vitamins, also water soluble, reflects dietary intake. The levels are affected acutely by maternal diet. Infantile beriberi is not unheard of in seemingly normal infants nursed by apparently well-nourished mothers with thiamin-deficient diets. The influence of maternal diet has been pointed out dramatically in the recently reported case of megaloblastic anemia and methylmalonic aciduria and homocystinuria in the breast-fed infant of a strict vegetarian. Vitamin B_{12} exists in all animal protein but not in vegetable protein. A strict vegetarian would require B_{12} supplements during pregnancy and lactation. B_{12} deficiency in infants has also been seen in New Delhi, where mothers had B_{12}-deficient milk. These infants also had megaloblastic anemia.

Thiamin (B_6) intake and milk levels were studied in healthy lactating women by West and Kirksey.[22] There were marked diurnal variations of B_6 levels, with peaks occurring in those mothers taking supplements 3 to 5 hr after a dose. Intakes of two to five times the recommended allowances did not increase the B_6 in the milk. Those taking less than 2.5 mg/day had much lower milk levels (129 $\mu g/L$).

Deodhar and Ramakrishnan[4] studied the effect of the stage of lactation on levels of vitamins B_1, B_2, B_3, B_{12}, and ascorbic acid. The values remained fairly constant throughout, except for those of B_3, which increased slightly over time. The relationship to socioeconomic group showed an increase in B_3 and B_6 levels with increased status. B_1 was higher in poorer mothers.

Fat-soluble vitamins. The concentration of fat-soluble vitamins is of concern because the levels in human milk are less easily improved by dietary changes. The low concentration of vitamin A in human milk is influenced by dietary inadequacies in this country as well as the developing countries. Levels may be marginal, and they may well vary seasonally. Since the levels of vitamin D in human milk appear to be marginal, maternal intake should be closely watched. Vitamin D and vitamin E levels in human milk are not raised by increasing their levels in the maternal diet. Vitamin E is in high levels in human milk, but vitamin D levels are thought to be low. Additional vitamin D has been identified in the aqueous fraction, but whether the aqueous levels are influenced by diet is yet to be determined.

Minerals

Calcium. Calcium has been associated with bone growth, and concern has been expressed because the total calcium in breast milk is low. The available information is inadequate to determine the requirement for lactation. Studies with radioactive calcium in the nonpregnant adult have shown that there are losses into the gut and through the kidney. Absorption and retention also depend on the reserves in the body. Long-term shortage causes economy of utilization and the apparent requirement is lower. In lactation, the absorption and retention is greater but not as great as during pregnancy. Atkinson and West[2] showed by scanning transmission techniques that lactating women mobilize about 2% of their skeletal calcium over 100 days of nursing. The calcium content of milk appears to be maintained despite markedly deficient intake, probably due to skeletal stores. The milk calcium levels are the same in mothers of rachitic and nonrachitic infants.

Sodium. The sodium content of milk depends on dietary intake, but unless there is a deliberately low sodium intake, values do not vary significantly.

Iron. The iron content of milk is not readily affected by the iron content of the diet or the maternal serum iron level. Increases in dietary iron that increase serum levels do not increase iron in the milk, according to Hytten and Thomson.[13] It is important, however, for the mother to replace her iron stores.

Phosphorus, magnesium, zinc, potassium, and copper. Phosphorus, magnesium, zinc, potassium, and copper levels in milk are not affected by dietary administration of these elements. Again, however, it is important for the mother to replenish her stores.

Iodine. Iodine in milk does depend on dietary content. The breast is able to raise the concentration of iodine in the milk above that in the blood, and thus there is an increased danger in giving radioactive iodine to the lactating woman.

Fluorine. The data are conflicting as to the impact of dietary fluorine on milk levels. Fluorine levels are low in milk, although it has been suggested that fluorine content may be higher than is reflected by present measuring techniques. Fluorine excretion in milk can be increased by giving sodium fluoride by mouth, but the rise is small relative to the dose, according to Hodge and Smith.[12]

RECOMMENDATIONS FOR NUTRITIONAL SUPPORT DURING LACTATION

In the previous section it was noted that the quantity, protein content, and calcium content of milk are relatively independent of maternal nutritional status and diet. Amino acids, lysine and methionine, certain fatty acids, and water-soluble vitamin contents vary with intake. It is important to point out that stores of calcium, minerals, and fat-soluble vitamins need to be replenished. Much of the data collected have varied, depending on the method used in collection. The daily intakes believed necessary for infants were determined by feeding infants processed human milk in a bottle, which is not a physiological standard. It is known, for example, that putting the entire sample in one container removes the natural variation in fat from beginning to end of the feeding.

The Committee on Recommended Dietary Allowances of the Food and Nutrition Board has recommended a balanced diet comparable to one for the nonlactating postpartum patient, with a few additions (Table 9-10). Although the calculated caloric cost of producing 1 L of milk is 940 kcal, it should be noted that during pregnancy most women store 2 to 4 kg of extra tissue in the physiological preparation for lactation. It is probably necessary, therefore, to add only 500 kcal to the diet, except in women with known high metabolic rates.

Preparation for lactation begins in pregnancy, if not before. The average gains in weight during pregnancy in various organs are noted in Table 9-10.

The recommended dietary allowances (RDA) for pregnancy are compared to the recommendations for an adult woman in Table 9-11. The major daily increases are 300 kcal, 20 g of protein, a 20% increase in all vitamins and minerals except

Table 9-10. Components of the average weight gained in normal pregnancy*

	Amount (g) gained			
Component	10 wk	20 wk	30 wk	40 wk
Total gain of body weight	650	4,000	8,500	12,500
Fetus	5	300	1,500	3,300
Placenta	20	170	430	650
Amniotic fluid	30	250	600	800
Increase of:				
Uterus	135	585	819	900
Mammary gland	34	180	360	405
Maternal blood	100	600	1,300	1,250
Total (rounded)	320	2,100	5,000	7,300
Weight not accounted for	330	1,900	3,500	5,200

*Reproduced from Committee on Maternal Nutrition, Food and Nutrition Board, National Research Council: Maternal nutrition and the course of pregnancy, Washington, D.C., 1970, Government Printing Office, p. 64, with the permission of the National Academy of Sciences.

Table 9-11. Recommended dietary allowances for adult women (ages 23 to 50 years)*

	Nonpregnant	Pregnant
Energy (kcal)	2000	2300
Protein (g)	46	76
Vitamin A		
RE†	800	1000
IU	4000	5000
Vitamin D (IU)		400
Vitamin E (IU)	12	15
Vitamin C (ascorbic acid) (mg)	45	60
Folic acid (μg)	400	800
Niacin (mg)	13	15
Riboflavin (mg)	1.2	1.5
Thiamin (mg)	1.0	1.4
Vitamin B_6 (mg)	2.0	2.5
Vitamin B_{12} (μg)	3.0	4.0
Calcium (mg)	800	1200
Phosphorus (mg)	800	1200
Iodine (μg)	100	125
Iron (mg)	18	18+
Magnesium (mg)	300	450
Zinc (mg)	15	20

*Reproduced from Food and Nutrition Board, National Research Council: Recommended dietary allowances, ed. 8, Washington, D.C., 1974, Government Printing Office, with the permission of the National Academy of Sciences.
†RE (retinol equivalent) replaces IU (international unit) as the standard measure of vitamin A activity.

Table 9-12. Recommended dietary allowances for lactation*

	Age (yr)			
	11-14	**15-18**	**19-22**	**23-50**
Body size				
Weight				
kg	44	54	58	58
lb	97	119	128	128
Height				
cm	155	162	162	162
in	62	65	65	65
Nutrients				
Energy (kcal)	2900	2600	2600	2500
Protein (g)	64	68	66	66
Vitamin A				
RE†	1200	1200	1200	1200
IU†	6000	6000	6000	6000
Vitamin D (IU)	400	400	400	400
Vitamin E activity (IU)	15	15	15	15
Ascorbic acid (mg)	80	80	80	80
Folacin (μg)	600	600	600	600
Niacin (mg)‡	20	18	18	17
Riboflavin (mg)	1.8	1.9	1.9	1.7
Thiamin (mg)	1.5	1.4	1.4	1.3
Vitamin B_6 (mg)	2.5	2.5	2.5	2.5
Vitamin B_{12} (μg)	4.0	4.0	4.0	4.0
Calcium (mg)	1200	1200	1200	1200
Phosphorus (mg)	1200	1200	1200	1200
Iodine (μg)	150	150	150	150
Iron (mg)	18	18	18	18
Magnesium (mg)	450	450	450	450
Zinc (mg)	25	25	25	25

*Modified from Food and Nutrition Board, National Research Council, National Academy of Sciences: Recommended Dietary Allowances, ed. 8, Washington, D.C., 1974, Government Printing Office, from Worthington, B. S.: Lactation, human milk, and nutritional considerations. In Worthington, B. S., Vermeersch, J., and Williams, S. R., editors: Nutrition in pregnancy and lactation, St. Louis, 1977, The C. V. Mosby Co.
†RE = Retinal equivalent: IU = international unit. The recommended unit of measure is RE. 1 RE = 10 IU.
‡Although allowances are expressed as niacin, it is recognized that on the average, 1 mg of niacin is derived from each 60 mg of dietary tryptophan.

folic acid, which is doubled, and a 33% increase in calcium, phosphorus, and magnesium. The RDA for lactation have been prepared for various age groups and are listed in Table 9-12. It should be noted in comparing the RDA for 19- to 22-year-old lactating women to nonlactating adult women that the increases suggested should provide ample nutrition and replace stores (Table 9-13).

When dietary supplements are suggested, there is concern about increased costs. Cost increases are modest for the standard diet and minimal for the low-budget diet, as demonstrated by Worthington.[23] The cost figures have been adjusted for 1979 levels (Tables 9-14 and 9-15). Although one rarely chooses breast-feeding or bottle-feeding on the basis of cost, one really needs to consider far more than the price of a few extra maternal kilocalories, and the cost of formula feeding makes a reassuring comparison. Hypoallergenic formulas are even more costly (Table 9-16).

Table 9-13. Dietary increases for lactation

Kilocalories	↑ 600
Protein (g)	↑ 20
Vitamin A (IU)	↑ 400
Vitamin D (IU)	0
Vitamin E activity	↑ 3
Vitamin C (mg)	↑ 35
Folacin (mg)	↑ 200
Niacin (mg)	↑ 5
Riboflavin (mg)	↑ 0.7
Thiamin (mg)	↑ 0.4
B_6 (mg)	↑ 0.14
B_{12} (mg)	↑ 1.0
Calcium (mg)	↑ 400
Phosphorus (mg)	↑ 400
Iodine (mg)	↑ 50
Iron (mg)	0
Magnesium	↑ 150
Zinc (mg)	↑ 10

Table 9-14. Nutrients, amounts, and estimated cost of foods needed to meet additional nutritional requirements of a lactating woman: standard (nonbudget) plan*

Suggested foods	Amount	Cost†	Kilo-cal-ories	Pro-tein	Vitamins					Cal-cium	Iron
					A	C	B_1	B_2	B_3		
Milk, fresh, 2%	2 cups	0.25	290	18	700		0.14	0.82	0.4	576	
Meat (round steak)	2 oz	0.26	150	13	35		0.04	0.11	2.8	6	1.7
Vegetable, dark green or yellow, cooked (broccoli)	½ cup ¾ cup	0.15	20	2.5	1990	70	0.07	0.15	0.6	68	0.6
Other vegetable or fruit (grapefruit)	½	0.20	45	1	10	44	0.05	0.02	0.2	19	0.5
Citrus fruit (orange juice)	½ cup	0.10	60	1	275	60	0.11	0.01	0.5	12	0.1
Enriched (or whole-grain) bread	1 slice	0.08	65	3			0.09	0.03	0.8	24	0.8
TOTAL		1.04	630	38.5	3010	174	0.50	1.14	5.3	705	3.7

*Modified from Worthington, B. S.: Lactation, human milk, and nutritional considerations. In Worthington, B. S., Vermeersch, J., and Williams, S. R., editors: Nutrition in pregnancy and lactation, St. Louis, 1977, The C. V. Mosby Co.

†Costs of Jan. 1979, Rochester, N.Y.

Table 9-15. Nutrients, amounts, and estimated cost of food needed to meet additional nutritional requirements of a lactating woman: budget plan*

| Suggested foods | | Cost† | Kilo-cal-ories | Pro-tein | Vitamins | | | | | Cal-cium | Iron |
					A	C	B₁	B₂	B₃		
Nonfat dry milk (prepared for drinking)	2 cups	0.07	180	18	20		0.18	0.88	0.40	592	
Peanut butter	2 oz	0.11	190	8			0.04	0.04	4.8	18	0.6
Vegetable, dark green or yellow, cooked (carrots)	½ cup ¾ cup	0.09	25	0.5	7610	4.5	0.04	0.03	0.04	24	0.45
Citrus fruit (tomato juice)	½ cup	0.06	25	1	970	20	0.06	0.04	0.95	86	1.1
Enriched (or whole grain) bread	2 slices	0.15	130	6			0.18	0.06	1.6	48	1.6
TOTAL		0.48	550	33.5	8600	24.5	0.50	1.05	7.79	768	3.75

*Modified from Worthington, B. S.: Lactation, human milk, and nutritional considerations. In Worthington, B. S., Vermeeroch, J., and Williams, S. R., editors: Nutrition in pregnancy and lactation, St. Louis, 1977, The C. V. Mosby Co.
†Costs of Jan. 1979, Rochester, N.Y.

Table 9-16. Cost per day of the most commonly used prepared formulas, basic equipment, and fuel*

Formula	Cost†		Average cost per day	
Formula, 13 oz can, double strength (formula, ready-to-feed, 1 qt)	$0.65	($0.95)	$0.65	($0.95)
12 unbreakable bottles with nipples at 63 cents each	$7.56		$0.05	$0.05
12 nipples at 3 for 55 cents	$2.20		$0.01	$0.01
Energy, electricity			$0.02	$0.02
TOTAL COST			$0.73	$1.03

*Modified from Worthington, B. S.: Lactation, human milk, and nutritional considerations. In Worthington, B. S., Vermeersch, J., and Williams, S. R., editors: Nutrition in pregnancy and lactation, St. Louis, 1977, The C. V. Mosby Co.
†Costs of June, 1979, Rochester, N.Y.

Malnutrition

Special supplementation for the lactating woman. It has been suggested that supplementing the diet of malnourished mothers with a special formula would be the best way to achieve nourishment for mother and child. The infant will then gain the additional advantages of human milk, such as protection against infection. Such formulas have been devised. Sosa and co-workers[20] have tried this approach in Guatemala.

Allergy

In families with a strong history of allergy, a hypoallergenic diet avoiding the common allergens such as wheat and eggs should be recommended. Further details are described in Chapter 15. An allergy prophylaxis scheme is described in Appendix K.

Vegetarian diet

B_{12} deficiency has been described in situations in which the resources of animal protein are limited. It is advisable to supplement the diet with B_{12}, up to 4 mg/day.

Supplementing the breast-fed infant's diet

For the newborn infant, human milk is the ideal food containing all the necessary nutrients. In establishing dietary norms for infants fed cow's milk, many nutrients identified as being needed in the diet were found to exist in greater amounts in cow's milk than in human milk. This does not consider the probability that the nutrient may be in a more bioavailable form in human milk. The specific items in question are protein, sodium, iron, vitamin D, and fluorine.

The Committee on Nutrition of the Academy of Pediatrics[3] has noted that iron deficiency is rare in breast-fed infants and attributes this to increased absorption and the absence of microscopic blood loss into the gastrointestinal tract, which is seen in bottle-fed infants. The committee recommends a source of iron in solid foods (fortified infant cereal) by 4 to 6 months of age for breast-fed infants.

Since rickets have been described in breast-fed infants, consideration should be given to the maternal intake of vitamin D and the exposure of the infant to sunshine. Foman[7] cautions against reliance on sunshine in the first year of life and advises providing infants with 400 IU of vitamin D. Individual discretion is appropriate, since infants of healthy mothers have not been observed to have rickets.

Fomon has stated that fluorine levels in breast milk are not adequate and therefore supplementation should be given. He provides the following dosage scale based on amounts of fluorine in the drinking water.

Fluorine concentration (ppm)	Dosage of fluorine (mg/day)
<0.3	0.5
0.3 to 0.7	0.5
0.8 to 1.1	0.5
> 1.1	0

Many breast-fed infants have done without fluorine supplementation and have had no adverse dental problems, but the decision should be based on individual determinants, including family dental history.

Dieting while breast-feeding

If one eats a balanced diet of nutritious food, one need not gain weight while nursing. If 940 kcal are used to nourish an average 3-month-old infant, then a mother could lose weight while nursing by not increasing her caloric intake. Weight loss by this method would require attention to selecting nourishing foods and avoiding junk food. With elimination of the "empty calorie" part of a diet, the infant will be provided with adequate nutrients. Fad diets are inappropriate. The high-protein low-carbohydrate diet is apt to increase a mother's blood urea nitrogen level, which would be passed into the milk. Since dieting involves mobilizing fat stores, it should not be pursued if there is a chance there are PBCs, DDT, or any other environmental toxin stored in the fat.

Foods to avoid

Some infants do not tolerate certain foods in the mother's diet, predominantly specific vegetables and fruits. Garlic and onions may cause colic in some infants. Cabbage, turnips, broccoli, or beans may also bother others, making them gassy and colicky for 24 hr. The same has been said of rhubarb, apricots, and prunes. If a mother questions the effect of a food, she should avoid it or document its effect carefully by watching for colic in the 24 hr following ingestion. In the summer, a heavy diet of melons, peaches, and other fresh fruits may cause colic and diarrhea in the infant.

REFERENCES

1. Anderson, T. W., et al., Enloe, C. F., and Hartley, H. L., moderators: To dose or megadose: a debate about vitamin C, Nutr. Today **13:**6, 1978.
2. Atkinson, P. J., and West, R. R.: Loss of skeletal calcium in lactating women, J. Obstet. Gynecol. Br. Commonwealth **77:**555, 1970.
3. Committee on Nutrition, Academy of Pediatrics: Iron supplementation for infants, Pediatrics **58:**765, 1976.
4. Deodhar, A. D., and Ramakrishnan, C. V.: Studies on human lactation, part II. Effect of socio-economic status on vitamin content of human milk, Indian J. Med. Res. **47:**352, 1959.
5. Edozien, J. C., Khan, M. A. R., and Waslien, C. I.: Human protein deficiency: results of a Nigerian village study, J. Nutr. **106:**312, 1976.
6. English, R. M., and Hitchcock, N. E.: Nutrient intakes during pregnancy, lactation and after the cessation of lactation in a group of Australian women, Br. J. Nutr. **22:**615, 1968.
7. Fomon, S. J.: Infant nutrition, ed. 2, Philadelphia, 1974, W. B. Saunders Co.
8. Food and Nutrition Board, National Research Council: Recommended dietary allowances, ed. 8, Washington, D.C., 1974, National Academy of Sciences.
9. Guthrie, H. A., Picciano, M. F., and Sheehe, D.: Fatty acid patterns of human milk, J. Pediatr. **90:**39, 1977.
10. Hambraeus, L.: Proprietary milk versus human breast milk in infant feeding. A critical approach from the nutritional point of view. In Neumann, C. G., and Jelliffe, D. B., editors: Symposium on nutrition in pediatrics, Pediat. Clin. North Am. **24:**17, 1977.
11. Hanafy, M. M., et al.: Maternal nutrition and lactation performance, J. Trop. Pediatr. **18:**187, 1972.
12. Hodge, H. C., and Smith, F. A.: Some public health aspects of water fluoridation. In Shaw, J. H., editor: Fluoridation as a public health measure, Washington, D.C., 1954, American Association for the Advancement of Science.
13. Hytten, F. E., and Thomson, A. M.: Nutrition of the lactating woman. In Kon, S. K., and Cowie, A. T., editors: Milk: the mammary gland and its secretion, vol. II, New York, 1961, Academic Press, Inc.
14. Jelliffe, D. B., and Jelliffe, E. F. P.: Human milk in the modern world, New York, 1978, Oxford University Press.
15. Jelliffe, E. F. P.: Maternal nutrition and lactation. In Ciba Foundation Symposium no. 45, breast feeding and the mother, Amsterdam, 1976, Elsevier Scientific Publ. Co.
16. Morrison, S. D.: Technical communication bulletin no. 18, London, 1952, Commonwealth Bureau of Animal Nutrition.
17. Pitkin, R. M.: Nutritional support in obstetrics and gynecology, Clin. Obstet. Gynecol. **19:**489, 1976.

18. Potter, J. M., and Nestel, P. J.: The effects of dietary fatty acids and cholesterol on the milk lipids of lactating women and the plasma cholesterol of breast-fed infants, Am. J. Clin. Nutr. **29:**54, 1976.
19. Sinclair, A. J., and Crawford, M. A.: The effect of a low-fat maternal diet on neonatal rats, Br. J. Nutr. **29:**127, 1973.
20. Sosa, R., Klaus, M., and Urrutia, J. J.: Feed the nursing mother, thereby the infant, J. Pediatr. **88:**668, 1976.
21. Von Muralt, A.: Maternal nutrition and lactation. In Ciba Foundation Symposium no. 45, breast feeding and the mother, Amsterdam, 1976, Elsevier Scientific Publ. Co.
22. West, K. D., and Kirksey, A.: Influence of vitamin B_6 intake on the content of the vitamin in human milk, Am. J. Clin. Nutr. **29:**961, 1976.
23. Worthington, B. S.: Lactation, human milk, and nutritional considerations. In Worthington, B. S., Vermeersch, J., and Williams, S. R., editors: Nutrition in pregnancy and lactation, St. Louis, 1977, The C. V. Mosby Co.

CHAPTER 10

Weaning

What does weaning mean? The textbooks on pediatrics and the mother's manuals all imply that it is the process by which one changes from one method of feeding to another. Raphael[5] states that the very first introduction of solid foods is the true beginning of weaning. If one consults the dictionary, however, one learns that to wean is to transfer the young of any animal from dependence on its mother's milk to another form of nourishment or to estrange from former habits or associations. A weanling is a child or animal who is newly weaned.

INFANT'S NEED

When discussing the process of weaning the human infant one might say it is the transfer of the infant from dependence on mother's milk to other sources of nourishment. If one were to determine the appropriate time for this to take place, it would be based on nutritional needs and developmental goals. Nutritionally, it is appropriate to begin iron-containing foods at 6 months, since that is the time the stores from birth are being diminished. The requirement at this age exceeds that supplied by human milk. An additional source of protein becomes necessary toward the end of the first year of life because the grams of protein per kilogram of body weight supplied by milk drop as the infant grows heavier. The content of protein in the milk begins to drop slightly after nine months of lactation. A human infant also needs bulk, or roughage, in the diet. The exact time this need becomes apparent is not known, but it is certainly by the end of the first year. Developmentally, he is ready to learn to chew solids instead of suckle liquids at about 6 months. Chewing is an entirely different motion of the tongue and mouth than sucking. The sucking fat pads in the cheeks begin to disappear at the end of the first year. The rooting reflex has been lost. Even though the teeth are not all in, the development of good dentition requires chewing exercise.

In summary, the infant is ready to explore new feeding experiences around 6 months. Feeding is an important social as well as nutritional encounter. Eating solids and learning to drink from a cup are important social achievements as well. That does not mean the infant is taken from the breast, but his diet is expanded and now includes solid foods, other liquids, and breast milk.

MOTHER'S RIGHTS

In practice, mothers are often the determinants of weaning time. Some mothers want to nurse for a few weeks and wean to a bottle to go to work. Other mothers wean at 3 months to be free again. Certainly any time spent breast-feeding is to the infant's advantage. The critical point in weaning is to make it a gradual adjustment for both the mother and infant.

WEANING PROCESS

Gradually replacing one feeding at a time with solids or a bottle or cup, depending on the infant's age and stage of development, is usually preferable.[1] After the adjustment has been made to one substitute feeding, then a second feeding is replaced with a substitute, usually at the opposite time of day. This process is continued until only the morning and night feedings remain. Then these two are stopped. The morning and night feedings can be maintained for some months and often an infant may be nursed beyond the second year, especially at these times. Mothers who wish to partially wean as early as 3 months may continue the morning and night nursing. This is especially suited to the working mother.

Emergency weaning

Occasionally there is a need for sudden weaning because of severe illness in the mother or some prolonged separation of mother and infant. (Sudden illness in the infant does not require weaning and, in fact, weaning would be contraindicated.) This is difficult for both. Depending on the age of the infant and his flexibility, it may take a patient surrogate mother a feeding or two to switch the infant to a bottle. In other cases the infant may take only solids and refuse other liquids for days. The mother may have considerable discomfort. Engorgement may be significant if it is only 4 to 6 weeks postpartum. The mother may experience milk fever at any time there is abrupt weaning. This illness is characterized by fever, chills, and malaise resembling a flulike syndrome. It is believed to be due to the sudden resorption of milk products into the system. Milk fever usually lasts 3 to 4 days and should not be confused with more serious illness.

The hormone change resulting from sudden weaning early in lactation is more definitive because the prolactin levels from suckling are higher immediately postpartum (Chapter 3). The hormone-withdrawal syndrome may be more marked with early weaning. Prolactin has been associated with a feeling of well-being, thus its decrease may be associated with relative depression. Patients with psychiatric disorders have been observed to cope by compensation postpartum until they wean the infant from the breast. It is important to provide an adequate support system during weaning for the mother who is prone to depression.

The normal, well-adjusted mother may experience some depression and sadness at the reality of the last feeding. It may be very difficult to face this last experience. It is important to recognize this as a physiological phenomenon as well as an emotional one. If a mother is forced by circumstances beyond her control to wean early, she may need a lot of understanding and encouragement to cope with the disappointment. If she has had pressure from friends or relatives to breast-feed, she may need to face what she considers failure and recognize that one can bottle-feed and still mother very well.

Historically, weaning has varied from strict to permissive schedules with the cultural styles of the day. Rigid feeding schedules were associated with early weaning. Weaning has varied from early denial to slow and gentle withdrawal. In this century, the time considered proper for weaning has gradually shortened from as much as 2 or 3 years to as little as 6 to 8 months, or less. Public opinion has overlooked the infant's needs in favor of what is considered the mother's rights. It is not necessary to have clearly in mind a specific plan for weaning in the early weeks of nursing unless there are some constraints on the mother's time. Weaning should be done with the infant's needs as a guide. If an infant under 1 year of age rejects the breast, it is unusual but not abnormal and should not be considered by the mother as a personal rejection. Some bottle-fed infants throw the bottle down at 9 months also.

Studies of weaning practices are few. Most observations are done on duration of feeding when the success rate is low. Jackson and associates[4] studied weaning times in mothers participating in the rooming-in project from 1942 to 1951 as compared to mothers who received traditional postpartum care at the New Haven Hospital during the same period. Rooming-in meant mother and infant were together in a special unit designed to accommodate both mothers and infants and managed as a pair by the same nursing staff. Infants were with their mothers as much as each mother wished. The rooming-in mothers nursed significantly longer. They averaged 3.5 to 3.8 months, whereas the controls weaned at 1.8 to 2.5 months postpartum. The incidence of breast-feeding decreases as the difficulty of the delivery increases. The number who breast-fed their infants did not differ by age, education, or race. Older mothers, better-educated mothers, and black mothers who breast-fed, however, nursed longer.

The patterns of weaning were studied in southern Brazil by Sousa and co-workers.[6] Brazil is also experiencing a decline in breast-feeding. The study was undertaken to understand the causes of early weaning to develop better means of encouraging longer breast-feeding and delaying weaning. The bottle was introduced at birth by 24%, by 2 months by 72.6%, and by 6 months by 88.0%. The main reasons given for weaning are shown in Table 10-1. A third of the mothers believed their milk was weak. The reasons the mothers thought their milk was thin are shown in Table 10-2. The researchers believed these data supported the hypothesis

Table 10-1. Main reasons for premature weaning

Reason	Number	Percentage
Not enough, inadequate, or "weak" milk	307	30.9
Child refused breast	177	17.8
Illness of child	159	16.0
Mother needed to go to work	149	15.0
"Correct age for bottle-feeding"	139	14.0
Other reasons	64	6.3
TOTAL	995	100.0

Table 10-2. Reasons for "milk inadequacy"

Reason	Number	Percentage
Milk is weak, thin, translucent	189	61.0
Infant cries after being breast-fed	59	18.7
Infant needs to be fed very often	35	11.2
Breast not adequately full	24	9.1
TOTAL	307	100.0

that the mothers did not understand the value of human milk and were influenced by advertisements about formulas and therefore compared their milk to formulas.

Weanling diarrhea

Most writings on weaning refer to the problems in underdeveloped countries when infants are weaned early to overdiluted cow's milk or formulas that cost money but do not contain the anti-infective properties of human milk for the human infant. Weanling diarrhea is well described by Gordon and Ingalls[2] as the clinical syndrome (weanling diarrhea is a collection of diseases) associated with weaning from the breast. In 1900 in New York City, the death rate from dysentery, diarrhea, and enteritis in children in the first year of life was 5,603/100,000 infants. This was largely attributed to weaning from the breast. Diarrheas are strongly associated with weaning not only because of the introduction of other foods, but also because of the loss of the protective properties of human milk. The diarrheas themselves contribute to the malnutrition seen in underdeveloped countries because of the resultant lack of appetite and increased metabolic losses. In third-world countries morbidity and mortality in infancy rise sharply at the time of weaning from human milk because of the rapid onset of infections. In well-nourished mothers and their infants, diarrhea does not occur from controlled gradual weaning unless there is a milk allergy or metabolic disorder in the infant.

WEANING AND THE WORKING MOTHER

There are mothers who will return to work. Whether the reasons are money, career, or personal satisfaction is not relevant to management. It takes tremendous commitment to work and breast-feed, but it can be done, it has been done, and it will be done. Usually the biggest problem a mother faces is coping with people who do not understand why she bothers. An understanding physician who provides the reassurance and support necessary to manage is a great asset. A mother may come home for a feeding in the middle of the day, pump milk to leave for the infant to have from a bottle, or give a substitute bottle. If there are occasional bottles of formula, the powder preparations are more economical and require only warming the water before adding the powder to assure rapid solution. Suggestions for collecting milk are in Chapter 18. Some infants quickly learn the mother's schedule and will sleep through while she is away and feed more frequently during the evening and night to make up for it. It takes some personal adjustment to plan ahead and a baby-sitter who is patient and cooperative. A mother needs to be alert to the infant's needs as well and may need to leave feedings ready when she is away even if she had hoped the infant would sleep through. If a mother works long hours or an inflexible schedule, it may be necessary to wean the infant to morning and night feedings at the breast. However, this arrangement still provides the special benefits of human milk as well as the closeness that an infant needs; thus it is worth the effort.

A mother may need to plan to pump her milk while she is at work because the breasts will fill and become uncomfortable. Daily engorgement, unless relieved, will serve to decrease the milk supply over a period of time. If possible, the mother can pump the milk by manual expression or various types of hand pumps and store in a sterile bottle under refrigeration. This milk can be used for the next day's feeding for the infant.

REFERENCES

1. Barnes, G. R., et al.: Management of breast feeding, J.A.M.A. **151:**192, 1953.
2. Gordon, J. E., and Ingalls, T. H.: Weanling diarrhea, Am. J. Med. Sci. Prev. Med. Epidemiol. **245:**345, 1963.
3. Jackson, E. B.: Pediatric and psychiatric aspects of the Yale Rooming-In Project, Conn. State Med. J. **14:**616, 1950.
4. Jackson, E. B., Wilkins, L. C., and Auerbach, H.: Statistical report on incidence and duration of breast feeding in relation to personal-social and hospital maternity factors, Pediatrics **17:**700, 1956.
5. Raphael, D.: The tender gift: breastfeeding, New York, 1976, Schocken Books.
6. Sousa, P. L. R., et al.: Patterns of weaning in South Brazil, J. Trop. Pediatr. **21:**210, 1975.

CHAPTER 11

Drugs in breast milk

Does a given drug pass into the breast milk? Can a patient take certain medications and still nurse her infant? Physicians are constantly perplexed by these questions because the data are meager and conflicting. In an analysis of 100 consecutive medical consultations about breast-feeding in Rochester, seventy were about medications needed for the mother, fifteen were about infants who where not thriving, ten were about sore or cracked nipples or mastitis, and five were miscellaneous in nature.

There are a number of general reviews of drugs in breast milk and dozens of articles about the effect of a specific medication in a particular infant. It is not appropriate to substitute wishful thinking for specific knowledge, yet it is equally inappropriate to discontinue breast-feeding when it is not medically necessary. Consideration of some of the pharmacokinetics will contribute to the understanding of the problems involved. Some of the data reported have been extrapolated from experiments performed on cows, goats, and rodents. Bovine experiments have been conducted using continuous infusions, which provide data on the passage of a drug into milk under certain circumstances of pH and plasma level.

Factors that influence the passage of a drug into the milk in humans include the size of the molecule, its solubility in lipids and water, whether it binds to protein, the drug's pH, and diffusion rates. Following is a summary of these factors:

    I. Drug
        A. Route of administration: oral, IM, or IV
        B. Absorption rate
        C. Half-life
        D. Dissociation constant
    II. Size of molecule
    III. Degree of ionization
    IV. pH of substrate (plasma 7.4, milk 6.8)
    V. Solubility
        A. In water
        B. In lipids
    VI. Protein binding more to plasma than to milk protein

Passive diffusion is the principal factor in the passage of a drug from plasma into milk. The drug may appear in an active form or as an inactive metabolite. The route of administration to the mother, the drug's half-life, and drug dissociation constants are also to be considered. Finally, a factor that has received relatively little attention is the infant. Will the infant absorb the chemical from the intestinal tract? If the infant absorbs the chemical, can the infant detoxify and excrete it or will minimal amounts in the milk build in the infant's system? Is the drug a material that could be safely given to an infant directly and at what risk? What dosages and blood levels are safe? It is these latter two questions that are more critical than the pharmacokinetic theory. The ultimate question faced by the physician is, "Can this infant be safely exposed to this chemical as it appears in breast milk without a risk that exceeds the tremendous benefits of being breast-fed?" Almost any drug present in mother's blood will appear to some degree in her milk.

CHARACTERISTICS OF THE DRUG
Protein binding

Drugs entering the circulation become protein bound or remain free in the circulation. The protein-bound component of the drug serves as an inactive reservoir of the drug that is in equilibrium with the free drug. Most drugs enter the mammary alveolar cells in the unbound form. Only those drug molecules that are free in solution can pass through the endothelial pores, either by diffusion or by reversed pinocytosis. Pinocytosis is the process whereby drug molecules that are dissolved in the interstitial fluid attach to receptors located at the surface of the cell membrane.[12] The cell membrane invaginates at the site of the drug attachment, bringing the drug into the cell. The membrane is pinched off, and the drug, surrounded by membrane, remains in the cell. Then the membrane is dissolved, leaving the drug molecule free in the cell. Reverse pinocytosis or apocrine secretion is the process by which the apical membrane evaginates after fusion of the intracellular membrane-bound secretion granules with the plasma membrane. The granules include lipids, proteins, lactose, drug molecules, and other cellular constituents. The evagination of the plasma membrane is pinched off and released into the alveolar lumen. Within the extravascular space, the drug may be bound to proteins in the interstitial fluid. Some agents in free solution can pass into the alveolar milk directly by way of the spaces between the mammary alveolar cells. These paracellular areas account for a major portion of the fluid changes across the epithelium. These spaces between adjacent alveolar cells serve to carry water-soluble drugs from the tissue into the milk.

Ionization

Depending on the pH of the solvent and the drug dissociation constant (pK_a), many weak electrolytes are more or less ionized in solution. Blood plasma and interstitial fluid are slightly alkaline (pH 7.4). Drugs that are weak acids are ionized to a greater extent in alkaline solution and are more extensively bound to protein. The amount of drug excreted from plasma (pH 7.4) to milk (pH 6.8 to 7.3, average 7.0) depends on the pH of the compound. Thus a weakly acidic compound has a higher concentration in plasma than in milk. Conversely, weakly alkaline compounds are in equal or higher levels in the milk than in the plasma (Table 11-1). The degree of drug ionization changes with the pH of the plasma and milk. Weak bases become more ionized with decreasing pH; thus the ionized component will increase in milk. The concentration in plasma and milk for the nonionized fraction will be the same, but the total amount of drug in the milk will be greater than in plasma. The sulfonamides demonstrate the effect of the pK_a on the concentration of drug that reaches the milk. Sulfacetamide, with a low pK_a, has a low milk/plasma (M/P) ratio, whereas sulfanilamide has a pK_a of 10.4 and an M/P ratio of 1.00 (Table 11-2).

Table 11-1. Concentration of various drugs in maternal blood and breast milk under normal pH conditions*

Drug administered (therapeutic dosage)	Drug levels (unit/100 ml)		Administered drug appearing in milk (%/day)
	Plasma or serum (pH 7.4)	Milk (pH 7.0)	
Aspirin	1-5 mg	1-3 mg	0.5
Bishydroxycoumarin	11-16.5 mg	0.2 mg	0.5
Chloral hydrate	0-3 mg	0-1.5 mg	0.6
Chloramphenicol	2.5-5 mg	1.5-2.5 mg	1.3
Chlorpromazine	0.1 mg	0.03 mg	0.07
Colistin sulfate	0.3-0.5 mg	0.05-0.09 mg	0.07
Cycloserine	1.5-2 mg	1-1.5 mg	0.6
Erythromycin	0.1-0.2 mg	0.3-0.5 mg	0.1
Ethanol	50-80 mg	50-80 mg	0.25
Ethyl biscoumacetate	2.7-14.5 mg	0-0.17 mg	0.1
Folic acid	3 μg	0.07 μg	0.1
[131]I	0.002 μCi	0.13 μCi	2-5
Imipramine hydrochloride	0.2-1.3 mg	0.1 mg	0.1
Isoniazid	0.6-1.2 mg	0.6-1.2 mg	0.75
Kanamycin sulfate	0.5-3.5 mg	0.2 mg	0.05
Lincomycin	0.3-1.5 mg	0.05-0.2 mg	0.025
Lithium carbonate	0.2-1.1 mg	0.07-0.4 mg	0.12
Meperidine hydrochloride	0.07-0.1 mg	trace (<0.1 mg)	<0.1
Methotrexate	3 μg	0.3 μg	0.01
Nalidixic acid	3-5 mg	0.4 mg	0.05
Novobiocin	1.2-5.2 mg	0.3-0.5 mg	0.15
Penicillin	6-120 μg	1.2-3.6 μg	0.03
Phenobarbital	0.6-1.8 mg	0.1-0.5 mg	1.5
Phenylbutazone	2-5 mg	0.2-0.6 mg	0.4
Phenytoin	0.3-4.5 mg	0.6-1.8 mg	1.4
Pyrilamine maleate	—	0.2 mg	0.6
Pyrimethamine	0.7-1.5 mg	0.3 mg	0.3
Quinine sulfate	0.7 mg	0.1 mg	0.05
Rifampin	0.5 mg	0.1-0.3 mg	0.05
Streptomycin sulfate	2-3 mg	1-3 mg	0.5
Sulfapyridine	3-13 mg	3-13 mg	0.12
Tetracycline hydrochloride	80-320 μg	50-260 μg	0.03
Thiouracil	3-4 mg	9-12 mg	5

*From Vorherr, H.: Postgrad. Med. **56**:98, 1974.

Table 11-2. Association between milk/plasma ratios and pK_a of sulfonamides*

Sulfonamide	Milk/plasma ratio	pK_a
Sulfacetamide	0.08	5.4
Sulfadiazine	0.21	6.5
Sulfathiazole	0.43	7.1
Sulfamethazine	0.51	7.4
Sulfapyridine	0.85	8.4
Sulfanilamide	1.00	10.4

*Modified from Lein, E. J., Kuwahara, J., and Koda, R. T.; from Gaginella, T. S.: U.S. Pharm. **3**:39, 1978.

The studies done in cows and goats with constant infusions demonstrate this principle more dramatically because the pH of bovine plasma is 7.4 to 7.5 and of bovine milk 6.5. Under normal circumstances, however, concentrations of drugs are rarely constant, and there is a delay in achieving a new equilibrium. During periods of rapidly decreasing blood levels there is some back diffusion into the plasma, according to Catz and Giacoia.[4]

Molecular weight

The passage of molecules into the milk also depends on the size of the molecule, or the molecular weight (mol wt). Water-filled membranal pores permit the movement of molecules of less than 200 mol wt. Due to action similar to the limitation of transport of certain large molecular chemicals across the placenta, insulin and heparin are not found in human milk, presumably because of the size of the molecule.

Solubility of the drug

The passage of drugs from the perialveolar interstitium into the milk has been likened by Vorherr[13] to the manner in which drugs penetrate the intestinal mucosa and reach the bloodstream. The alveolar epithelium is a lipid barrier that is most permeable in the first few days of lactation, when colostrum is being produced. The solubility of a compound in water and in lipid is a determining factor in its transfer. Un-ionized drugs, which are lipid soluble, usually dissolve and descend in the lipid phase of the membrane. The solubility is closely linked to the manner in which the drug crosses the membranes (Table 11-3). The membrane of the alveolar epithelial cells is composed of lipoprotein, glycolipid, phospholipid, and free lipids, as described in Chapter 2. The transfer of water-soluble drugs and ions is inhibited by this hydrophobic barrier. Water-soluble materials pass through pores in the basement membrane and paracellular spaces.

Mechanisms of transport

Drugs pass into milk by simple diffusion, carrier-mediated diffusion, or active transport. Following is a summary of the methods of transport:

Simple diffusion—concentration gradient decreases
Carrier-mediated diffusion—concentration gradient decreases
Active transport—concentration gradient increases
Pinocytosis
Reverse pinocytosis (apocrine secretion)

Table 11-3. Predicted distribution ratios of drug concentrations in milk and plasma*

	Milk/plasma ratio
Highly lipid-soluble drugs	~1
Small (mol wt <200) water-soluble drugs	~1
Weak acids	≤1
Weak bases	≥1
Actively transported drugs	>1

*From Gaginella, T. S.: U.S. Pharm. **3:**39, 1978.

The concentration of the drug in the circulation of the mother depends on the mode of administration (oral, intramuscular, or intravenous) and the distribution, protein binding, and metabolism of the drug by the mother. Nonelectrolytes such as ethanol, urea, and antipyrine enter the milk by diffusion through the lipid membrane barrier and may reach the same concentrations in the milk as in the plasma, irrespective of the pH. The main entrance site of molecules is at the basement laminal membrane, where water-soluble materials pass through the alveolar pores. Un-ionized drugs cross the membrane more easily than ionized ones because of the structure of the membrane. The nonionized drugs pass through the membrane by diffusion. When simple diffusion takes place, the ratio between the concentration in the milk and in the plasma (the M/P ratio) is 1.0. Passive diffusion provides the same ratio regardless of the plasma concentrations of the drug or the volume of milk secreted. Different M/P ratios depend on the binding to protein and are a measure of the protein-free fraction. The dissimilar ratios for the sulfa drugs (Table 11-2) are due to the difference in protein binding.

Large molecules depend on their lipid solubility and ionization to cross the membrane, since they pass in a lipid-soluble nonionized form. The M/P ratio is determined when there is equilibrium in the amount of nonionized drug in the aqueous phase on both sides of the membrane. When drugs are only partially ionized, it is the nonionized fraction that determines the concentration that crosses the membrane. The drugs whose nonionized fraction is not very lipid soluble will pass only in limited degree into breast milk.

Passive drug transport may occur in the form of facilitated diffusion. The active compound is transported across the cell membrane by a carrier enzyme or protein. The gradient is toward a lesser or equal concentration in both simple diffusion and facilitated diffusion and is controlled by chemical activity gradients. Facilitated diffusion usually involves a water-soluble substance too large to pass through the membrane pores.

Active transport mechanisms provide a process whereby the gradient is "uphill," or higher, in the milk. The process is similar to facilitated diffusion except that metabolic energy is required to overcome the gradient. Examples of substances actively transported include glucose, amino acids, calcium, magnesium, and sodium. Pinocytosis and reverse pinocytosis, as described previously, are involved in the transport of very large molecules and proteins. Chloride ions are secreted into milk via an active apical membrane pump, whereas sodium and potassium are diffused by electrical gradient. Since the level of sodium is kept low, there may be an active return of sodium into the plasma.

A summary of the steps in the passage of drugs into breast milk follows[14]:

1. Mammary alveolar epithelium represents a lipid barrier with water-filled pores and is most permeable for drugs during colostral phase of milk secretion (first week postpartum).
2. Drug excretion into milk depends on the drug's degree of ionization, molecular weight, solubility in fat and water, and relation of pH of plasma (7.4) to pH of milk (7.0).
3. Drugs preferably enter mammary cells basally in the un-ionized, non-protein-bound form by diffusion or active transport.
4. Water-soluble drugs of mol wt below 200 pass through water-filled membranal pores.

5. Drugs leave mammary alveolar cells apically by diffusion, active transport, and apocrine secretion.
6. Drugs may enter milk via spaces between mammary alveolar cells.
7. Most ingested drugs appear in milk; drug levels in milk usually do not exceed 1% of ingested dosage and are independent of milk volume.
8. Drugs are bound much less to milk proteins than to plasma proteins.
9. Drug-metabolizing capacity of mammary epithelium is not understood.

EFFECT ON THE NURSING INFANT
Absorption from the gastrointestinal tract

Although one is concerned about the amount of a given agent in the breast milk, of greater importance is the amount that is absorbed into the infant's bloodstream. There is no accurate way to measure this because other factors also affect the level in the infant's bloodstream. The tolerance of the chemical to the pH of the stomach and the enzymatic activity of the intestinal tract is significant. The volume of milk consumed is a factor as well.

Infant's ability to detoxify and excrete the agent

Any drug that is given to an infant by any route has to be evaluated according to the infant's ability to detoxify or conjugate the chemical in the liver and/or excrete it in the urine or stool. Some compounds that appear in milk in very low levels are not well excreted by the infant and therefore accumulate in the infant's system to the point of toxicity.

Drugs that depend on the liver for conjugation such as acetaminophen are theoretical risks because of the limited reserve of the neonatal hepatic detoxification system. When a single dose of a drug is given to a mother and the level is measured in her milk and in her infant, it does not give a clear picture of the potential for accumulation in the infant's system. The competition for binding of a drug to protein is also important. Some drugs such as sulfadiazine compete for binding sites that might normally bind bilirubin in the first week or so of life. This puts the infant in jeopardy of kernicterus at a given bilirubin level because of an increase in the fraction of unbound bilirubin even though the indirect bilirubin level appears to be below the dangerous level.

The chronological age of the infant and the infant's gestational age play a part in the interpretation of risks. An infant who is premature handles most drugs less well and may have immature activity of liver enzymes and other mechanisms that normally detoxify, inactivate, or excrete such agents. Prematures also have lower albumin levels, and thus have fewer available binding sites in protein.

The age of the infant makes a difference in the total volume of milk consumed, and in the older child there are other items in the diet so that milk does not comprise the total intake. Age makes a difference because the more mature infant can metabolize drugs more effectively; thus sulfa drugs, for instance, can be given to infants after the first month of life.

If the agent is fat soluble, the fat content of the milk may be significant. The fat content at any feeding increases over time; thus the so-called fore milk is low in fat and the hindmilk is rich in fat and serves to satisfy the appetite toward the end of a feeding. The total amount of fat in a given feeding is less in the morning, peaks at midday, and drops off in the evening even though the total amount of fat will be about the same each 24 hr period. The concentrations in fat of different members of the barbital family are influenced by the lipid fraction. Pentobarbital and secobarbital are found in the lipid phase, whereas phenobarbital is found in the aqueous phase.

The agent may appear in low levels in a mother's serum, but mammary blood flow during lactation is 500 ml/min and a mother produces about 60 ml of milk/hr. The agent that appears in minimal concentrations in the milk may present a significant problem when one considers that 1000 ml of milk may be consumed in a day by an infant. During the colostral phase of lactation, the breast is more permeable to drugs.

EVALUATING THE DATA ABOUT A GIVEN DRUG

Although it should be theoretically possible to determine how much of a specific drug reaches the infant in his mother's milk if one knew all the properties of the drug, including its pH, pK_a, lipid solubility, protein-binding activity, and rate of detoxification in the maternal system, there is sufficient variation in the levels that reach the infant and how he deals with the agent to make it necessary to have specific data about a specific drug. Thus a few simple steps in the decision-making process are helpful in determining risk.

Safety of drug for an infant

Is this a drug that can be given to the infant directly if necessary? Antibiotics such as penicillin, for instance, that one could give the infant are in this category; whereas an antibiotic one would not give the infant under ordinary circumstances, such as chloramphenicol, should be avoided in the nursing mother. The toxicity of chloramphenicol in the infant is dose related and associated with an unpredictable accumulation of the drug.

If the drug in question can be given to the infant, is there any risk to the infant in the amount in the milk? Phenobarbital can be given to infants for various reasons, thus the question is whether enough will reach the infant to cause difficulty. The infant should be watched for symptoms of depression. This is most quickly determined by a change in feeding and sleeping pattern. If the infant is sleeping long periods and feeding less than usual (specifically, less than five or six times a day), then the medication may be at fault. Phenobarbital is a significant drug for the mother with seizures; therefore a careful review of the risk-to-benefit ratio to the mother as well as to the infant should be undertaken. In anepileptic dosages it has not been reported as a problem. Barbiturates vary in their effect in young infants because the newborn does not handle the short-acting barbiturates, which are readily detoxified in the adult liver, as well, whereas phenobarbital depends more on the kidney for excretion. If one can safely give the drug to an infant, then it is only a question of watching for any symptoms of excessive accumulation that might develop.

When the drug in question is one that is not normally given to an infant of his particular age, weight, or degree of maturity, then a more difficult decision has to be made. Specific information about the amount of the drug that appears in the milk is essential in decision making. Often conflicting information is available. Many lists of drug-milk levels have perpetuated the same errors in calculation, thus having more than one reference may not provide confirmed information.

If the medication will have to be taken for weeks or months, such as some of the cardiovascular drugs, the drug has greater potential impact than when it will only be taken for a few days.

Sensitization

Is there risk of sensitization, even in the small dosages of a drug that might pass into the milk? This question arises most frequently around the use of antibiotics, and use of penicillin is most frequently questioned. Certainly if there is a strong history of drug sensitization in the family, it should be considered. In that case, however, it should be questioned for the mother as well. Whether infants are put at risk of developing resistant strains of bacteria in their systems by small amounts of antibiotic in their feedings is a serious question and, of course, is pertinent for the dairy and meat industry as well as the humans who consume these products.

Correlation of drug safety in pregnancy and lactation

Very rarely is valid information on the appearance of a drug in milk available on the package insert, since the pharmaceutical companies usually merely indicate it should not be taken during pregnancy and lactation. Agents that may be safe in pregnancy may not be so in lactation because during pregnancy the maternal liver and kidney are serving as detoxification and excretion resources for the fetus via the placenta, whereas during lactation the infant has to handle the drug totally on his own once it has reached his circulation. The infant in utero receives the drug in greater quantity via the circulation, whereas the nursing infant receives only what reaches the milk. One should be cautious about translating data pertaining to these two states back and forth.

MINIMIZING THE EFFECT OF MATERNAL MEDICATION

If a mother needs a specific medication and the hazards to the infant are minimal, the following important adjustments can be made to minimize the effects:
1. Do not use the long-acting form of the drug because the infant has even more difficulty in excreting these agents, which usually require detoxification in the liver. Accumulation in the infant is then a genuine concern.
2. Schedule the doses so the least amount gets into the milk. Given the usual absorption rates and peak blood levels of most drugs, having the mother take the medication immediately after a breast-feeding is the safest time for the infant.
3. Watch the infant for any unusual signs or symptoms such as change in feeding pattern or sleeping habits, fussiness, or rash.
4. When possible choose the drug that produces the least amount in the milk (Table 11-2).

SPECIFIC DRUG GROUPS

The information that is available about specific individual drugs has been provided in Appendix F. It is hoped that the increase in the incidence of breast-feeding will be accompanied by an increase in information and specific data about such factors as the appearance of a drug in milk. Considerably more information is needed to provide proper insight into the question than that obtained by giving a single specific dose of a medication to a mother and measuring the level in her milk without also measuring her serum level and identifying the peak level and half-life in her serum and milk and in her infant.

Analgesics

Drugs such as heroin have been known for decades to appear in milk, and at one time withdrawal symptoms in the neonate were prevented or treated by breast-feeding and then gradual weaning. Codeine, meperidine (Demerol), and pentazocine (Talwin) appear in milk at low levels. Individual variation is common, and neonates can be depressed by the medication; therefore care should be taken to monitor the infant carefully. For example, a breast-fed newborn was transferred to the special-care nursery at Rochester because of unusual floppiness and poor muscle tone. His mother was taking dextropropoxyphene (Darvon) every 4 hr. Temporarily stopping the nursing until the mother's drug level dropped and discontinuing use of the drug produced dramatic improvement, which persisted when the infant went back to nursing. Diazepam (Valium) has caused sleepiness, mild depression, and decreased intake in some infants.

Antibiotics

Levels in milk vary with the pH of the drugs and their pK_a. The risks vary among groups of antibiotics. Penicillins are not usually toxic but theoretically, can cause sensitivity. Sulfa drugs should not be used in the first month of life because they can interfere with the binding of bilirubin to protein. The risk diminishes with age, and infants are given sulfa drugs directly at 6 to 8 weeks of age. Infants with G6PD deficiency should never receive sulfa drugs. Chloramphenicol is contraindicated in nursing very young infants because of the risk of accumulation of the drug even from small amounts in milk. Tetracycline causes staining of teeth and abnormalities of bone growth when given directly to children for a week or more. Infants breast-fed by mothers taking tetracycline for mastitis may have stained and mottled first and second teeth when therapy exceeds 10 days. The amount in milk is half that in the mother's plasma.

Erythromycin appears in higher amounts in milk than in plasma. When given intravenously to the mother, the levels are ten times higher. When the infant is old enough to receive erythromycin directly, the mother can take it as well. Kanamycin appears in breast milk; therefore the infant should be monitored. Maintenance of kanamycin therapy longer than 10 days can be related to toxicity in the auditory nerve and disturbance of the renal function.

Metronidazole (Flagyl) does appear in milk at levels equal to those in serum. Most researchers consider the risk to the infant to be sufficient to suggest alternative therapy for the mother. Symptoms include decreased appetite and vomiting and, occasionally, blood dyscrasia.

Cephalexin, cephalothin, chloroquine, oxacillin, and para-aminosalicylic acid are reported by O'Brien[9] to be safe because they are not excreted in milk.

Anticholinergics

Anticholinergic drugs include atropine, scopolamine (hyoscine), and synthetic quaternary ammonium derivatives, some of which are available in over-the-counter medications. Some atropine does enter the milk. Infants are particularly sensitive to this drug; therefore the infant involved should be watched for tachycardia and thermal changes, which are more easily measured in infants. There may be a decrease in milk secretion in the mother, and constipation and urinary retention may occur in the infant. The quaternary anticholinergics should not appear in milk in any degree because, as cations, they do not pass into the acidic milk. Mepenzolate methylbromide (Cantil) has been reported by both O'Brien[9] and Gaginella[5] not to appear in milk.

Anticoagulants

Heparin does not pass into milk, but it is not a drug that can be given orally to the mother or without close monitoring of prothrombin times. Coumarin anticoagulants appear in breast milk and have been reported to prolong prothrombin times, not only in the mother, but also in the infant. Infants nursed by coumarin-taking mothers have been sustained with 1 mg of vitamin K daily. Because of the competition for conjugation in the glucuronidase system, extra vitamin K is not recommended in the first few weeks of life. Knowles has reviewed the literature thoroughly on coumarin drugs and specifically bis-3′:3′-(4-oxycoumarinyl) ethyl acetate (Tromexan). Although infants nursed by mothers taking the drug had been observed to hemorrhage, they had improvement of their prothrombin times. Infants given the drug directly in milk had poorer prothrombin times. It is believed the drug is altered by maternal metabolism. The drug has also been observed to cause changes in capillary resistance, especially when there has been previous vascular damage. Vitamin K has no effect on the hemorrhagic tendencies in these infants. When the mother was taking phenindione (an indandione derivative), hemorrhaging in the nursing newborn has been associated with trauma. Ethyl biscoumacetate has also been found in mother's milk by Illingworth and Finch.[6a]

Analysis of the milk of mothers using warfarin, however, did not reveal any drug in the milks or in the infants. The infants' prothrombin times remained normal. From this it has been suggested that warfarin is the drug of choice in the lactating mother who requires anticoagulant therapy and wishes to continue breast-feeding.

Antithyroid drugs

Iodide has been known for generations to pass into the milk and has been recorded to cause symptoms in infants not only when used for hyperthyroidism but also in asthma preparations and cough medicines. Iodides have been noted to be goitrogenic and to sensitize the thyroid gland to other drugs such as lithium, chlorpromazine, and methylxanthines.

Thiouracil is actively transported into the milk and appears in higher concentration in milk than in blood or urine, being reported at three to twelve times higher in milk than blood. It has the potential of causing goiter-suppressing thyroid activity or agranulocytes. It has been suggested that the infant could be medicated with small amounts of thyroid extract while breast-feeding but there are no published reports of such a procedure and such a plan should not be undertaken without careful monitoring of the infant. The availability of microdeterminations for T_3, T_4, and TSH improve the quality of monitoring.

Methimazole (Tapazole) presents risks to the nursing infant similar to those seen with thiouracil, that is, thyroid suppression and goiter. Giving 0.125 grain of thyroid extract to an infant may not adequately protect him, and careful monitoring of neonatal thyroid function would be mandatory.

Caffeine and other stimulants

Caffeine ingestion has been singled out for discussion because it is a frequent concern, yet the data provided in most reviews are misleading. Although with a given dose of caffeine that is comparable to a cup of coffee, the level in the milk is low (1% of level in mother) and in the infant's plasma is also low, caffeine does accumulate in the infant. Prior to the availability of the laboratory test for caffeine, cases were managed on clinical symptoms alone. It had been recognized by many clinicians and documented in my Rochester series[8a] of nursing mothers that wakeful, hyperactive infants were often the victims of caffeine stimulation. If a mother drank more than six to eight cups of any caffeine-containing beverage in a day's time, her infant could accumulate symptomatic amounts of caffeine. It was often the soft drinks such as colas and even the white "un-cola" drinks (such as Mountain Dew) that contributed to the caffeine build-up. When the situation was identified—a wide-eyed, active, alert infant who never slept for long—it was suggested that the mother try caffeine-free beverages, both hot and cold drinks. Often the infant settled down to a reasonable sleep pattern after a few days with no caffeine. Since information on milk and plasma levels has become available, researchers[8a] have identified three cases of caffeine excess in breast-fed infants, one of whom Rivera-Calimlin[12] reported. The infants all had measurable levels of caffeine in the plasma, which disappeared over a week's time after the caffeine was discontinued. The corresponding milk levels were as previously reported, about 1% of the mother's level, which supports the hypothesis that it accumulates in the infant. The infants do not need to be hospitalized, and verification of blood caffeine levels is helpful but not mandatory, since clinical trial will suffice. Smoking has been observed to augment the caffeine effect.

Reports on amphetamines have also varied; some published reports have claimed the drug does not appear in the milk, whereas others have reported measurable amounts. The symptoms reported are tremors, jitteriness, and wakefulness in the infant. If a mother is taking amphetamines for significant therapeutic reasons, then careful observation of the infant will indicate if there are problems from accumulation of the drug. The difference in observed reports may well be due to dosage, frequency of medication, and individual variation. In two identified cases when amphetamines were used for weight loss in over-the-counter diet preparations (dextroamphetamine [Dexedrine], 5 to 10 mg daily), the infants were jittery and wakeful and responded to withdrawal of the drug. Theophylline has also been observed to reach the breast-fed infant, causing irritability.

Cardiovascular drugs and diuretics

Digitalis is given to infants, but only for serious reasons. Cardiovascular drugs do appear in breast milk in small amounts. There is sufficient experience accumulated to date to conclude that mothers taking sustaining doses of digitalis preparations may nurse their infants without any harm to the infant.

Propranolol was found in trace amounts in the milk of a mother in Rochester but has since been reported by others as not appearing in milk samples. It does not appear to accumulate in the infant. Thus experienced cardiologists have permitted mothers taking propranolol to nurse their infants without any ill effect being observed in the infants. In 1973, Levitan and Manion[8b] reported significant quantities of propranolol in breast milk. β-adrenergic blockade effects have been described, including hypoglycemia, in an infant breast-fed by a mother taking propranolol. Since the reports are conflicting, it would be necessary to carefully monitor the breast-fed infant when the mother is taking propranolol. Monitoring plasma levels of the infant may be helpful if there is any question.

Reserpine, on the other hand, has been reported to cause nasal stuffiness, bradycardia, and respiratory difficulty with increased tracheobronchial secretion and is contraindicated in both pregnancy and lactation. Use of diuretics requires careful observation because they have the potential for causing a diuresis in the neonate that could be markedly dehydrating. Although diuretics such as furosemide (Lasix) are given to neonates, it is done only when fluid and electrolyte levels can be followed closely.

A mother who is lactating may actually require substantially less medication, particularly diuretics. Close monitoring of the mother while lactating to try to reduce her medications may provide a therapeutic balance that is good for the mother and safe for the infant.

Central nervous system drugs

Phenobarbital can be given to infants and is usually safe, but careful observation of the infant for variation in sleeping habits is important.

Phenytoin in the breast milk has been associated with vomiting, tremors, rash, blood dyscrasia (rarely), and methemoglobinemia but not with drowsiness and lethargy. Many mothers have nursed without apparent incident while taking phenobarbital and phenytoin. Fetal hydantoin syndrome has been described; therefore any possible correlation with further exposure during nursing should be considered. Where infant plasma level determinations are available, it might be advisable to check the plasma level after 1 or 2 weeks of nursing, providing an opportunity to evaluate possible accumulation.

Psychotherapeutic agents

Lithium is the one drug in this group with a clear risk of toxicity in the neonate as well as clear evidence that it reaches the breast milk. Lithium is contraindicated in pregnancy as well as in lactation. Infants have been reported to be hypotonic, flaccid, and "depressed" when the nursing mother is taking lithium.

Chlorpromazine or phenothiazine appears in the milk in small amounts but does not appear to accumulate. Doses of 100 mg/day do not appear to cause symptoms in the infants. It has been the practice in Rochester to permit breast-feeding while the mother is taking phenothiazines, considering it an important part of the treatment of the mother. All infants so nursed gained well and were not dehydrated or unusually depressed. Diazepam (Valium) has been detected in milk and in breast-fed infant's serum and urine. It has caused depression and poor feeding with weight loss in the infant. Chlordiazepoxide (Librium) and clorazepate (Tranxene) do reach the milk and may cause drowsiness and poor suckling. These substances' metabolites are also active, and therefore the half-life of therapeutic activity is prolonged. Meprobamate (Miltown, Equanil) has an M/P ratio greater than 1 and has been identified in milk. Infants whose mothers are taking meprobamate may become drowsy, but dosage adjustment may be indicated if the risk-benefit ratio is significant.

Tricyclic antidepressants such as imipramine have not been identified in the breast milk after 5 days of medication, according to Knowles[7]; thus cautious use may well be appropriate. Amitriptyline (Elavil) was not found in milk according to Ayd.[2]

Pesticides and pollutants

Human milk has been known to contain insecticides. Chlorinated hydrocarbons such as DDT and its metabolites dieldrin, aldrin, and related compounds are the best known. The major reason these compounds appear in breast milk is because they are deposited in body lipid stores and move with lipid. It has been pointed out that the fetus receives his greatest dose in utero and that adult body fat has approximately thirty times the concentration in milk.

Polychlorinated biphenyls (PCBs) in heavily contaminated pregnant Japanese women produced small for gestational age infants who had transient darkening of the skin ("cola babies"). Polybrominated biphenyls (PBBs) are similar compounds associated with a heavy exposure to farm animals and contaminated cattle fed in the lower Michigan Peninsula. The only women in the United States who have any risk of high exposure to PCBs or PBBs are those who have worked with or eaten fish in excess (i.e., at least once a week) that was caught by sports fishing in contaminated waters. Unless there is heavy exposure, there is no contraindication to breast-feeding. When there is a question, the state health department can be consulted for specific advice or to measure plasma and milk levels.

In most cases, the levels of pesticides in human milk have been less than those in cow's milk. The accumulated amounts have not exceeded safe allowable limits. Thus, unless the circumstances are unusual, breast-feeding should not be abandoned on the basis of insecticide contamination.

Most common air pollutants are not found in human milk.

Radioactive materials

Because of the increasing number of diagnostic tests available today with radioactive materials, it is not uncommon for a nursing mother to face such a procedure.

Radioactive iodine (^{125}I and ^{131}I) passes into milk at levels as high as 5% of the dose. When used for diagnostic purposes, breast-feeding should be discontinued for 24 hr. The excretion by the breast may alter the validity of the test result. If radioactive iodine is to be used therapeutically, breast-feeding must be discontinued until the iodine has cleared the system, which may be 1 to 3 weeks. A carefully collected sample of milk can be tested for radioactivity so that the period that the infant is off the breast is not unnecessarily long. If more than a 30 μci dose of ^{131}I is used, nursing should not be resumed until the milk is clear. If the infant is older and getting other foods, time can be altered accordingly.

Galium-67 citrate appears in significant amounts in the milk. It does clear the body quickly and is relatively safe for use in patients. Breast-feeding should be discontinued for at least 72 hr.

Technetium-99 is reported to clear the milk in 6 to 48 hr. The stage of lactation, whether or not the breast is emptied prior to receiving the dose, and the method of clearing the breast may well be responsible for the inconsistent results. Discontinuing breast-feeding for at least 24 hr is advisable.

With the advent of ultrasound examination, CAT scanning, and other techniques, occasionally there is an alternative to use of radioactive material.

IMMUNIZATIONS
Immunizing the breast-fed infant

Questions often arise as to whether a breast-fed infant should be immunized on a different schedule because of the protective maternal antibodies that might interfere with the infant's response to antigen stimulation. Following are some brief guidelines on the more common situations of concern:

1. DPT vaccination is not altered by breast-feeding, and the regular schedule should be followed for the infant.
2. Since poliovirus vaccine is an oral live virus vaccine there is concern that the maternal antibodies would inactivate the live virus. The recommendation is that the same schedule be followed, but that breast-feeding be postponed at least 30 min following the administration of the oral vaccine. A booster should be given as soon as the infant is weaned, 1 year later, and before the child enters kindergarten.
3. Rubella, mumps, and measles vaccines should be given at the regularly scheduled times.

Immunizing the nursing mother

Smallpox. Smallpox vaccination is inadvisable for the mother of any infant under 1 year of age, nursing or not. It is the personal contact, not the breast-feeding, that causes the risk; therefore there is no advantage to weaning if vaccination is necessary.

Rh_oGAM. Only rare trace amounts of anti-Rh are present in colostrum and none in mature milk of women given large doses of Rh_oGAM immediately postpartum. No adverse response was noted even with these high dosages. It has been thought that any Rh antibodies in the mother's milk were inactivated by the gastric juices. Rh_oGAM or Rh sensitization is not a contraindication to breast-feeding.

Rubella. Following is the recommendation of the American College of Obstetrics and Gynecology with respect to rubella:

1. In the adult female population, approximately 85% to 90% of the individuals are thought to have a high level of naturally acquired immunity and only 10% to 15% are considered to be susceptible to rubella infection.
2. Vaccination of pregnant women is contraindicated under all circumstances.
3. No woman of childbearing age should be vaccinated without having been first tested for immunity.
4. If the test is negative, the woman may be vaccinated if there is reasonable assurance that she will not become pregnant for at least 2 months.
5. At present the duration of immunity acquired from vaccination remains in question. It is possible that adult women vaccinated in childhood may be susceptible and might acquire an active rubella infection, which may go undetected.

REFERENCES

1. Arena, J. M.: Drugs and breast feeding, Clin. Pediatr. **5**:472, 1966.
2. Ayd, F.: Excretion of psychotropic drugs in human breast milk, Int. Drug Ther. Nlett. **8**:33, 1973.
3. Breastfeeding and drugs, Vet. Hum. Toxicol. **20**:346, 1978.
4. Catz, C. S., and Giacoia, G. P.: Drugs and breast milk, Pediatr. Clin. North Am. **19**:151, 1972.
5. Gaginella, T. S.: Drugs and the nursing mother-infant, U.S. Pharm. **3**:39, 1978.

6. Hervada, A. R., Feit, E., and Sagraves, R.: Drugs in breast milk, Perinat. Care **2:**19, 1978.

6a. Illingworth, R. S., and Finch, E.: Ethyl discoumacetate (Tromexan) in human milk, J. Obstet. Gynecol. Br. Empire **66:**487, 1959.

7. Knowles, J. A.: Excretion of drugs in milk: a review, J. Pediatr. **66:**1068, 1965.

8. Knowles, J. A.: Breast milk: a source of more than nutrition for the neonate, Clin. Toxicol. **7:**69, 1974.

8a. Lawrence, R.: Unpublished data.

8b. Levitan, A. A., and Manion, J. C.: Propranolol therapy during pregnancy and lactation, Am. J. Cardiol. **32:**2, 1973.

9. O'Brien, T. E.: Excretion of drugs in human milk, Am. J. Hosp. Pharm. **31:**844, 1974.

10. Rasmussen, F.: Mammary excretion of benzyl penicillin, erythromycin and penethamate hydriodide, Acta Pharmacol. Toxicol. (Kbh) **16:**194, 1959.

11. Rasmussen, F.: Mammary excretion of antipyryne ethanol and urea, Acta Vet. Scand. **2:**151, 1961.

12. Rivera-Calimlim, L.: Drugs in breast milk, Drug Ther. **2:**20, Dec., 1977.

13. Vorherr, H.: Drug excretion in breast milk, Postgrad. Med. **56:**97, 1974.

14. Vorherr, H.: The breast, morphology, physiology and lactation, New York, 1974, Academic Press, Inc.

CHAPTER 12

Normal growth, failure to thrive, and obesity in the breast-fed infant

NORMAL GROWTH

Bottle-fed infants gain more rapidly in weight and length during the first months of life than do breast-fed infants. Therefore evaluating an infant's physical growth by standards set by bottle-fed infants predisposes one to the diagnosis of failure to thrive. Fomon and colleagues[4] reported a longitudinal study of breast-fed and bottle-fed infants during the first few months of life that demonstrated that the 10th and 90th percentile values for weight and length of the two groups were similar at birth, and the 10th percentile values of the two groups were similar at age 112 days. The significant difference was in the values for the 90th percentile, which showed the bottle-fed infants to be substantially greater (Table 12-1). These differences were attributed to caloric intake rather than the difference in composition of the diet. Similar differences have been noted by other investigators, including Mellander and co-workers[9] in the 1959 Norbotten study of Swedish infants. Mellander and associates recorded a weight gain of 3.34 kg for 162 breast-fed infants and 3.53 kg for 143 bottle-fed infants at age 4½ months.

A study of "well-born" American infants reported by Jackson and associates[6] showed no difference between breast-fed and bottle-fed infants in the first 4 months of life in either weight or length. Between 4 and 6 months of life they observed the gain in weight and length was less rapid in the breast-fed infants. Fomon and colleagues[5] have shown that not only did the bottle-fed infant gain more in weight and length but also he gained more weight for a unit of length. This reflects the overfeeding of the bottle-fed infants. Whether this contributes to subsequent obesity is an important issue.

In assessing the normal growth of the breast-fed infant, the tables devised by Fomon and co-workers,[4] Jackson and colleagues,[6] or Mellander and associates[9] will serve better than the standard tables (Appendix A). It is appropriate to compare a breast-fed infant to standards set by healthy breast-fed infants. Increments of gain in weight and length per day and week can also be found in Appendix A.

Gain in physical growth is not as critical as gain in brain growth, but measurements of brain growth are only indirectly implied from growth of the head. In evaluating any infant's progress, head circumference is an important consideration, especially in the first year of life (Tables 12-2 and 12-3). Deceleration in the rate of increase in head circumference occurs over the first year. The head circum-

Table 12-1. Size of breast-fed infants and those fed milk-based formulas: percentile values*

Age (days)	Per-cen-tile	Weight (kg)				Length (cm)			
		Males		Females		Males		Females	
		Fed milk-based formulas (65)†	Breast-fed (58)	Fed milk-based formulas (77)	Breast-fed (46)	Fed milk-based formulas (65)	Breast-fed (58)	Fed milk-based formulas (77)	Breast-fed (46)
Birth	10	2870	2947	2816	2798				
	25	3125	3216	3135	2994				
	50	3410	3470	3350	3188				
	75	3705	3642	3615	3520				
	90	3804	3916	3964	3730				
8	10	2878	2881	2903	2746	48.9	49.5	48.8	48.5
	25	3248	3216	3274	2978	50.1	50.4	49.9	49.5
	50	3502	3459	3401	3260	51.7	51.2	51.1	50.7
	75	3688	3642	3698	3465	52.6	52.3	52.0	51.4
	90	3906	3839	4031	3555	53.4	52.8	53.2	52.2
14	10	3132	3089	3124	2990	49.8	50.6	49.4	49.7
	25	3399	3375	3426	3199	50.9	51.5	50.7	50.4
	50	3665	3681	3575	3500	52.6	52.4	52.0	51.6
	75	3876	3881	3894	3630	53.4	53.3	53.0	52.2
	90	4089	4065	4127	3698	54.1	54.2	54.1	53.4
28	10	3636	3406	3605	3511	51.6	52.0	51.5	51.6
	25	3970	3960	3824	3763	52.8	53.3	52.4	52.0
	50	4235	4271	4134	3935	54.6	54.2	53.8	53.3
	75	4470	4507	4440	4148	55.3	55.1	55.1	53.9
	90	4761	4692	4593	4230	55.9	55.7	56.0	55.0
42	10	4250	3962	4028	3930	53.0	53.8	53.0	53.2
	25	4506	4466	4275	4136	54.8	54.8	54.0	53.7
	50	4828	4808	4579	4360	56.2	56.0	55.2	54.7
	75	5080	5040	4915	4600	57.3	56.8	56.5	55.5
	90	5437	5312	5060	4692	57.7	57.5	57.6	56.6
56	10	4685	4387	4441	4243	54.3	55.2	54.6	54.6
	25	4967	4933	4603	4498	56.3	56.3	55.3	55.1
	50	5255	5250	4953	4758	57.6	57.6	56.8	56.3
	75	5599	5550	5308	4959	58.7	58.4	58.1	56.9
	90	5918	5791	5500	5161	59.3	59.4	59.2	57.7
84	10	5292	5320	5000	4707	57.8	58.3	57.0	57.2
	25	5740	5589	5388	5161	59.3	59.0	58.2	57.7
	50	5973	5955	5675	5424	60.8	59.9	59.5	58.6
	75	6501	6236	6027	5654	61.6	61.0	60.8	59.7
	90	7015	6773	6357	5800	62.6	61.9	61.7	60.2
112	10	5949	5933	5568	5282	60.1	61.1	59.6	59.7
	25	6305	6186	5976	5582	61.4	61.8	60.3	60.0
	50	6697	6482	6288	5987	63.0	62.6	61.9	60.9
	75	7253	7051	6669	6204	64.5	63.8	63.2	62.2
	90	7993	7306	7018	6428	65.4	64.2	64.0	63.1

*From Fomon, S. J., et al.: Acta Paediatr. Scand. suppl. 223:1, 1971.
†Values in parentheses are number of subjects.

Table 12-2. Increment in head circumference in various age intervals*

Age interval (mo)	Percentiles	SD	Increment in head circumference (cm)	
			Males	Females
0–1		−2	1.0	0.8
	10		2.0	1.5
	25		2.5	2.6
	50		3.6	3.3
	75		4.3	4.0
	90		5.3	4.7
		+2	6.2	5.6
1–3		−2	1.9	1.9
	10		2.4	2.5
	25		2.8	2.6
	50		3.3	3.1
	75		3.7	3.4
	90		4.2	3.8
		+2	4.7	4.3
3–6		−2	1.7	1.8
	10		2.2	2.3
	25		2.6	2.5
	50		3.0	2.9
	75		3.3	3.2
	90		4.0	3.4
		+2	4.5	3.8
6–9		−2	1.1	0.9
	10		1.3	1.4
	25		1.6	1.6
	50		1.9	1.9
	75		2.1	2.2
	90		2.3	2.5
		+2	2.7	2.9
9–12		−2	0.5	0.4
	10		0.8	0.8
	25		1.0	1.0
	50		1.3	1.2
	75		1.6	1.6
	90		1.8	1.7
		+2	2.1	2.0
12–18		−2	0.6	0.4
	10		1.0	0.7
	25		1.3	1.1
	50		1.6	1.5
	75		1.8	1.7
	90		2.1	1.9
		+2	2.6	2.4
18–24		−2	0.0	0.0
	10		0.2	0.5
	25		0.6	0.7
	50		0.9	0.9
	75		1.3	1.2
	90		1.7	1.5
		+2	2.0	2.0

*From Fomon, S. J.: Infant nutrition, ed. 2, Philadelphia, 1974, W. B. Saunders Co.

Table 12-2. Increment in head circumference in various age intervals—cont'd

Age interval (mo)	Percentiles	SD	Increment in head circumference (cm)	
			Males	**Females**
24–36		−2	0.0	−0.5
	10		0.5	0.5
	25		0.7	0.8
	50		1.0	1.1
	75		1.3	1.3
	90		1.5	1.6
		+2	2.0	2.7

Table 12-3. Head circumference at various ages*

Age (mo)	Percentiles	SD	Head circumference (cm)	
			Males	**Females**
1		−2	34.4	34.2
	10		35.2	35.0
	25		36.2	35.6
	50		37.0	36.2
	75		37.8	36.7
	90		38.6	37.6
		+2	39.6	38.2
3		−2	37.9	37.3
	10		38.6	37.9
	25		39.5	38.7
	50		40.3	39.5
	75		41.0	39.8
	90		41.7	40.4
		+2	42.3	41.3
6		−2	40.9	40.1
	10		41.9	40.9
	25		42.7	41.5
	50		43.3	42.2
	75		44.0	42.8
	90		44.8	43.4
		+2	45.7	44.1
9		−2	42.8	42.0
	10		43.7	42.7
	25		44.5	43.3
	50		45.0	44.0
	75		45.8	44.5
	90		46.6	45.5
		+2	47.6	46.0
12		−2	44.3	43.3
	10		45.0	44.0
	25		45.8	44.5
	50		46.5	45.3
	75		47.2	45.9
	90		47.7	46.6
		+2	48.7	47.3

*From Fomon, S. J.: Infant nutrition, ed. 2, Philadelphia, 1974, W. B. Saunders Co.

Continued.

Table 12-3. Head circumference at various ages—cont'd

Age (mo)	Percentiles	SD	Head circumference (cm)	
			Males	Females
18		−2	45.4	44.6
	10		46.4	45.4
	25		47.1	45.9
	50		48.1	46.7
	75		49.0	47.3
	90		49.6	48.2
		+2	50.6	48.6
24		−2	46.4	44.8
	10		47.3	46.4
	25		48.1	46.8
	50		49.0	47.8
	75		49.7	48.3
	90		50.5	49.0
		+2	51.6	50.4
36		−2	47.4	46.5
	10		48.0	47.1
	25		49.3	47.8
	50		50.0	48.8
	75		50.9	49.5
	90		51.7	50.1
		+2	52.6	50.9

ference increases about 3 inches in the first year of life and another 3 inches in the next 16 years of life. When growth failure includes failure of head growth, the failure is severe. Many other factors independent of body growth influence head growth, however.

Initially after birth, the normal infant loses 5% of his body weight before starting to gain, whether breast- or bottle-fed. In a study of infants at the University of Rochester, it was noted that breast-fed infants who were given added water or added formula to force fluids in the first few days of life lost more weight and were less likely to start gaining prior to discharge than infants who were entirely breast-fed or who were bottle-fed.

The human infant requires at least 100 days to double his birth weight, whereas the calf with the high protein, ash, calcium, and phosphorus contents of cow's milk requires only 50 days. If a reference infant at the 50th percentile is followed, it is estimated the birth weight will double at about 110 days for the breast-fed infant.

FAILURE TO THRIVE
Definition

The term failure to thrive has been loosely used to include all infants who show some degree of growth failure. For the breast-fed infant it may be a matter of comparing a slower gainer to the excessive weight-gain patterns of the bottle-fed infant. The definition offered by Fomon[3] states that "failure to thrive [should] be defined as a rate of gain in length and/or weight less than the value corresponding to two standard deviations below the mean during an interval of at least 56 days for infants less than five months of age and during an interval of at least three months for older infants.'' The values for 2 standard deviations (SD) below the mean in gains in length and weight for various age intervals are given in Appendix A. Fomon further suggests that infants gaining in length and weight at rates less than the 10th percentile values be suspected of failing to thrive. Certainly in managing the breast-fed infant, more careful and frequent medical evaluation should be provided for the infant who drops to the tenth percentile for weight, fails to gain weight, or continues to lose after the tenth day of life, rather than waiting for 56 days to establish the trend unquestionably. For the sake of this discussion, therefore, an infant should be evaluated for possible failure to thrive or slow weight gain when he continues to lose weight after 10 days of life, does not regain birth weight by 3 weeks of age, or gains at a rate below the 10th percentile for weight gain beyond 1 month of age. Unlike the bottle-fed infant who can then be placed in the hospital where professionals can feed him, the breast-fed infant needs to be evaluated in the home setting, nursing at the breast.

Diagnosis of failure to thrive

The problem of slow or inadequate weight gain has confounded even the physicians most committed to breast-feeding. It should be approached with the same orderly diagnostic process that one uses to attack any medical problem. Thus a complete history, a physical examination of the infant, an examination of the maternal breast, observation of the feeding, and appropriate laboratory work are indicated. Organizing the data amassed by this process will help identify the facts that do appear. Fleiss and Frantz[2] have 3 years of experience with a questionnaire they developed to analyze the breast-fed infant who is failing to grow. The questionnaire has been modified slightly to assemble questions about the mother and the infant separately; it appears in Appendix D.

A schema for classifying failure to thrive at the breast is suggested in Fig. 12-1. Here the causes associated with infant behavior and problems are distinguished from those due to problems in the mother. The causes in the infant can be further evaluated by looking at intake, which is the cause, in association with poor feeding, poor net intake due to additional losses, and high energy needs. The maternal causes can be divided into poor production of milk and poor release of milk. When a poor let-down reflex acts long enough, it will eventually cause a decrease in milk production. There may be several factors affecting the outcome, thus more than one management change may be indicated.

Evaluation of the infant. Examination of the infant should suggest any underlying physical problems such as hypothyroidism, congenital heart disease, or mechanical abnormalities of the mouth such as cleft palate, or major neurological disturbances. The infant's ability to root, suck, and coordinate swallowing should be observed. There is a greater risk today of missing subtle structural problems because infants spend much of their hospital life out of the newborn nursery away from the watchful eyes of experienced nurses and then are discharged before problems become manifest. The first office visit should be at 2 weeks of age or earlier and include a complete inspection whether there are complaints from the parents or not. A small number of infants will be identified with physical abnormalities that need medical attention (Table 12-4).

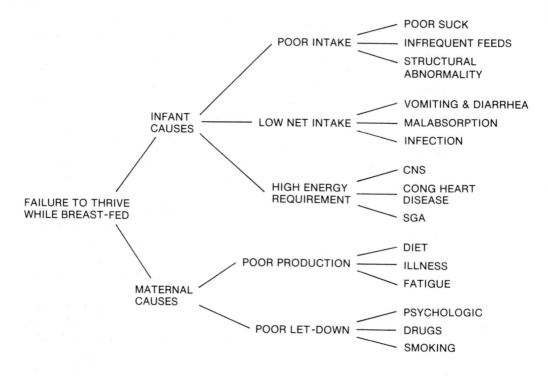

DIAGNOSTIC FLOW CHART FOR FAILURE TO THRIVE

Fig. 12-1. Diagnostic flow chart for failure to thrive.

Table 12-4. Conditions associated with or causing disorders of sucking and swallowing*

Absent or diminished suck	Mechanical factors interfering with sucking	Disorders of the swallowing mechanism (not including esophageal abnormalities)
Maternal anesthesia or analgesia	Macroglossia	Choanal atresia
Anoxia or hypoxia	Cleft lip	Cleft palate
Prematurity	Fusion of gums	Micrognathia
Trisomy 21	Tumors of mouth or gums	Postintubation dysphagia
Trisomy 13-15	Temporomandibular ankylosis	Palatal paralysis
Hypothyroidism	or hypoplasia	Pharyngeal tumors
Neuromuscular abnormalities		Pharyngeal diverticula
Kernicterus		Familial dysautonomia
Werdnig-Hoffmann disease		
Neonatal myasthenia gravis		
Congenital muscular dystrophy		
Infections of the CNS		
Toxoplasmosis		
Cytomegalovirus infection		
Bacterial meningitis		

*Modified from Gryboski, J.: Gastrointestinal problems in the infant, Philadelphia, 1975, W. B. Saunders Co.; from Behrman, R. E., Driscoll, J. M., Jr., and Seeds, A. E., editors: Neonatal-perinatal medicine: diseases of the fetus and infant, ed. 2, St. Louis, 1977, The C. V. Mosby Co.

SMALL FOR GESTATIONAL AGE INFANT. The small for gestational age (SGA) infant will be identified if gestational age and birth weight are scrutinized. This infant is small at birth despite full gestational time in utero. The SGA infant has a large nutritional deficit to make up from his intrauterine failure to grow. The cause of his intrauterine problem should be assessed (placental insufficiency, maternal disease, toxemia, heavy smoking, or intrauterine infection such as toxoplasmosis). SGA infants are difficult to feed initially by any method and often require tube feedings for a few days. Their caloric needs parallel the needs of an infant of appropriate weight for gestation rather than their actual low weight. The SGA infant should be placed on frequent feedings, every 2 to 3 hr by day and every 4 hr at night. He should be awakened for feedings if he sleeps long periods of time. If he has not been nursing well, the breast has not been stimulated to produce to its full capability. The successful nursing of an SGA infant may require extended effort on the part of the mother to assure adequate growth. On the other hand, such effort is well worth the trouble if one considers the impact of intrauterine growth failure on the central nervous system. It would be to the infant's advantage to have the critical amino acids such as taurine and the lipids of human milk with which to "catch up" brain growth.

JAUNDICE. Hyperbilirubinemia is discussed in Chapter 13, but an infant with an elevated bilirubin level from any cause may be depressed and lethargic and therefore may not nurse well. If the infant appears jaundiced, laboratory evaluation in search of the cause and its appropriate treatment should be undertaken.

METABOLIC SCREEN. Most hospitals provide, often because the law mandates it, screening for metabolic disorders including galactosemia, phenylketonuria, maple sugar urine disease, and disorders of metabolism of other amino acids. If these simple screening tests were not performed or their validity is in doubt, they should be done again. Usually the service is available in the state or county laboratory. Thyroid screening for abnormal T_4 and/or TSH should also be performed. Mass screening programs for neonatal thyroid disease have identified cases of deficiency that even in retrospect show none of the characteristic findings of hypothyroidism, such as thick, coarse features, hoarse cry, slow pulse, macroglossia, umbilical hernia, or jaundice. In the neonate hypothyroidism is often associated with failure to thrive, if undiagnosed.

Galactosemia. Galactosemia, which is a hereditary disorder of the metabolism of galactose-1-phosphate, is manifested by renal disease and liver dysfunction following the ingestion of galactose. The lack of galactose-1-phosphate uridyltransferase may be relative or partial. The clinical symptoms may be fulminating with severe jaundice, hepatosplenomegaly, vomiting, and diarrhea or may be more subtle. Cataracts are not invariably present. In mild cases, failure to thrive may be the presenting symptom. A screen of the urine for reducing substances (by Clinitest and not just Dextrostix, which will only identify glucose) should be done on all infants who fail to thrive, especially if there is hepatomegaly and/or jaundice. The definitive diagnosis is the identification of absence or near absence of galactose-1-phosphate uridyltransferase in red blood cell hemolysates. A screen of the urine should be considered even though an initial metabolic screen for galactosemia was done on the second or third day of life by hospital routine. The treatment is a galactose-free diet, which would mandate prompt weaning from breast milk to prevent further insult to the liver and kidneys. This is one of the few indications for prompt weaning from human milk. A formula free of lactose such as Isomil or Nutramigen is indicated. (Refer to pediatric texts on neonatal metabolic disorders for a full description of the disease.)

VOMITING AND DIARRHEA. Vomiting and diarrhea are very unusual in a breast-fed infant. Spitting up small amounts of milk after feedings is sometimes observed in otherwise normal infants and is of no consequence if it does not affect overall weight gain. Although pyloric stenosis is reportedly less common in breast-fed infants, this phenomenon should be ruled out in any infant who vomits consistently after feeding, has diminished urine and stools, shows no weight gain or actually loses weight, and has reverse peristalsis. Usually these infants do well initially, and the vomiting becomes progressive.

Vomiting may be a presenting symptom for various metabolic disorders. Thus metabolic disorders should be considered in the differential diagnosis. The usual causes of vomiting should be considered as well as the causes peculiar to breast milk. Maternal diet should be checked for unusual foods. In families at high risk for allergy, intake by the mother of known family food allergens may cause symptoms in the infant. Diarrhea may be due to foods in the mother's diet or the use of cathartics by the mother such as phenolphthalein (Ex-Lax).

INFECTION. Chronic intrauterine infection, which predisposes a small for gestational age infant to intrauterine growth failure, may continue to cause problems of growth in the presence of adequate kilocalories.

Acute infections. An infant who is not growing well may have an infection in the gastrointestinal tract, therefore the nature of the stools is important. The urinary tract may be another source of infection not readily identified. If, however, the initial evaluation includes a urinalysis with microscopic evaluation and a white blood cell count and differential count, this will be ruled out.

HIGH ENERGY REQUIREMENTS. When the metabolic rate of the infant is increased, the weight gain will be diminished or absent. When the infant is hyperactive with a strong startle reflex and sleeps poorly, consideration should be given to stimulants present in the milk as well as to neurological disorders. When a mother drinks coffee, tea, cola, or other carbonated beverages with added caffeine (such as Mountain Dew), the accumulated caffeine may be sufficient to make the infant very irritable and hyperactive. The best treatment is to replace the caffeine-containing beverages (Chapter 11). CNS disorders are associated with hyperactivity. Infants with severe congenital heart disease are constantly exercising to breathe and oxygenate and have markedly increased metabolic rates. For management of these special infants at the breast see Chapter 14.

Observation of nursing process. When it has been established that there are no obvious physical or metabolic reasons for the failure to gain weight, the infant should be observed suckling at the breast. Does the infant get a good grasp and suck vigorously? If not, what interferes? A receding chin, a weak suck, lack of coordination, the breast obstructing breathing, or mouthing the nipple or other ineffectual sucking techniques are some of the possibilities. If the problem is the suckling process, the infant may need retraining. This cause is more common with infants who have had some experience with bottles or rubber nipples or who use a pacifier. Small or slightly premature infants who were started on bottle-feedings have trouble relearning the proper sucking motion with the tongue (Figs. 6-6, 6-7, and 6-9). Bottle-feedings and pacifiers may have to be discontinued until the infant is more experienced at the breast. This will require a program of manually expressing milk to soften the areola, having milk at the nipple to entice the infant, and gently offering the nipple and areola well compressed between two fingers. If the infant has a receding chin or a relaxed jaw, it may help to have the mother hold the lower jaw forward by supporting the angle of the jaw with her thumb.

The five general types of nursing patterns described in Chapter 8 should be kept in mind. If the mother understands that it is acceptable for the infant to drop off to sleep and snack later, she may not hesitate to follow his lead, thus providing a more adequate feeding.

Simple changes in position can be suggested. Some infants will not settle down and nurse well if there is too much activity or noise. Some need to be tightly swaddled, others fall asleep and need to be unwrapped and stimulated to provide adequate suckling time. Frequent feedings, using both breasts, may be the answer in some cases. In others there may be too many ineffective feedings, which are wearing the mother out; a change that lengthens the time between feedings but also lengthens the time at the breast may help.

Maternal causes for failure to thrive. The special questionnaire by Fleiss and Frantz[2] includes questions about the mother's health, her dietary habits, sleep pattern, smoking habits, medication intake, the events that occur during nursing, and the psychosocial atmosphere in the home.

POOR MILK PRODUCTION

Diets. Although it has been demonstrated that malnourished mothers can produce milk for their infants, marginal diets in Western cultures do affect some mothers' ability to nourish an infant. If the mother is restricting intake deliberately or inadvertently, she should be instructed to meet the dietary requirement for lactating women (Chapter 9). One does not have to drink milk to make milk, but the necessary dietary constituents should be in the diet through cheese, eggs, ice cream, or other sources of calcium and protein. Prescribing brewer's yeast as a dietary supplement has been observed to provide improvement in milk production beyond that accounted for by mere addition of the same nutrients. Some mothers report a feeling of well-being from taking yeast that they do not obtain from taking daily vitamins.

Maternal illness. The presence of infection or other illness in the mother may affect milk production, and the cause of the illness should be identified and treated. Urinary tract infection, endometritis, or upper respiratory infection may need treatment with antibiotics. The antibiotic prescribed should be appropriate for the infant as well, since it will pass into the milk.

Fatigue. The most common cause of inadequate milk supply is fatigue. Fatigue may be lack of sleep because the infant demands considerable attention at night, but generally it is more subtle. The pressures of the rest of the family for meals or services or the self-inflicted demands of a job, career, or social commitments may be the cause. The mother must be placed on a medically mandated strict rest regime that is respected by family and friends. In the first month, while lactation is being established, fatigue is devastating to production. The infant then becomes hungry more often, cries and demands more frequent feeding, thus the vicious cycle is established. In later months of lactation, a mother becomes quickly aware of the impact of protracted fatigue on the nursing experience and usually will take steps to increase her rest.

POOR RELEASE OF MILK. Interference with the let-down reflex may cause a well-

nourished lactating mother to fail to satisfy her infant. The collecting ducts may be full but if the let-down or ejection reflex is not triggered the process will be at a standstill. The infant becomes frustrated and pulls away crying or screaming. Interference with the ejection reflex is predominantly iatrogenic and rarely hormonal (Fig. 7-10).

Smoking may interfere with the let-down reflex, and if this is the case, a mother who wants to smoke while nursing should wait to light up until the infant is sucking vigorously and the ejection is well established.

Experimentally, alcohol has been shown to interfere with oxytocin release in laboratory animals, but the dosage used collates with moderate to heavy drinking in humans. Therapeutically, alcohol has been recognized as an excellent adjunct to nursing if used judiciously. A glass of wine, a mug of beer, or a cocktail, especially in the early evening when some mothers may be under tension to feed the infant and family, will provide the relaxation necessary to permit adequate let-down response to take place. In countries where wine and beer are common beverages they have been recognized for centuries as important tonics for lactation. Alcohol's medical uses have been obscured by the concern for the disease of alcoholism, but the small amount of alcohol that would reach the milk is a sedative and muscle relaxant for the frantic infant.*

Medications that the mother may be taking should be evaluated. Although L-dopa and ergot preparations are known to inhibit prolactin release, other medications less well identified may have the same effect.

The most common cause for the failure of the ejection reflex is psychological inhibition. In a few cases the cause of the psychological stress may be obvious, such as a husband or mother who openly disapproves of breast-feeding, but in most cases the nursing mother has already considered this possibility and reassures the physician that she is relaxed and calm. It will require carefully taking the mother's history to "tease out" the source of stress. This is the time at which a home visit by the nurse practitioner from the physician's office or an experienced public health nurse will be valuable. The nurse may observe what is overlooked by the mother: construction for a new building next door, incessant barking from the neighbor's dog, or marital discord.

No obvious cause. Even though no obvious cause for failure to thrive is identified, the treatment may have to include establishing a positive attitude. Jelliffe[7] has often referred to nursing as a "confidence game." It becomes necessary to instill confidence in the mother rather than fear. Threatening the mother with stopping breast-feeding and switching to formula does not instill confidence. The physician should prescribe a positive plan for number and length of feedings, suggest diet and rest for the mother, and set reachable goals for growth.

If the let-down reflex is the crux of the problem and simple adjustments have not changed the ejection quality, oxytocin as a nasal spray (Pitocin), described in Chapter 6, should be prescribed. It is available only by prescription and should be used under the physician's guidance, although it is not dangerous. It does not

---

*An excellent treatment for colic is a few drops of alcohol in warm water or via the breast milk. An elixir is 25% alcohol, and it is often the elixir that sedates the infant, not the drug that it serves as the vehicle for. Thus elixir of phenobarbital is more sedating to the infant than the same dose of phenobarbital alone.

affect the milk or the infant. It is contraindicated only in pregnancy or hypersensitivity.

The rare infant who does not respond to this management protocol may have a malabsorption or metabolic disease as yet undiagnosed that will not become overt until cow's milk is introduced. Infants with strong family history of cystic fibrosis, milk allergy, or malabsorption should have careful diagnostic work-up before abandoning human milk, which may be the most physiological feeding available for the infant.

OBESITY

The best definition of obesity should be based on the percentage of body weight accounted for by fat. What percentage would be detrimental and how it could easily be measured is not known. Fomon[3] suggests, however, that until that is possible a clinical definition that circumvents clinical impressions would be useful. He suggests that "values greater than +2 standard deviation value for triceps and subscapsular skinfold thickness be considered evidence of obesity" (Table 12-5). Fomon also recognizes the difficulty of obtaining skinfold measurements on young infants and offers as a less satisfactory alternative the relation of body weight to stature (Table 12-6). The infant with a heavy bone structure and musculature but without excessive fat may appear to be obese based on this table. Therefore some discretion is advised when using these criteria for obesity.

The concern for obesity rests with the long-range outcome as an obese adult. There is a problem that obesity in infancy predisposes the child to immobility and inactivity; thus an obese infant lags on the developmental curve. The question of whether obesity in infancy predisposes the child to obesity in adult life has not been resolved satisfactorily. There are retrospective studies that support both sides of the question.

Breast-fed infants are rarely obese. The usual cause is adding solids early. Solids often provide excessive kilocalories. The obese breast-fed infant should have his diet and the feeding pattern scrutinized. If necessary, some restriction of prolong feeding should be suggested. In the normal course of a breast-feeding, the fat content of the milk increases over time and satisfies the infant after 10 to 15 min of nursing.

Table 12-5. Increments in skinfold thickness at various age intervals*

Age interval (mo)	Per-centiles	SD	Triceps (mm)		Subscapular (mm)	
			Males	Females	Males	Females
1–3		−2	−0.6	−0.9	−1.8	−1.4
	10		0.7	0.1	−0.5	−0.7
	25		1.5	1.4	0.2	0.5
	50		2.5	2.5	1.4	1.6
	75		3.6	3.4	2.2	2.6
	90		4.7	4.4	3.1	3.4
		+2	5.8	5.9	4.6	4.6

*From Fomon, S. J.: Infant nutrition, ed. 2, Philadephia, 1974, W. B. Saunders Co.

Continued.

Table 12-5. Increments in skinfold thickness at various age intervals—cont'd

Age interval (mo)	Per-centiles	SD	Triceps (mm)		Subscapular (mm)	
			Males	Females	Males	Females
3–6		−2	−1.5	−1.7	−3.3	−2.3
	10		−0.1	−0.1	−1.5	−1.2
	25		0.8	0.7	−0.7	−0.6
	50		1.8	2.1	0.2	0.2
	75		2.8	3.3	1.2	1.1
	90		3.6	4.4	2.3	2.0
		+2	5.3	5.9	3.9	2.9
6–9		−2	−3.0	−3.5	−2.9	−3.3
	10		−1.7	−2.2	−1.5	−2.0
	25		−0.7	−1.1	−0.8	−1.1
	50		0.2	−0.2	0.0	−0.2
	75		1.4	0.8	0.8	0.5
	90		2.6	1.6	1.9	1.2
		+2	3.8	3.3	3.1	2.7
9–12		−2	−3.7	−3.6	−3.2	−2.5
	10		−2.4	−2.4	−1.4	−1.6
	25		−1.5	−1.4	−0.6	−1.0
	50		0.0	−0.2	0.0	−0.3
	75		1.2	1.0	0.7	0.4
	90		2.4	2.1	1.8	1.1
		+2	3.5	3.2	3.2	1.9
12–18		−2	−3.2	−3.0	−3.3	−3.1
	10		−2.0	−2.2	−2.1	−2.1
	25		−1.0	−0.9	−1.0	−1.3
	50		−0.1	0.2	−0.4	−0.6
	75		1.4	1.3	0.4	0.2
	90		2.3	2.1	1.3	1.5
		+2	3.6	3.4	2.7	2.1
18–24		−2	−3.4	−3.0	−3.2	−2.7
	10		−2.0	−2.0	−1.7	−1.6
	25		−1.3	−0.8	−1.2	−1.1
	50		0.0	0.1	−0.5	−0.6
	75		1.2	1.2	0.2	0.2
	90		2.4	2.5	0.9	0.9
		+2	3.4	3.4	2.4	1.7
24–36		−2	−3.5	−4.2	−2.9	−3.5
	10		−2.3	−2.7	−1.9	−1.8
	25		−1.2	−1.2	−1.2	−0.9
	50		−0.2	0.3	−0.6	−0.4
	75		1.2	1.3	0.0	0.3
	90		2.3	2.3	0.4	1.2
		+2	3.3	4.2	1.5	3.3

Table 12-6. Tentative definition of obesity* †

	Males		Females	
Age (mo)	Length (cm) less than	Weight (kg) more than	Length (cm) less than	Weight (kg) more than
1	51.8	4.2	51.5	4.0
	53.0	4.5	52.2	4.3
	54.2	4.7	53.5	4.6
	55.2	5.1	54.6	4.8
3	58.0	6.0	57.1	5.6
	59.2	6.4	58.0	5.9
	60.2	6.9	59.2	6.2
	61.5	7.3	60.2	6.6
6	65.6	7.7	63.3	7.5
	66.5	8.2	65.2	8.0
	67.8	9.0	66.3	8.4
	69.2	9.6	67.8	8.9
9	70.0	9.1	68.2	8.9
	70.9	9.7	69.5	9.4
	72.3	10.7	71.1	9.9
	73.6	11.2	73.1	10.4
12	73.6	10.2	72.5	9.9
	74.7	10.9	73.2	10.5
	76.4	11.6	75.1	11.1
	78.0	12.5	76.9	11.6
18	80.0	11.6	78.7	11.1
	81.7	12.6	80.2	11.8
	83.2	13.3	82.0	12.7
	85.3	14.4	84.2	13.2
24	85.0	12.8	84.2	12.3
	87.3	13.9	85.8	13.1
	88.8	14.5	87.5	14.2
	90.9	16.0	90.3	14.9
36	93.4	14.8	92.1	14.3
	95.3	15.7	94.2	15.3
	97.3	16.8	96.2	17.0
	100.6	18.6	99.0	17.7

*From Fomon, S. J.: Infant nutrition. ed. 2, Philadelphia, 1974, W. B. Saunders Co.
†The table is based on data of Fomon et al. (1970, 1971, 1973) for ages 1 and 3 months, and on the data of Karlberg et al. (1968) for subsequent ages. At each age, the values for length for each sex are the 10th, 25th, 50th and 75th percentiles, while the values for weight are the 50th, 75th and 90th percentiles, and the mean +2 standard deviations.

REFERENCES

1. Behrman, R. E., Driscall, J. M., Jr., and Seeds, A. E., editors: Neonatal-perinatal medicine: diseases of the fetus and infant, ed. 2, St. Louis, 1977, The C. V. Mosby Co.
2. Fleiss, P. M., and Frantz, K. B.: Management of slow gaining breast fed infants, Keeping Abreast, J Hum. Nurt. (in press).
3. Fomon, S. J.: Infant nutrition, ed. 2, Philadelphia, 1974, W. B. Saunders Co.
4. Fomon, S. J., et al.: Growth and serum chemical values of normal breast fed infants, Acta Paediatr. Scand. suppl. 202:1, 1970.
5. Fomon, S. J., et al.: Food consumption and growth of normal infants fed milk-based formulas, Acta Paediatr. Scand. suppl. 223:1, 1971.
6. Jackson, R. L., et al.: Growth of "well-born" American infants fed human and cow's milk, Pediatrics 33:642, 1964.
7. Jelliffe, D. B., and Jelliffe, E. F. P.: Human milk in the modern world, Oxford, 1978, Oxford University Press.
8. Karlberg, P., et al.: The development of children in a Swedish urban community. A prospective longitudinal study, III. Physical growth during the first three years of life, Acta Paediatr. Scand. suppl. 187:1, 1968.
9. Mellander, O., et al.: Breast feeding and artificial feeding: a clinical, serological, and biochemical study of 402 infants with survey of the literature. The Norbotten study, Acta Paediatr. 48 (suppl. 116):1, 1959.

CHAPTER 13

Breast-feeding the infant
with a problem

A normal full-term infant can usually be breast-fed with only minor adjustment problems even without the support of medical expertise. The infant with a medical or surgical problem presents special concerns that cannot be conquered simply by a strong-willed mother who is determined to overcome all obstacles to breast-feed her infant. An understanding of the medical problem of the infant, his special nutritional needs, and the mechanical obstacles to feeding and nutritional absorption will be necessary before a rational judgment can be made regarding breast-feeding. When the infant cannot nurse directly at the breast, would providing mother's milk be appropriate? What is the overall prognosis in terms of ever feeding at the breast or perhaps for survival itself? Parents are so awed by the medical staff of special and intensive care nurseries that they are often afraid to bring up the subject of breast-feeding. In addition, the nursery staff may be so busy balancing electrolytes and adjusting respirators that they have not thought to ask what plans the mother might have had for feeding before the infant developed a problem. There are absolute contraindications to breast-feeding infants with certain problems. Those problems are few in number and rare in occurrence. Each medical problem will be dealt with separately. General information on establishing a milk supply without the stimulus of the infant's suckling will be provided in Chapter 16.

LOW–BIRTH WEIGHT INFANTS

Infants who are born weighing less than average, or less than 2500 g, will be referred to as low–birth weight infants. If the infants are less than 37 weeks of gestation, they are premature; if they are full term and low birth weight, they are small for gestational age (SGA).

Premature infants

The prognosis for survival of infants who are less than 37 weeks of gestation at birth depends on the gestational age, weight, respiratory status, and presence of any other complicating factors. For instance, if the infant develops hyaline membrane disease requiring respiratory support with continuous positive airway pressure (CPAP) or a respirator, the survival rate is decreased compared to an infant of the same weight and age without hyaline membrane disease.

A 2001 to 2500 infant without complications may be weaned from the incubator to an open crib within 24 hr. Although his suck reflex may be poor, he can usually

Table 13-1. Protein, calcium, and sodium requirements by growing premature infants and composition of human milk*

	Protein (g/100 kcal)	Calcium (mg/100 kcal)	Sodium (mEq/100 kcal)
Estimated requirements for hypothetical growing premature infants†	2.54	132‡	2.3
Composition of banked human milk	1.50	43	0.8

*From Fomon, S. J., Ziegler, E. E., and Vazquez, H. D.: Am. J. Dis. Child. **131**:463, 1977, copyright 1977, American Medical Association.
†Assumed body weight is 1200 g; weight gain, 20 g/day; energy intake, 120 kcal/kg/day. The basis for estimating requirements is described in the text.
‡This estimate does not apply to infants fed formulas from which calcium absorption is less than 65% of intake.

be nipple fed. If he is vigorous enough, he can be tried at the breast. If he can stimulate the breast briefly and obtain the rich, antibody-containing, cell-filled colostrum, it will protect against infection while providing a small amount of nutrition. If the infant cannot suck and must be tube fed, any colostrum the mother can manually express or pump from the breast can be given by gavage tube along with the prescribed formula necessary for nourishment. The value of colostrum to the infant has been thoroughly reviewed in Chapter 5. A recent study in Guatemala that was repeated in the special care nursery of the Rainbow Children's Hospital in Cleveland showed that the infection rate among sick and premature newborns was greatly diminished by providing 15 ml of human colostrum contributed by random donors daily.[29] These findings were especially dramatic in Guatemala, where the mortality from infection in the nursery is extremely high.

Protein requirements. The major concern of nutritionists in contemplating the use of human milk for low–birth weight infants has been based on the protein concentration. Calculations made from information extrapolated from intrauterine growth curves indicate that the premature infant requires more protein than can be provided by human milk. There is no easy way to determine the availability of this protein for absorption, although it is agreed that more of the protein in human milk is utilizable than that in formulas derived from a cow's milk base. Fomon and co-workers[15] have provided calculations to demonstrate the needs of the premature infant and the nutrients supplied by an appropriate amount of human milk (Table 13-1).

These determinations are made by using a reference infant, who has been described for various ages and weights and the daily increment of body content of protein. Allowances are made for inevitable losses and the degree of intestinal absorption; the total of these is the requirement. For the premature infant, the body content of a fetus of his gestational age is considered ideal, and the ideal growth curve is presumed to be that achieved in normal intrauterine growth. Fomon and colleagues point out that for the reference fetus between 28 and 32 weeks of gestation, protein accounts for 12.2% of the weight gained. They took a 1200 g premature infant gaining 20 g/day, of which 12.2% is protein, and determined that the increment in body protein will be 2.44 g. There is additional protein necessary for metabolism or "nongrowth" that averages 0.5 g/kg/day. Thus the total requirement for protein absorbed by the body is 3.04 g (2.44 g + [1.2 × 0.5]).

Table 13-2. Intake of protein and calories of the formulas compared to pooled human milk*

Nutrient	True protein (g/kg/day)	Calories† (kcal/kg/day)	Protein kcal ratio (g/100/kcal)	Distribution (%) of calories		
				Protein	Fat	Carbo-hydrate
Pooled human milk	1.63	114	1.4	6	51	43
1.5% (60:40)	2.25	118	1.9	8	50	42
3.0% (60:40)	4.5	116	3.8	17	51	32
1.5% (18:82)	2.25	118	1.9	8	50	42
3.0% (18:82)	4.5	116	3.8	17	51	32

*From Räihä, N. C. R., et al.: Pediatrics **57**:661, 1976, copyright American Academy of Pediatrics.
†Caloric intake calculated on the basis of combustion fuel values of 4.4 for protein, 9.4 for fat, and 3.95 for carbohydrate.

If only 83% of the dietary protein ingested is absorbed, 3.66 g of protein is required in the diet. If the dietary requirement for kilocalories is 120 kcal/kg/day, then conclude Fomon and Ziegler,[13] the 1200 g infant needs 144 kcal/day from human milk, or 2.54 g of protein/100 kcal, or 216 ml of human milk (180 ml/kg).

EXPERIENCE FEEDING HUMAN MILK TO PREMATURES. Räihä and others[20,36-38] have approached the question of feeding prematures by performing a controlled study in which a group of premature infants were fed human milk and other groups of premature infants were fed formulations of cow's milk altered to provide different ratios of casein and whey and total protein. They reported their studies in a series of four articles highlighting metabolic responses, effect on growth, effects on aliphatic amino acids and sulfur-containing amino acids, and effects on tyrosine and phenylalanine in plasma and urine. The premature infants were from one of three groups weighing less than 2100 g; T_1 was 28 to 30 weeks, T_2 was 31 to 33 weeks, and T_3 was 34 to 36 weeks. The infants were randomly assigned to one of five feeding groups including breast milk or an isocaloric formula varying in the quality and quantity of protein but not in fat or mineral content (Table 13-2). Caloric intake was 117 kcal in 150 ml/kg/day for formulas and 170 ml/kg/day for human milk (to obtain the same caloric intake per kilogram as the formulas provide).

Räihä and associates found no significant differences in rate of growth, in crown to rump length, in femoral length, in head circumference, or in rate of gain in weight from time of regaining birth weight to time of discharge at 2400 g. Their data also demonstrate that the blood urea nitrogen, urine osmolarity, total serum protein, serum albumin, and serum globulin levels varied directly with the quantity of protein in the diet. Blood ammonia concentration also varied with the quantity and quality of the protein in the diet: the more protein and the more casein, the higher the ammonia concentration. Metabolic acidosis in this study was more frequent, more severe, and more prolonged in the infant fed casein-predominant formulas than in those fed whey protein or breast milk (Fig. 13-1 to 13-4). Investigations on specific amino acids showed that the plasma amino acid concentrations of infants fed formulas high in protein and in casein had high levels of methionine and phenylalanine compared to those fed breast milk. Räihä and co-workers suggest that the human preterm infant has limited capacity to convert methionine to cystine.

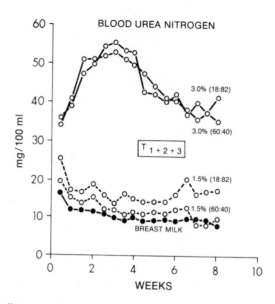

Fig. 13-1. Effect of dietary regimen on mean concentration of blood urea nitrogen. Data for all gestational age groups combined. Whey-predominant protein formulas are indicated by *1.5% (60:40)* and *3.0% (60:40)* and casein predominant formulas by *1.5% (18:82)* and *3.0% (18:82)*. (Modified from Räihä, N. C. R., et al.: Pediatrics **57**:659, 1976.)

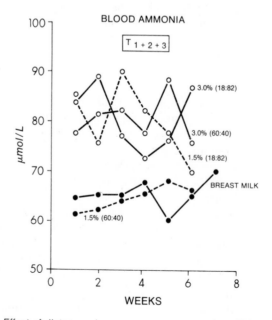

Fig. 13-2. Effect of dietary regimen on mean concentration of blood ammonia.

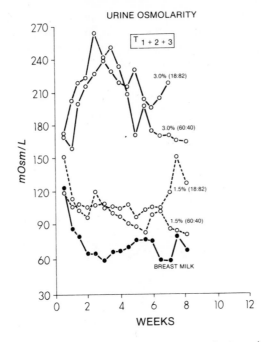

Fig. 13-3. Effect of dietary regimen on mean urine osmolarity.

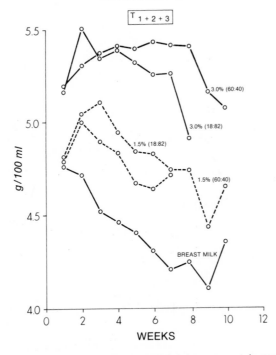

Fig. 13-4. Effect of dietary regimen on mean total serum protein concentration.

ESSENTIAL AMINO ACIDS. Important exceptions to the finding that high-protein formulas producing high–plasma protein levels were the findings on cystine and taurine. Taurine, which is present as a free amino acid in human milk and many mammal milks with the exception of the cow, was in highest concentration in infants fed human milk. Infants fed formulas low in taurine had reduced concentrations of taurine in the urine and plasma. Räihä and co-workers[36] suggested that the

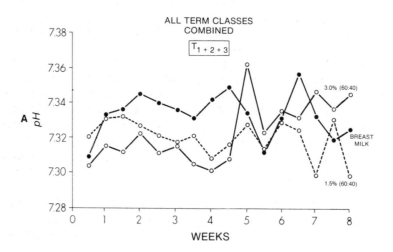

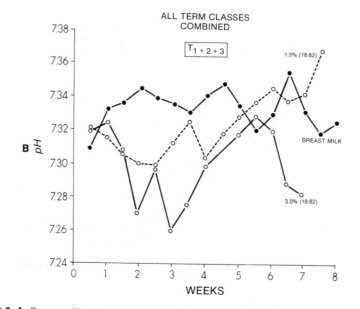

Fig. 13-5. A, Breast milk compared to 60:40 milk preparations with pH of 1.5% and 3.0%. **B,** Breast milk compared to 18:82 milk preparations with pH of 1.5% and 3.0%.

ability of the infant to convert cystine to taurine via cysteine sulfinic acid decarboxylase is limited. They found the enzyme in only trace amounts in fetal and mature
human liver. The levels of this enzyme in the human are a small fraction of levels
found in other mammals such as rat (1/1000), cat (1/10) or monkey (1/10). Infants
who receive low-protein casein-predominant formulas with half the cystine of
human milk and almost no taurine had urinary excretion of cystine and taurine
reduced significantly in 2 weeks. The plasma taurine levels fell steadily. When fed
high-protein casein-predominant formulas, they maintained cystine levels but the
plasma taurine level dropped steadily. This work suggests a dietary requirement
for taurine (Figs. 13-5 and 13-6). Taurine has been shown to be of special importance in the developing nervous system in the human and other mammals such as
the rat, rabbit, cat, and monkey.

In-depth study of tyrosine and phenylalanine by these researchers[38] provides
additional evidence that the immature infant is ill-prepared to metabolize these
aromatic amino acids. Plasma and urine concentrations of tyrosine and phenylalanine were higher in infants fed high-protein formulas than in infants fed breast
milk. The role of high protein intakes and resultant metabolic inbalances on brain
development have not yet been prospectively reported. Even the appropriate
physiological mean serum levels of tyrosine are not agreed on. It should be noted
that no infant fed breast milk had a tyrosine level over 20 μmol/100 ml (Figs. 13-6
to 13-10).

Snyderman[42] considers tyrosine an essential amino acid for the low–birth
weight infant and has determined that the minimum daily requirement is 50 mg/kg
of body weight. Plasma levels are 1 mg/100 ml or 5.5 μmol/100 ml. Filer and

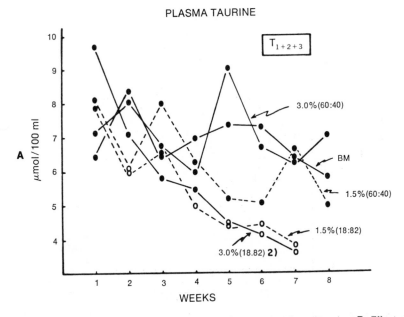

Fig. 13-6. A, Effect of dietary regimen on mean plasma concentration of taurine. **B,** Effect of dietary
regimen on mean urine concentration of taurine. (From Gaull, G. E., et al.: J. Pediatr. **90:**348, 1977.)

Continued.

URINE TAURINE

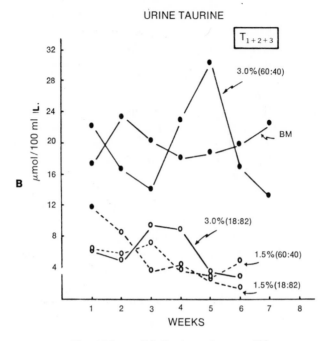

Fig. 13-6, cont'd. For legend see p. 193.

PLASMA PHENYLALANINE

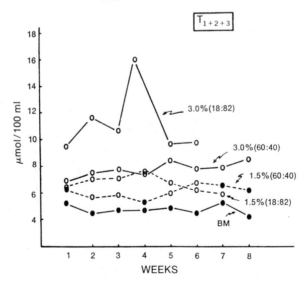

Fig. 13-7. Effect of dietary regimen on the mean plasma concentration of phenylalanine.

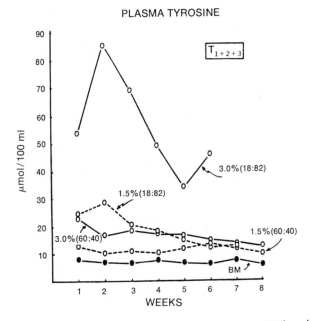

Fig. 13-8. Effect of dietary regimen on the mean plasma concentration of tyrosine.

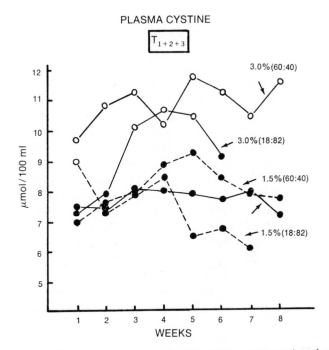

Fig. 13-9. Effect of dietary regimen on the mean plasma concentration of cystine.

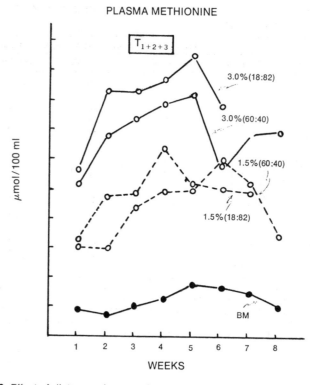

PLASMA METHIONINE

Fig. 13-10. Effect of dietary regimen on the mean plasma concentration of methionine.

associates[11] confirmed these findings. Gaull and colleagues[19,20] have concluded that cystine is an essential amino acid for prematures and newborns.

Sodium and calcium requirements. Nutritionally, the ash content, specifically sodium and calcium, required for the premature infant is also calculated to be greater than can be provided by human milk. According to Fomon and Ziegler,[14] for the reference fetus between 28 and 32 weeks of gestation, 617 mg of calcium is added to the body for each 100 g of weight gained. Nongrowth requirements for calcium are insignificant. Fomon and Ziegler calculated that if 65% of the calcium is absorbed from human milk, then there is a need for 190 mg/day or 132 mg/100 kcal. If 65% of the calcium is absorbed from human milk, then the premature infant would require 190 mg/day or 132 mg/100 kcal. As noted in Table 13-1, human milk provides only 43 mg of calcium/100 kcal. Forbes[16] makes similar observations by mathematical calculations of an increase in body weight of 30 g in a 1500 g infant consuming 120 kcal/kg/day. Human milk would provide 85 mg of calcium, whereas 250 mg is calculated to be needed. Forbes has shown the weight of the infant, regardless of gestational age, to advance on a logarithmic curve and the rate of increase in calcium to be equal to the rate of change in weight times a power of the weight (a 1000 g infant who gains 30 g needs 229 mg of calcium for proper growth during that gain).

Similar calculations have been made for sodium, demonstrating that the same reference fetus of 28 to 32 weeks has 7.4 mEq of body sodium. When 20 g/day is

Table 13-3. Accumulation of various components during the last trimester of pregnancy*

Component	Accumulation during various stages of gestation				
	26–31 wk	31–33 wk	33–35 wk	35–38 wk	38–40 wk
Body weight (g)†	500	500	500	500	500
Water (g)	410	350	320	240	220
Fat (g)	25	65	85	175	200
Nitrogen (g)	11	12	12	6	7
Calcium (g)	4	5	5	5	5
Phosphorus (g)	2.2	2.6	2.8	3.0	3.0
Magnesium (mg)	130	110	120	120	80
Sodium (mEq)	35	25	40	40	40
Potassium (mEq)	19	24	26	20	20
Chloride (mEq)	30	24	10	20	10
Iron (mg)	36	60	60	40	20
Copper (mg)	2.1	2.4	2.0	2.0	2.0
Zinc (mg)	9.0	10.0	8.0	7.0	3.0

*Modified from data of Widdowson; reproduced with permission from Heird, W. C., and Anderson, T. L.: Nutritional requirements and methods of feeding low birth weight infants. In Gluck, L., et al., editors: Current problems in pediatrics, vol. VII, no. 8, Chicago, 1977, Year Book Medical Publishers, Inc., copyright © 1977.
†Body weight of the 26-week fetus is 1000 g; that of the 40-week fetus is 3000 g.

gained in weight there is a retention of 1.48 mEq of sodium. Considering a urinary loss of 1.0 mEq/kg and 0.2 mEq/kg via the skin, there is a total loss of 1.44 mEq/kg/day. With 87% absorption from dietary sources, the requirement is 3.36 mEq/day or 2.3 mEq/100 kcal, according to Fomon and associates.[15] Human milk provides 0.8 mEq/100 kcal.

• • •

Fomon and co-workers[15] conclude that human milk is inadequate in meeting the nutritional requirement of the small premature infant. In the larger premature infant of 1800 g or more, the requirements, except for calcium, would just barely be met by human milk, if he only gained 20 g/day (Table 13-3). However, a workshop was held by the Office for Maternal and Child Health of the Department of Health, Education, and Welfare to determine the benefits and risks of feeding human milk to premature infants. Representatives of the major organizations interested in infant nutrition as well as key representatives of the research in this field attended the December 1975 workshop. They concluded that it is safe to feed human milk to human premature infants with the possible exception of fresh human milk from a donor other than the mother. Most participants believed that risk of nutritional inadequacy was small in relation to possible benefits. It was thought important to know the chemical composition of the food and to monitor the nutritional status of the infant.

Milk of mothers who deliver prematurely. Human milk was noted to differ chemically and immunologically from woman to woman but also may differ in the same woman from feeding to feeding (Chapter 2). Fresh milk from the infant's own

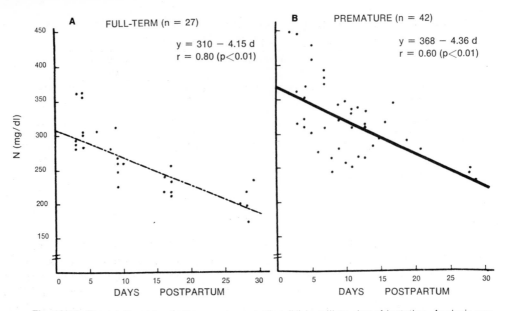

Fig. 13-11. The relationship of nitrogen concentration *(N)* in milk to day of lactation. Analysis performed to define regression lines as indicated for **A,** full-term and **B,** premature infant. (From Atkinson, S. A., Bryan, M. H., and Anderson, G. H.: J. Pediatr. **93:**67, 1978.)

mother may offer advantages. This point was demonstrated by studies done by Atkinson and co-workers[3] on the nitrogen concentrations of milk from mothers of term and premature infants. The data demonstrated that for a given volume of milk, the premature would receive 20% more nitrogen than would the full-term infant if both were fed their own mother's milk. The significance of the higher nitrogen concentration in the premature infant's own mother's milk will be even greater when compared to the same volume of intake of mature breast milk from a third-party donor or pooled milks. The researchers point out that if there is a similar distribution between protein and nonprotein nitrogen in the milk of mothers of both mature and immature infants, the premature infant would receive at least twice as much protein and utilizable nitrogen from an equal volume of his own mother's milk during early lactation (Fig. 13-11 and Table 13-4).

In response to this unique observation, Fomon and Ziegler[14] editorialize on the question as to whether this is a result of manual expression to obtain samples. They asked if this increased concentration of nutrients in the milk of mothers who deliver prematurely also included levels of carbohydrate and fat. If so the protein energy ratio of the milk of mothers of premature infants would not be higher than that of mothers of term infants. Investigation is necessary to confirm the findings of increased nitrogen and protein levels and explore the levels of carbohydrate, fat, and minerals under the same circumstances.

The question remains to be answered regarding what is the normal growth pattern for the premature infant. The growth curves that have been used have been derived from the curves of intrauterine growth of the fetus. Whether this is actually ideal for the infant in extrauterine life, obtaining nutrients via the gastrointestinal

Table 13-4. Comparsion of mean nitrogen (N) concentration in milk from mothers of premature (PT) and full-term (FT) infants* †

Milk group	Number	N concentration (mg/dl)	
		Observed	Adjusted‡
FT	27	260.6 ± 8.9§	267.5 ± 8.7
PT	42	315.5 ± 8.4	312.3 ± 8.3
FT vs PT		P < 0.001	P < 0.001

*From Atkinson, S. A., Bryan, M. H., and Anderson, G. H.: J. Pediatr. **93**:67, 1978.
†Adjusted values were obtained by covariance analysis to correct for effect of day and volume.
‡N adj = $\overline{N}$ − day error − volume error.
§Mean ± SE.

tract rather than the placenta, has not been resolved. Gaull and co-workers[19] indicate that the premature infant is a new biological entity with uncertain standards of normal growth and normal biochemical measurements. Further studies are necessary to determine whether, when, and how the premature infant may require supplementation if nourished by human milk. Gaull and associates question whether or not increased growth rate is desirable if it produces potentially dangerous metabolic imbalances.

Feeding the premature infant at the breast. Large premature infants of 36 weeks of gestation or older may be nursed at the breast if otherwise stable. Particular care should be given to assist the mother in getting the infant to suckle, especially if the breast and/or nipples are large or engorged. Weight should be followed closely to prevent excessive weight loss. In our experience, infants who receive sugar water and formula supplements lose more weight than those who are nursed frequently at the breast without supplementation. If breast-feeding is going well, the infant could be discharged with his mother from the hospital as soon as he begins to gain substantially.

Small for gestational age infants

Infants who are below the 10th percentile or 2 SD in weight for their gestational age are termed small for gestational age, or SGA. These infants may also be shorter in length and have smaller heads, depending on when in the gestational life the insult to their growth occurred. The more general the growth failure, the earlier the intrauterine effect. For example, rubella in the first trimester causes total growth retardation, whereas hypertension in the mother in the third trimester predominantly affects weight. The more profound the growth retardation, the more difficult the nutritional problems.

SGA infants are prone to be hypocalcemic; however, if they can be provided with adequate breast milk early, this complication may be avoided. Other problems, including hypothermia and hypoglycemia, which lead to a vicious circle of acidosis and associated problems, can be triggered by unmonitored exposure of the infant to thermal stress in the first hours of life and failure to identify the hypoglycemia early. Thus the perinatal nursery staff may appear to be obstructive to breast-feeding when they hover over this infant or even insist on his transfer to the nursery. Initially breast-feeding at delivery is permissible if adequate external heat is provided. Testing with Dextrostix should be performed in the delivery room recovery area and the infant sent to the nursery if hypoglycemia or hypothermia cannot be controlled. Frequent breast-feeding can be initiated unless the blood sugar level is too low (below 30 mg/100 ml or unresponsive to oral treatment). It may not be possible for even an actively lactating multipara to sustain an SGA infant initially, but the infant should be put to breast at least every 3 hours and given IV glucose in addition. SGA infants often have a poor suck and poor coordination with the swallow reflex. There may be considerable mucus with gagging and spitting. A simple lavage of the stomach with a number 8 feeding tube (or 5, if the infant weighs less than 2600 g) and warmed glucose water usually relieves the gagging. Once this SGA infant begins to eat, he will do well and will require sufficient kilocalories to meet the needs of an infant who is appropriate for gestational age.

•   •   •

Infants who are less than 1800 g at birth and have to be gavaged or infants of any weight who are acutely ill present a complex problem. The mother should be instructed to manually express her milk initially and contribute any colostrum she produces. This can be given by gastric or nasojejunal tube. An Egnell pump is effective in helping a mother increase the volume produced. When the infant is born at 1000 g, requires respirator support for days, and is not discharged for 8 weeks, it is difficult to maintain a large volume of milk by pumping. When the infant is strong enough he may nurse at the breast while still in the hospital. When the infant is sent home, the breast milk may be limited in volume or the infant may refuse the breast because he has to work harder to obtain the milk after becoming accustomed to soft premature rubber nipples in the hospital. He becomes frustrated and may even turn away screaming.

A mother reported when seen in the follow-up clinic at the University of Rochester that it took her 4 days to break her premature into breast-feeding and she gave him nothing but the breast during that seige. She thought he might have to starve first! One can see that the reserves of the premature are limited if one studies the absolute and relative body composition of infants at birth (Fig. 13-12). If one considers how long it takes to starve a premature compared to a full-term infant, the risks of starving a premature infant while he adapts to nursing at the breast are real (Fig. 13-13). The solution to the problem is to provide nourishment while the infant stimulates maternal milk production by suckling at the breast. There is equipment called Lact-Aid that will provide this set-up very effectively. It was developed to provide nourishment for the adopted infant that is being nursed by a mother who has not been pregnant or has ever lactated and sustains the infant while the mother's milk supply develops. The same effect can be provided for the premature or sick infant who has not nursed at the breast since birth and needs nourishment while the mother's supply develops. Experience to date at the University of Rochester with six mothers who have taken home infants 4 to 12 weeks of age to nurse has been good. The infant can continue to gain weight while stimulating the breast. The volume required from the Lact-Aid dropped continually in all but one case so that the infants were on the breast alone after a week. In one case the infant required the Lact-Aid for a month. Chapter 16 gives

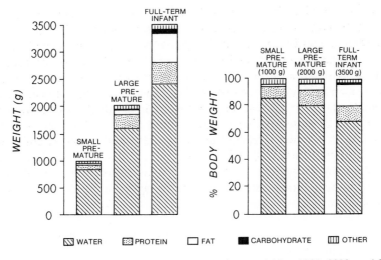

Fig. 13-12. Absolute and relative body composition of infants weighing 1000, 2000, and 3000 g at birth. (Reproduced with permission from Heird, W. C., and Anderson, T. L.: Nutritional requirements and methods of feeding low birth weight infants. In Gluck, L., et al., editors: Current problems in pediatrics, vol. VII, no. 8, Chicago, 1977, Year Book Medical Publishers, Inc., copyright © 1977.)

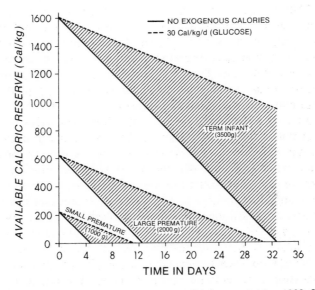

Fig. 13-13. Estimated survival of starved and semistarved infants weighing 1000, 2000, and 3500 g at birth.

details of the equipment. Lact-Aid provides a simple means of assuring adequate nourishment while adapting to the breast. It is preferable to using supplemental bottles because the infant is not confused by the rubber nipple, which requires a different mechanism of sucking than the human nipple. Furthermore, the suckling of the human nipple provides continued stimulus for milk production.

POSTMATURE INFANTS

Postmature infants are full-grown mature infants who have stayed in utero beyond the full vigor of the placenta and began to lose weight in utero. They are usually "older looking" and look around wide eyed. Their skin is dry and peeling, and subcutaneous tissue diminished; thus the skin appears too big. These infants have lost subcutaneous fat and lack glycogen stores. Initially they may be hypoglycemic and require early feedings to maintain blood glucose levels of 45 mg/100 ml or higher. If breast-fed, the infant should go to the breast early, giving care to maintain body temperature, which is quite labile. Blood sugar levels should be followed. These infants may feed poorly initially and require considerable prodding to suckle. If the infant becomes hypoglycemic despite careful management, consideration should be given to a feeding of 10% glucose in water. In extreme cases of hypoglycemia an intravenous infusion may be necessary, and management should follow guidelines for any infant who has hypoglycemia that is resistant to routine early feedings. Calcium problems, on the other hand, although common in these infants, generally are uncommon if the infant is adequately breast-fed early. This is due to the physiological ratio of calcium and phosphorus in breast milk. Once a postmature infant begins to feed well, he is apt to catch up quickly and continue to adapt very well. Problems with hyperbilirubinemia are uncommon.

MULTIPLE BIRTHS

It is possible to nurse twins and triplets. There are many case reports to support this fact. That a single mother can provide adequate nourishment for more than one infant has been documented for centuries. In the seventeenth century in France, wet nurses were allowed to nurse up to six infants at one time. Foundling homes provided wet nurses for every three to six infants. The key deterrent to nursing twins is not usually the milk supply, but time. If the mother can nurse both infants simultaneously, the time factor is minimized. Many tricks have been suggested to achieve this feat. As the infants become larger and more active, it may be difficult to keep them simultaneously nursing with only two hands to cope. If the mother has help at home who can assist with feedings, it can be accomplished. The first year of life for the mother of a set of twins is an extremely busy one and really requires additional help, particularly if the mother is going to breast-feed. She will need time for adequate rest and nourishment.

FULL-TERM INFANTS WITH MEDICAL PROBLEMS

Infants who have self-limited acute illnesses, such as fever, upper respiratory infection, colds, diarrhea, or contagious diseases like chickenpox, do best if breast-feeding is maintained. Because of breast milk's low solute load, an infant can be kept well hydrated despite fever or other increased fluid losses. If respiratory symptoms are significant, an infant seems to nurse well at the breast and poorly with a bottle. This observation has been documented many times when nursing mothers have "roomed-in" with their sick infants in the hospital. The studies of Johnson and Salisbury[28a] on the synchrony of respirations in breast-feeding in contrast to the periodic breathing or gasping apnea pattern of the normal bottle-fed infant may well be the underlying explanation for the phenomenon of an acutely ill infant continuing to nurse at the breast.

In addition to the appropriateness of the human milk for a sick infant, there is the added comfort of nursing because of the closeness with the mother. If the infant is suddenly weaned, psychological trauma is added to the stress of the illness.

It may become difficult to distinguish the effect of the trauma of acute weaning from the symptoms of the primary illness, such as poor feeding or lethargy, if the acutely weaned infant fails to respond to adequate treatment. Going back to breast-feeding may be the answer because the stress of acute weaning will be removed.

It is not appropriate to give the mother medicine intended to treat the infant, especially antibiotics. This has been tried to the detriment of the child, since variable amounts of the drug reach the infant, depending on the dosage, dosage schedule, and amount of milk consumed.

Gastrointestinal disease

Bouts of diarrhea and intestinal tract disease are much less common in breast-fed infants than bottle-fed infants, but when they occur, the infant should be maintained on the breast if possible. Human milk is a physiological solution that causes neither dehydration or hypernatremia. Occasionally an infant will have diarrhea or an intestinal upset because of something in the mother's diet. It is usually self-limited and the best treatment is to continue to nurse at the breast. If the mother has been taking a laxative that is absorbed or has been eating laxative foods such as fruits in excess, she should adjust her diet. Intractable diarrhea should be evaluated as it would be in any infant. Allergy to mother's milk is extremely rare and would require substantial evidence to support the diagnosis. Milk lactase deficiency may be manifest by chronic diarrhea. The only cure is a lactose-free diet. Some chronic diseases are better controlled on breast milk, and symptoms become more severe with weaning. Should an infant be weaned and do poorly on formula, relactation of the mother might be considered. With the availability of the Lact-Aid device, this possibility is no longer remote (Chapter 16).

Respiratory illness

Infants who develop respiratory illnesses should be maintained at the breast. The added advantages of antibodies and anti-infective properties are valuable to the infant. A sick infant can nurse more easily than cope with a bottle. Furthermore, the comfort of having his mother nearby is important whenever the infant has a crisis, but weaning during illness may be devastating.

Young infants who have older siblings may well be exposed to some virulent viruses and bacteria. Developing croup or chickenpox, for instance, may make the infant seriously ill. Hydration can be maintained by frequent, short breast-feedings. Studies have shown that respirations are maintained more easily when feeding on human milk than on cow's milk. Nursing at the breast permits regular respirations, whereas bottle-feeding is associated with a more gasping pattern. Thus breast-fed infants continue to nurse when they are ill. If the infant is hospitalized, every effort should be made to maintain the breast-feeding if he can be fed at all. One should provide rooming-in for the mother if a care-by-parent ward is not available.

Galactosemia

Galactosemia, which is due to the deficiency of red cell uridyltransferase, is a rare circumstance in which the infant is unable to metabolize lactose and must be placed on a lactose-free diet. The disease can be rapidly fatal in the severe form. The infant may have severe and/or persistent jaundice, vomiting, diarrhea, electrolyte imbalances, cerebral signs, and weight loss. This does necessitate weaning from the breast to a special formula because human milk contains high levels of lactose.

Inborn errors of metabolism

Other metabolic deficiency syndromes are usually only apparent as mild failure to thrive syndrome until the infant is weaned from the breast and the symptoms become severe. This particularly applies to inborn errors of metabolism due to an inability to handle one or more of the essential amino acids. Infection is often a complication early in the lives of these infants with inborn errors. In the process of treating the acute infection the infant may be weaned, and the metabolic disorder then becomes apparent precipitously.

An infant in a coma was transferred to the intensive care unit of the University of Rochester Medical Center from another hospital where he had been admitted at 7 weeks of age. He had been entirely well until 3 weeks of age when he was abruptly weaned from the breast because he developed sepsis and possible meningitis. He became acutely acidotic, then comatose with shock symptoms. On transfer he had a blood ammonia level of $1600 \mu mol/L$. He was ultimately diagnosed postmortem, after heroic efforts to bring the ammonia to normal levels. The disease, propionic acidemia, was incompatible with life, but the parents were able to console themselves in their loss because the child had had a few apparently "healthy, happy weeks" while being breast-fed.

If one refers to Table 4-9, it will be observed that there is significantly less of certain amino acids in human milk than in cow's milk, such as phenylalanine, methionine, leucine, isoleucine, and others associated with metabolic disorders. Management of an amino acid metabolic disorder while breast-feeding would depend on careful monitoring of blood and urine levels of the specific amino acids involved. Since these are essential amino acids, a certain amount is necessary in the diet of all infants, including those with the disease. An appropriate combination of breast-feeding and a milk free of the offending amino acid could be developed. The care of such infants should be in consultation with a pediatric endocrinologist. Transient neonatal tyrosinemia, which has been reported to occur in a high percentage (up to 80%) of bottle-fed neonates, is associated with blood tyrosine levels ten times those of adults. Wong and associates[46] have associated severe cases with learning disabilities in later years.

Acrodermatitis enteropathica (Danbolt-Closs syndrome)

Acrodermatitis enteropathica is a rare but unique disease in that feeding with human milk may be life saving. It is inherited as an autosomal recessive trait. It is characterized by a symmetrical rash around the mouth, genitalia, and periphery of the extremities. The rash is an acute vesicobullous and eczematous eruption often secondarily infected with *Candida albicans*. It may be seen by the third week of life or not until later infancy and has been associated with weaning from the breast. Failure to thrive, hair loss, irritability, and chronic severe intractable diarrhea are often life threatening. The disease has been associated with extremely low plasma zinc levels. Oral zinc sulfate has produced remission of the disease.

Human milk contains less zinc than bovine milk, with zinc concentrations of both decreasing throughout lactation. Eckhert and colleagues[9] studied the zinc binding in human and cow's milk and noted that the low–molecular weight binding ligand isolated from human milk may enhance absorption of zinc in these patients. Gel chromatography indicated that most of the zinc in cow's milk was associated with high–molecular weight fractions, whereas zinc in human milk was associated with low–molecular weight fractions. The copper/zinc ratio may also be of significance, since the ratio is lower in cow's milk.

The zinc binding ligand from human milk was further identified as prostaglandin E by chromatography, ultrafiltration, and infrared spectroscopy by Evans and Johnson.[10] These patients have low arachidonic acid levels. Arachidonic acid is a precursor of prostaglandin. The efficacy of human milk in the treatment of acrodermatitis enteropathica results from the presence of the zinc-prostaglandin complex.

The clinical significance of the relationship of human milk to onset of the disease and its treatment is in developing lactation in the mother of such an infant, rare as the disease may be. Delayed lactation or relactation is possible and should be offered as an option to the mother of such an infant (Chapter 16).

Down's syndrome

The infant with Down's syndrome or other trisomies is usually difficult to feed. When they are breast-fed it takes patience on the part of the mother to teach this infant to suck with sufficient vigor to initiate the let-down reflex and to stimulate adequate production of milk. Manual expression to start flow and holding the breast firmly for the infant so that the nipple does not drop out of the mouth when the infant stops suckling will assist the process.

The birth of an infant with a major genetic abnormality is a shock even to the strongest parents. If the mother wants to breast-feed she should be offered all the encouragement and support necessary. Usually she needs to talk with someone just to express her anguish about the infant, not the feeding per se. A sympathetic nurse practitioner can be invaluable in providing the support as well as the expertise necessary to help with the management problems. Three mothers in the Rochester area that have come to our attention have each successfully nursed an infant with a trisomy.

Hypothyroidism

It has been reported by Bode and co-workers[6] that an infant with congenital cretinism was spared the severe effects of the disease because he was breast-fed. This was attributed to significant quantities of thyroid hormone in the milk. Sack and associates[40] measured thyroxine concentrations in human milk and found it to be present in significant amounts. Varma and colleagues[44] have reported the study of thyroxine, triiodothyronine, and reverse triiodothyronine concentrations in human milk in seventy-seven healthy euthyroid mothers from the day of delivery to 148 days postpartum. They calculated from their data that if an infant received 900 to 1200 ml of milk/day, he would receive 2.1 to 2.6 μg of thyroxine/day, based on 238.1 ng/dl of milk after the first week. This amount of T_3 is much less than the recommended dose for the treatment of hypothyroidism (18.8 to 25 μg/day of levo-triiodothyronine). T_3 in human milk may partially alleviate or mask hyperthyroidism in some infants. T_4 was essentially unmeasurable in the milk sampled. No definite relationship between the levels of T_3 and rT_3 could be found. It is therefore suggested that neonatal screening for thyroid disease may be even more urgent if the clinical symptoms are apt to be masked in a breast-fed infant. There is no contraindication to breast-feeding when the infant is hypothyroid, and it may well be beneficial. Appropriate therapy should also be instituted.

Hyperbilirubinemia and jaundice

Jaundice in the newborn has become a source of considerable misinformation, confusion, and anxiety in recent years. There is a higher incidence of jaundice in full-term infants than a decade ago. More physicians are paying attention to the development of hyperbilirubinemia in newborns. These two factors serve to increase the frequency of the question of the role of breast-feeding in the development of hyperbilirubinemia. Some of the confusion and inconsistencies associated with the management can be attributed to the indecisive terminology. An attempt will be made to clarify the issues and outline the causes and effects of hyperbilirubinemia.

Why the concern about jaundice. Bilirubin is a cell toxin, as can be demonstrated dramatically by adding a little bilirubin to a tissue culture, which will be quickly destroyed. Excessive bilirubin causes concern because when there is free, unbound, unconjugated bilirubin in the system it can be deposited in various tissues, ultimately causing necrosis of the cells. The brain and brain cells, if destroyed by bilirubin deposits, do not regenerate. The full-blown end result is bilirubin encephalopathy or kernicterus, which is essentially a pathological diagnosis that depends on identifying the yellow pigmentation and necrosis in the brain, especially the basal ganglion, hippocampal cortex, and subthalamic nuclei. About 50% of the infants with kernicterus at autopsy also have other lesions due to bilirubin toxicity. There may be necrosis of the renal tubular cells, intestinal mucosa, or pancreatic cells or associated gastrointestinal hemorrhage. The classic clinical manifestations of bilirubin encephalopathy are characterized by progressive lethargy, rigidity, opisthotonos, high-pitched cry, fever, and convulsions. The mortality is 50%. Survivors usually have choreoathetoid cerebral palsy, high-frequency deafness, and mental retardation. Premature infants are particularly susceptible to bilirubin-related brain damage and may have kernicterus at autopsy without the typical clinical syndrome. Classic full-blown kernicterus rarely occurs today, but what may well develop are mild effects on the brain that will be manifest clinically in later life as incoordination, hypertonicity, and mental retardation or perhaps learning disabilities, symptoms sometimes collectively called minimal brain damage.

Mechanism of bilirubin production in the neonate. The normal full-term infant has a hematocrit in utero of 50% to 65%. Because of the low oxygen tension delivered to the fetus via the placenta, the fetus requires more hemoglobin to carry the oxygen. As soon as the infant is born and begins to breathe room air the need is gone. The infant bone marrow does not make more cells, and excess cells are destroyed and not replaced. The life span of a fetal red blood cell is 70 to 90 days instead of the adult's 120 days. Normally when red cells are destroyed, the released hemoglobin is broken down to heme in the reticuloendothelial system (RES). The reticuloendothelial cells contain a microsomal enzyme, heme oxygenase, which is capable of oxidizing the alpha-methene bridge carbon of the heme molecule after the loss of the iron and the globin to form biliverdin, a green pigment, according to Gartner and Lee.[18] Biliverdin is water soluble and is rapidly degraded to bilirubin. A gram of hemoglobulin will produce 34 mg of bilirubin.

The reticuloendothelial cell releases the bilirubin into the circulation, where it is rapidly bound to albumin. Bilirubin is essentially insoluble (less than 0.01 mg/100 ml soluble). Adult albumin can bind two molecules of bilirubin, the first more tightly than the second. Newborn albumin has reduced molar binding capacities.

Unconjugated bilirubin is removed from the circulation by the hepatocyte, which converts it by conjugation of each molecule of bilirubin with two molecules of glucuronic acid into direct bilirubin. Direct bilirubin is water soluble and is excreted via the bile to the stools. The balance between hepatic cell uptake of bilirubin and the rate of bilirubin production determines the serum unconjugated bilirubin concentration.

Evaluation and management. Normal full-term newborns have serial bilirubin tests to determine the range of values. Many have observed that the cord bilirubin level may be as high as 2.0 mg/100 ml and rise over the first 72 hr to 5 to 6 mg/100 ml, which is barely in the visible range, and gradually taper off, assuming adult levels of 1.0 mg/100 ml after 10 days. Less than 50% of normal infants are visibly jaundiced in the first week of life. Why any normal infant is visibly jaundiced is not known, although it has been suggested by Gartner and Lee[18] that it is due to insufficient enzyme synthesis, inhibition of enzymatic activity by naturally occurring substances, deficient synthesis of the glucuronide donor UDPGA, or a combination of factors. This would suggest the jaundice is idiopathic, not physiological. The acceptable level of bilirubin depends on a number of factors. In some premature infants, even bilirubin levels under 10 mg/100 ml may be of concern.

FACTORS THAT INFLUENCE SIGNIFICANCE. For a given level of bilirubin several associated factors may need to be considered. If there has been acidosis, anoxia, asphyxia, hypothermia, hypoglycemia, or infection, even lower levels of bilirubin may have a significant risk of causing deposition in the brain cells. These factors increase the susceptibility of the brain to bilirubin deposition: prematurity, asphyxia, hypoxia, hypoglycemia, hypothermia, acidosis, and infection. There is an increased incidence of elevated bilirubin levels in certain races and populations. Oriental populations, including Chinese, Japanese, and Korean, and American Indians may have bilirubin levels averaging between 10 and 14 mg/100 ml. There is also a higher incidence of autopsy-identified kernicterus. It does not seem to be related to G6PD deficiency, which is also common in these groups.

DETERMINATION OF CAUSE OF JAUNDICE. If one follows the chain of events from the red cell and its destruction in the newborn through to the final excretion of conjugated bilirubin in the stools, it simplifies understanding the cause of a specific case of jaundice. Causes include (1) increased destruction of red cells, (2) decreased conjugation in the glucuronidase system, (3) decreased albumin binding, and (4) increased reabsorption from the gastrointestinal tract. Conditions associated with increased destruction of red cells can be outlined as follows:

    I. Isoimmunization
       A. Rh incompatibility

    B. ABO incompatibility
    C. Subgroup and private antigen incompatibility
  II. Elevated hematocrit levels
    A. Chronic intrauterine hypoxia
    B. Maternal smoking
    C. Twin-to-twin transfusion
    D. Intrauterine growth failure
    E. Cord stripping
  III. Sequestered blood
    A. Cephalohematomas, scalp hemorrhage, subdural hematomas
    B. Ecchymoses, especially in breech delivery
    C. Extensive hemangiomas
  IV. Red cell defects
    A. G6PD deficiency
    B. Pyruvate kinase deficiency
    C. Hexokinase deficiency
    D. Congenital erythropoietic porphyria
  V. Structural abnormalities of red cells
    A. Hereditary spherocytosis
    B. Hereditary elliptocytosis
    C. Pyknocytosis
  VI. Infection
    A. Bacterial (sepsis, meningitis)
    B. Viral (cytomegalovirus)
    C. Protozoal (toxoplasmosis)

Causes of decreased conjugation of bilirubin in the hepatic cells are as follows:
  I. Inherited defects
    A. Glucuronyltransferase deficiency, type I, (Crigler-Najjor syndrome)
    B. Gilbert's syndrome
    C. Glucuronyltransferase deficiency, type II
  II. Transient familial neonatal hyperbilirubinemia
  III. Drugs that compete in the conjugation system (such as vitamin K and novobiocin)
  IV. Prematurity (and therefore prematurity of the liver and its enzyme systems)
  V. Breast-milk jaundice

    When albumin binding is altered, the visibility of the jaundice is not affected. The bilirubin level may not be very high, but the substance is not bound to albumin and is available at lower levels to pass into the brain cells. Premature infants have much lower albumin levels and thus have fewer binding sites. Drugs that also bind to albumin compete for binding sites. These drugs include aspirin and sulfadiazine, for instance. A lower level of bilirubin puts the infant who has these medications in his system at risk because the bilirubin is unbound and available to enter tissue cells, including brain cells.

    Reabsorption from the gastrointestinal tract can increase the bilirubin level. This occurs when the conjugated bilirubin that was excreted into the colon is unconjugated by the action of intestinal bacteria and reabsorbed, which happens when stools are decreased or slowed in passage. Poor feedings, pyloric stenosis,

Table 13-5. Correlation of weight to safe peak indirect bilirubin levels

Weight (g)	Indirect bilirubin level (mg/100 ml)
2500	20
2000	20
1500	15
1200	12
1100	11
1000	10

and other forms of intestinal obstruction are common causes. Some bacteria are more apt to have this effect on conjugated bilirubin than others.

SAFE LEVELS OF BILIRUBIN. Safe levels of bilirubin depend on a number of factors noted previously, including acidosis, hypoxia or anoxia, and sepsis. A handy rule of thumb is the correlation of birth weight in the premature infant and the indirect bilirubin level, using a value 2 to 3 mg lower when the infant has multiple problems (Table 13-5).

Any value of 20 mg/100 ml or over warrants treatment. Phototherapy is generally used when the bilirubin is roughly 5 mg/ml below the exchange level. Jaundice that is visible under 24 hr of age is of special concern because it is usually associated with an incompatibility or infection. Rapidly rising bilirubin levels are also of concern, and a 0.5 mg/100 ml rise/hr is also an indication for treatment, usually an exchange transfusion.

TREATMENT. Treatment depends on identifying the cause. Blood incompatibilities should be treated by exchange transfusion if severe enough (i.e., bilirubin 20 mg/100 ml or rising at 0.5 mg/100 ml/hr or dropping hematocrit). The exchange transfusion removes affected red blood cells (RBC) and antibodies and improves excessive bilirubin levels. If the cause is sepsis, the infection should be treated as well as the bilirubin problem. About half the cases of jaundice will not have an identified cause and may be classified as idiopathic rather than physiological jaundice. Refer to standard texts of pediatrics and neonatology for more extensive discussions of neonatal hyperbilirubinemia.

Breast-milk jaundice. A small group of infants estimated by Gartner and Lee[18] to be less than 1 in 200 breast-fed infants will develop jaundice directly associated with breast milk. Drew[8] reported only one case of proven breast-milk jaundice in a review of 13,102 consecutively born infants; 878 (6.7%) of these infants had pathological jaundice.

The pattern of this jaundice is distinctly different. Normally idiopathic jaundice peaks on the third day and then begins to drop. Breast-milk jaundice, however, becomes apparent or continues to rise after the third day, and bilirubin levels may peak any time from the seventh to the tenth day, with untreated cases being reported to peak as late as the fifteenth day. Values have ranged from 10 to 27 mg/100 ml during this time. There is no correlation with weight loss or gain, and stools are normal.

The syndrome of breast-milk jaundice has been attributed by Arias and co-workers[1,2] to a substance in the milk of some mothers that inhibits the hepatic enzyme glucuronyltransferase, preventing the conjugation of bilirubin. The substance has been identified as 5β-pregnane-$3\alpha,20\beta$-diol, a breakdown product of progesterone and an isomer of pregnanediol that is not usually found in milk, but occurs normally in about 10% of the lactating population. The pregnanediol isomer is found in the breast milk and urine of these lactating women. When they are not lactating, none of this metabolite is found in the urine even when large doses of progesterone are given orally. Gartner and Lee[18] have assumed this metabolite is synthesized in the mammary gland tissue during periods of active lactation. It has no other known significance, and these females are not discernible in any other way.

Arias and Gartner[1] administered 5β-pregnane-$3\alpha,20\beta$-diol to full-term newborns and produced unconjugated hyperbilirubinemia that subsided as soon as the material was discontinued. Older infants and an adult given the same material did not become jaundiced. It did demonstrate that unconjugated hyperbilirubinemia can be produced in very young full-term infants by oral doses of 5β-pregnane-$3\alpha,20\beta$-diol in amounts equivalent to that isolated from inhibitory human milk. This material has also been isolated from the milk and serum of mothers whose infants were jaundiced. Foliot and associates[12] showed that pathological breast milk from mothers of jaundiced infants will inhibit bromsulphalein (BSP)-Z protein binding only when stored under conditions that also cause the appearance of the capacity to inhibit bilirubin conjugation in vitro, as well as causing the liberation of nonesterified fatty acids. They conclude that the appearance of this inhibitory capacity in vitro seems linked to the lipolytic activity peculiar to pathological milks.

It has been reported by Luzeau and associates[31,32] that milks with inhibitory activity contain increased concentrations of free fatty acids. These simple forms of fat are presumed to be derived by the enzymatic breakdown of the triglycerides normally present in milk, suggesting a greater lipase activity. Some type of synergistic effect between pregnanediol and free fatty acids may be responsible for the clinical syndrome of breast-milk jaundice.

Diagnosis depends on circumstantial evidence, since there is no easy rapid laboratory test. All other causes, including infection, should be ruled out in the usual manner and a thorough history taken, including medications and family history. If the mother has nursed other infants, were they jaundiced? Usually 70% of the previous children of a given mother whose infant has "breast-milk jaundice" have been jaundiced. The difference may be related to the greater maturity of the liver of a given infant who then is able to handle the increased demands on the glucuronyltransferase system. If the mother had a previous infant who was jaundiced but bottle-fed, this should raise a question about the diagnosis of breast-milk jaundice. To establish the diagnosis firmly, and this is necessary when the bilirubin level is above 15 mg/100 ml for more than 24 hr, a bilirubin reading should be obtained 2 hr after a breast-feeding and then breast-feeding discontinued for at least 12 hr. The infant must be fed fluids and calories, preferably a 60:40, lactalbumin/casein milk. In some cases, a mother of a nonjaundiced infant is available to nurse the child or provide breast milk. The infant's mother should be assisted in pumping her breasts to maintain her supply. Even more urgent is providing the mother with a sympathetic explanation of the problem and the process. After at least 12 hr without mother's milk, the bilirubin level should be measured. If there is a significant drop of more than 2 mg/100 ml, then the infant can be put to breast. Bilirubin levels should be obtained to determine if the bilirubin rises again and, if so, how much. In most cases, in the time not breast-feeding the infant's body equilibrates the levels sufficiently, so there is only a slight increase in bilirubin on return to breast-feeding followed by a slow but steady drop. If that is the case, breast-feeding can continue. The bilirubin level should be checked at 10 days and 14 days to be certain the bilirubin is truly clearing.

If the bilirubin has not dropped significantly after 12 hr off the breast, the time off the breast should be extended to 18 to 24 hr, measuring bilirubin levels every 4 to 6 hr. If the bilirubin rises while off the breast, it is clearly not the breast milk; breast-feeding should be resumed and other causes for the jaundice be re-evaluated.

PHOTOTHERAPY AND BREAST-MILK JAUNDICE. Phototherapy is the use of light energy from a fluorescent light source, which provides light in the white to blue range of the photo spectrum. Fluorescent lamps (20W), daylight, cool white, or blue, are usually used and provide 420 to 500 nm. A fluorescent bulb provides this light energy for only about 400 hr of its usual 14,000 hr life. Standard lamps are available for use with plexiglass screens to filter out the small amount of ultraviolet light and protect the infant should the bulb break. They should be at least 16 inches (40 cm) from the unclothed infant. Phototherapy can destroy the retina in 12 hr, thus protecting the eyes with opaque eye covers is mandatory. Lights should be turned off to collect blood samples. The infant should be fed with the lights and eye covers off to provide a cycle of light and dark for the establishment of normal circadian rhythms. For discussion of the "bronze baby" syndrome, congenital erythro-poietic porphyria, and other complications of phototherapy, refer to standard neonatology texts.

If one is attempting to establish the diagnosis of breast-milk jaundice, photo-therapy should not be used while breast milk is being discontinued. If establishing the diagnosis is not necessary (perhaps because of the same diagnosis in older siblings), phototherapy can be used to bring the values to a more acceptable range, that is, under 12 mg/100 ml. When phototherapy is discontinued it is most impor-tant to establish that there is no rebound. In addition, it will be important to follow the infant at home after discharge through at least 14 days of life, or longer if the values are not below 12 mg/100 ml. It should not be assumed that the diagnosis is breast-milk jaundice when breast-feeding has been stopped and phototherapy initiated simultaneously.

LATE DIAGNOSIS OF BREAST-MILK JAUNDICE. With the frequency of early discharge from the hospital, especially for families enjoying the birthing center concept, breast-fed infants are often discharged before jaundice for any reason has devel-oped. Since breast-milk jaundice is apt to be delayed to the fourth or fifth day, peaking at 10 to 14 days of age, most normal infants are already home. Occasional-ly an infant is observed in the pediatrician's office at 10 days of age or older with a bilirubin level over 20 mg/100 ml, often 23 to 25 mg/ml (highest, 27 mg/ml). This is a medical emergency. It necessitates the admission of this infant to the hospital for a complete bilirubin workup. It is important to recognize that other causes of hyperbilirubinemia must be ruled out, including incompatibilities. At this age it is also necessary to rule out biliary obstruction and hepatitis, which might have a high direct or conjugated bilirubin level. There is conflicting opinion as to whether it is appropriate to perform an immediate exchange transfusion or to discontinue breast milk and use phototherapy for 4 to 6 hours to establish whether this therapy will be effective in dropping the level sufficiently. It has been our approach to stop breast-feeding and start phototherapy immediately on admission while the diagnostic workup is being performed. (The bilirubin level should be obtained first, but the result need not be reported before initiating therapy if the infant is 7 days or older as long as an exchange transfusion for a blood type incompatibility is not omitted because of the temporary effect of phototherapy.) It usually takes about 4 hours to do the diagnostic workup and prepare compatible blood for an exchange transfusion, thus actually no time is lost. Only once have we had to do an exchange transfusion in what appeared to be a "breast-milk jaundice" infant.

PERSISTENT JAUNDICE IN THE BREAST-FED INFANT. It has been acknowledged that breast-milk jaundice is extremely rare but in that rare case, the infant will be observed to maintain a bilirubin level over 12 mg/100 ml if breast-fed. Pediatricians[23] in Rochester have reported that this persists beyond 6 weeks of age and is only altered by giving one or two feedings of formula a day to dilute the effect of the breast milk or by discontinuing breast-feeding altogether. There are no prospective studies of a 7-year long-range nature to confirm that this is a benign condition. It has been the policy to give enough formula feeding to keep the bilirubin level under 12 mg/100 ml (preferably 10 mg/100 ml), which is actually arbitrarily selected. Occasionally levels will hover at 15 mg/100 ml or higher with some formula feeding, at which point breast-feeding is discontinued (two cases in 5 years). An exchange transfusion might be an alternative to drop the bilirubin significantly and continue breast-feeding. The physician needs to weigh the advantages and risks with the family and document the final care plan. Rechecking the direct bilirubin level and the color of the urine and stools to rule out hepatitis and biliary obstruction is also appropriate. Phenobarbital has not been effective in the postnatal period.

Breast-feeding and hyperbilirubinemia. Not all breast-fed infants who are jaundiced have "breast-milk jaundice." When the bilirubin curves of bottle- and breast-fed infants are compared, it should be observed that the bilirubin levels are the same in the first 3 days of life. It has been suggested that the breast-fed infant is dehydrated and that is why the bilirubin is elevated, but the hematocrit, urine volume, and urine specific gravity are within normal range. In a study by Dahms and colleagues[7] of 199 breast-fed and bottle-fed infants followed for the first 4 days of life, the mean bilirubin values were found to be similar, regardless of the feeding regimen. They observed an 8% mean weight loss in infants breast-fed without supplements compared to a 4% weight loss in all other infants. Hyperbilirubinemia was not related to weight loss. The percentage of infants having serum bilirubin concentrations greater than 15 mg/100 ml was the same for both breast-fed and bottle-fed infants. The hematocrit was stable for any given infant even when the weight changed significantly. The reticulocyte count was between 7% and 8% at 48 hr.

The researchers concluded that breast-feeding per se is not associated with hyperbilirubinemia. Previous literature has been divided on this point, but no series of statistics shows a clear-cut difference. This study points out that the demand feeding group of breast-fed infants lost more weight than controls and 12% of the group developed low-grade fever that responded to feeding of water or formula. Fever, however, was not associated with hyperbilirubinemia. A retrospective study of 200 infants in Rochester who were chart screened for weight loss, intake, bilirubin, and body temperature showed that breast-fed infants who were supplemented with water did less well, lost more weight than those who were not supplemented, and had more problems nursing beyond 4 days of life. Further data are necessary to clarify the issues of early supplementation and ad-lib breast-feeding.

It is interesting to note that Wong and Wood[47] reported that among the breast-fed infants in the normal lying-in wards of a maternity hospital, a significantly higher incidence of "idiopathic" jaundice was found in infants of mothers who had been receiving the contraceptive pill before the present pregnancy than in the infants whose mothers never took the pill. This included mothers who had oral estrogen-progesterone only for contraceptive purposes and for at least 21 days.

INFANTS WITH PROBLEMS REQUIRING SURGERY
The immediate neonatal period

First arch disorders. Feeding of any sort may be greatly hindered by abnormalities of the jaw, nose, and mouth. A receding chin may be a minor problem and only require positioning the jaw forward. A mother can hook the angle of the jaw with her finger and draw it forward. If the tongue is too large for the jaw, the infant will actually nurse better at the breast than bottle because the human nipple fits into the mouth with less bulk. Infants with first arch abnormalities usually require considerable help in feeding. A cleft palate may also be present. It may be necessary to insert semipermanent nasal tubes so that the infant can be fed orally until he is older; definitive surgery may be necessary later. Once the nasal tubes are in place the infant can manage at the breast. Feeding by any technique, however, is never easy.

Cleft lip. A solitary cleft lip is usually repaired in the first few weeks of life. Prior to surgery the infant will need some help, but he can nurse at the breast if a seal around the areola can be developed. Actually the breast may fill the defect, and suckling will go well. It is important to encourage the infant to suck to strengthen the tongue and jaw muscles. If all else fails, a breast shield can be tried, affixing a special cleft-lip nipple to the shield.

The mother may have to express or pump milk and offer it by dropper or other means if sucking is ineffective. The pediatrician, plastic surgeon, and parents should work together as a team from the time of birth to determine a coordinated plan of treatment. Some surgeons have special protocols before and after surgery to assure optimal healing. It is important to make all plans for feeding around the surgical plan. There are reports in the literature of individual mothers' experiences nursing infants with lip defects. The major caution in sharing these experiences is to consider that the supportive surgical approach may differ from those reported in the cases in the literature.

Cleft palate. The prognosis for successful feeding of an infant with a cleft palate depends on the size and position of the defect (soft palate, hard palate) as well as the associated lesions. Lubit[30] recommends the application of an orthopedic appliance to the neonatal maxilla to close the gap, thus aiding nursing, stimulating orofacial development, developing the palatal shelves, preventing tongue distortions, preventing nasal septum irritation, and decreasing the number of ear infections. This will aid the plastic surgeon and help the mother psychologically as well. Lubit further relates that a cleft involving the secondary palate can interfere with normal nursing. For the infant to suckle, the nose must be sealed off from the mouth, creating a negative pressure in the oral cavity. The milk may also run out the nose. The absence of the palatal tissue can prevent expulsion of milk from the nipple. The orthopedic appliance prosthetically restores the anatomy of the palate, permitting normal suckling.

Since the purpose of the negative pressure in the mouth is to hold the nipple and areola in place and not to extract milk from the breast, a seal is needed to keep the pressure. One mother was able to perform the positioning task by holding the breast to her infant's mouth firmly between two fingers, as in Fig. 8-8.[45] The infant was then able to milk the areola and nipple with the tongue pressing it against the roof of the mouth, even with the cleft. The breast had to be held in position much as a bottle would be held throughout the feeding.

It has been noted in Chapter 8 that breast-fed infants have fewer bouts with otitis media, which has been attributed to the position of the infant while feeding at the breast as well as the anti-infective properties of the milk. It is certainly an important consideration in infants with cleft palates, who have been identified as having more ear infections in general than other infants.

Feeding infants with oral defects requires extra effort. Each infant is slightly different. Usually mothers learn to feed their own infants more effectively, even when bottle-feeding, than the skilled professional can. This amplifies the fact that it requires a special patience and knack. Breast-feeding can be successful. Infants with cleft lip and/or palate should be managed as normal infants. They should be brought to the mother to feed and for rooming-in, as with any infant. Reinforcing the fact that the infant is normal and merely needs some reconstructive surgery is important in helping the parents adjust. Here parent-to-parent programs are most helpful.

Intestinal tract. Infants with anomalies of the gastrointestinal tract that cause obstruction develop symptoms that depend on the location of the problem in the intestinal tract.

TRACHEOESOPHAGEAL FISTULA. Tracheoesophageal (T-E) fistula is apparent early and, depending on the exact anatomy of the lesions, shows respiratory symptoms and signs of obstruction. This is a surgical emergency. If no feedings have been given or no milk has been aspirated, surgery can be done as soon as possible. If pneumonia intervenes, the course is protracted and the infant may have to be maintained on peripheral venous alimentation until surgery can be done and healing takes place.

A mother who wishes to breast-feed an infant with a T-E fistula can manually express milk and/or pump, saving all samples in the freezer until the infant can take oral milk feedings. If the infant has a gastrostomy tube in place, small feedings may be started fairly early postoperatively, and human milk is ideal if available because of its easy digestibility and anti-infective properties. If there is initially a need to partially supplement the milk with intravenous fluids, the fluids can be calculated to make up the difference between needs and nutrients supplied by the orally taken breast milk. As nutrition progresses, if supply does not keep up with requirements, feedings can be supplemented with other nutrients. When ready for oral feedings, a full-term or large premature infant can nurse at the breast. Unless the mother is able to spend most of the day and night at the hospital, the infant will have to receive bottle feedings as well. If the mother has been able to store up enough milk, the infant may be able to fulfill his needs from breast milk. Once the infant is discharged and begins to nurse at the breast every feeding for a few days, the supply will increase immediately. If there is concern for nutritional lag between needs and production, the Lact-Aid device can be used briefly to stimulate the breast without starving and exhausting the infant (Chapter 16).

PYLORIC STENOSIS. Pyloric stenosis occurs in about 2 to 5/1000 live births. There is a family tendency, but the disease is more common in first-born males. Usually it occurs between the second and sixth weeks of life, although it can occur anytime after birth. Vomiting is characteristic. It is intermittent at first and progresses to include evey feeding and is often projectile. These infants are eager feeders and go back for more milk until the weight loss and dehydration makes them anxious and irritable. In the investigation of vomiting, it is important to keep in mind that overfeeding can cause spitting and vomiting, even projectile vomiting, but it is not associated with weight loss, decreased urine and stools, and dehydration. Therapy consists of pyloromyotomy following correction of the dehydration and associated electrolyte abnormalities. If the procedure is uncomplicated, the infant can go back to the breast in 6 to 8 hr after a trial of water at 4 hr shows the infant is alert and sucking well. The breast-fed infant may be discharged in 24 hr if nursing has gone well. If the duodenum is entered at the time of surgery, gastric decompression and intravenous fluids will be necessary and oral feeding delayed several days until signs of healing occur. A breast-fed infant may resume nursing earlier than a bottle infant returns to formula because of the rapid emptying time of the stomach and the zero curd tension of the milk.

DISORDERS OF THE SMALL INTESTINE. Disorders of the small intestine, including duodenal obstruction, malrotation, jejunoileal obstruction and duplications, require surgery. Depending on the extent of the lesion, whether or not the bowel wall is opened, if bowel segments are removed, and if there are associated lesions such as annular pancreas, the infant will need postoperative maintenance on intravenous fluids and possibly alimentation. The mother who wishes to breast-feed may or may not have ever nursed the infant, depending on the time of onset of symptoms and their severity. The mother should be counseled about the prognosis and encouraged to manually express and pump if it appears feasible for her to eventually breast-feed. The decision should be made with the parents, surgeon, neonatologist, and pediatrician. Frequently infants with atresias are also small or premature.

DISORDERS OF THE COLON. Disorders of the colon occur more commonly in full-term infants. Hirschsprung's disease or congenital aganglionic megacolon is the most common lesion. There is usually delayed passage of meconium; however, only 10% to 15% of all children with delayed passage of meconium have Hirschsprung's disease. Constipation and abdominal distention are the most frequent initial symptoms. They may begin during the first few days of life and gradually progress to include bilious vomiting. The clinical picture may be indistinguishable from meconium ileus, ileal atresia, or large bowel obstruction. In any infant with perforation of the colon, ileum, or appendix, Hirschsprung's disease should be considered. The breast-fed infant may have milder symptoms and delayed onset of real stress because the breast milk stools are normally loose and seedy and easily passed. The pH and flora of the intestinal tract are also different, leading to less distention. Enterocolitis may occur at any age and is the major cause of death.

No data have been located to distinguish the incidence of this complication in breast- and bottle-fed infants, although an argument could be mounted regarding the projected value of secretory IgA and intestinal flora of the breast-fed infant. The treatment depends on the symptoms, x-ray findings, and results of biopsy for the identification of the aganglionic segment. Usually colostomy is done on diagnosis and definitive surgery done later in the first year of life. Feedings can be resumed as soon as the infant is stable, after the colostomy has healed sufficiently to permit bowel activity. Human milk has the same advantages for early postoperative feeding in this disease as well because of its anti-infective properties and easy digestibility.

MECONIUM PLUG SYNDROME AND MECONIUM ILEUS. Meconium plug syndrome and meconium ileus are less common and less severe in breast-fed infants who have received a full measure of colostrum. Colostrum has a cathartic effect and stimulates the passage of meconium. Should either disorder be diagnosed, the infant should continue to nurse in addition to any other treatment.

NECROTIZING ENTEROCOLITIS. Although necrotizing enterocolitis (NEC) has been known of for 100 years, it has only been since 1960 that it has been identified with any frequency, which suggests an iatrogenic component. It is most common in premature infants and infants compromised by asphyxia. It has been associated with umbilical catheters, exchange transfusions, polycythemia, hyperosmolar feedings, and infection. Its cause is not clear. Work with animals has suggested that human breast milk, specifically colostrum, provides protection against the disease. A good control study to evaluate this in human infants has not been reported. A "dose or two" of human milk may not be enough. There are cases of NEC reported that have occurred so early in life that no feedings were given. Present regimens of treatment call for cessation of all oral feedings and use of oral and systemic gentamycin, gastric decompression, plasma and/or blood transfusions, and rigorous monitoring for progression or perforation with serial x-ray studies as well as a septic workup. Further study is necessary to determine cause and possible prevention and the role colostrum or breast milk might play.

The organisms generally associated with NEC are gram-negative organisms such as *Bacteroides, E. coli,* and especially *Klebsiella.* Brown and colleagues[6a] reported that 89% of the infants with NEC had received cow's milk formulas and that gram-negative bacteria and endotoxins were present in the stool. Colonization of breast-fed infants with *Klebsiella* does not occur, and *L. bifidus* predominates, according to Mata and Urrutia.[33] The uncommon occurrence of NEC in Helsinki, at the University of Helsinki Children's Hospital intensive care nursery is remarkable. Jelliffe and Jelliffe[26] report that all the premature infants are routinely fed with colostrum and breast milk in Helsinki.

IMPERFORATE ANUS. Defects in the rectum and anal sphincter are usually diagnosed in the first few hours on physical examination or because a rectal thermometer cannot be passed. When the blind pouch is more generous, diagnosis may depend on the evaluation of failure to stool. Depending on associated lesions and fistulas to bladder or vagina, the surgical decompression can be performed. Until this time, oral feedings are withheld. High lesions require an immediate colostomy with later final repair, whereas low lesions may be repaired at the primary procedure through a perineal approach. Infants may be breast-fed as soon as any bowel activity can be permitted, often 2 to 3 days postoperatively.

GASTROINTESTINAL BLEEDING. The most common cause of vomiting blood or passing blood via the rectum in a breast-fed infant is a bleeding nipple in the mother, which may or may not be painful. Any time fresh blood is found in the vomitus or stool of any newborn, the blood should be tested for adult or fetal hemoglobin. If it is adult hemoglobin it indicates the source is maternal. This is done by a qualitative test, the APT test. (Mix blood with 2 to 3 ml normal saline solution, add 2 to 3 ml of 10% NaOH [0.25M]. Mix gently. Observe for color change. Fetal hemoglobin is stable in alkali and will remain pink, whereas adult hemoglobin turns brown. Use a known adult sample as a color control.) If the blood is adult hemoglobin in a breast-fed infant, the possibility of a cracked and bleeding nipple should be ruled out by inspection of the maternal breast (p. 124).

If the blood is fetal hemoglobin, the differential diagnosis for bleeding in any neonate should be followed. Breast-feeding can be maintained meanwhile unless a lesion requiring surgery is identified. More than 50% of the cases of gastrointestinal bleeding in the neonate go undiagnosed. Anorectal fissure is uncommon as a cause in breast-fed infants. Allergy to human milk is unreported as a cause of intestinal bleeding. The distribution of causes of intestinal bleeding in the neonate, without selection for type of feeding are: idiopathic, 50%; hemorrhagic disorders, 20%; swallowed maternal blood, 10%; anorectal fissures, 10%; intestinal ischemia, 5%; and colitis, 5%.

Malformations of the central nervous system. Malformations of the central nervous system (CNS) that are diagnosed at birth include the clinical spectrum from anencephaly and complete craniorachischisis to dermal sinuses. Defects of the spinal column run from complete spinal rachischisis to spina bifida occulta. Those which are incompatible with life or are inoperable present the additional problem to the mother who had planned to breast-feed of coping with her desire to nurse her infant. If the infant is to be given normal newborn care and the mother desires to nurse this infant, breast-feeding should be discussed by the pediatrician and parents together. It has been well demonstrated that parents grieve more physiologically if they have contact with their abnormal infants, but their imaginations are more vicious than some abnormalities of development. The professional's personal bias as to how to deal with this infant should not overshadow the discussion with the parents. If the mother chooses to nurse the infant who has no life expectancy and the infant is to be fed at all by mouth, she should have that choice.

Infants with CNS abnormalities requiring surgery can be breast-fed until the operation and postoperatively as soon as oral intake is permitted. In these cases in which the gastrointestinal tract is not involved, breast-feeding can be initiated 6 to 8 hr postoperatively, at the surgeon's discretion. The risk of lung irritation from breast milk is minimal. The rapid emptying time of the stomach and other anti-infective factors serve as advantages in the postoperative course.

Surgery or rehospitalization beyond the neonatal period

The infant who requires surgery or rehospitalization can and should be breast-fed postoperatively in most cases. The gravity of the surgery and the length of the recovery phase will determine the time necessary for the mother to pump and manually express her milk to keep her supply available. The infant who is hospitalized is already traumatized by the separation, the strange surroundings and people, and the underlying discomfort of the disease process itself. If he is to be fed orally, it should be at the breast as much as possible. If the mother can room-in or the hospital has a care-by-parent ward, this works out well. If obligations to other family members make it impossible for mother to stay around the clock, she can pump her milk and bring it in fresh day by day or frozen if the time interval between visits is longer than a day. Freezing will destroy the cellular content, but that is not a major problem beyond the immediate neonatal period. The infant should not be subjected to the added trauma of being weaned from the breast when he needs the security and intimacy of nursing most unless it is absolutely unavoidable.

The medical profession needs to be aware of this infant and mother and their special needs for support. An opportunity to discuss the breast-feeding aspect of the infant's management should be offered by the physician. The parents should not have to fight for the right to maintain breast-feeding. Plans for pumping and saving milk should be discussed and provided for. If the infant is housed in an open ward or even a room with other infants and their parents without adequate privacy, a separate room should be provided for the mother to nurse or pump her milk. This room should be clean, neat, adequately illuminated, and equipped with a sink for washing hands. If a mechanical pump is to be used, it should be kept clean, sterile, and operable. Store rooms, broom closets, and staff dressing rooms are inappropriate.

Arrangements for providing sterile containers for collecting milk and storing it should be discussed (Chapter 18). Occasionally a mother may become so concerned about the adequacy of her milk for her infant that she may nurse far too frequently. Actually her child will need much more nonnutritive cuddling and holding than usual. The physician may need to reassure the mother when pointing this out. The father should also be encouraged to understand all the tubes, bandages, and appliances the infant may have attached. He is an important member of the parenting team and should provide some of the cuddling and soothing as well.

REFERENCES

1. Arias, I. M., and Gartner, L. M.: Production of unconjugated hyperbilirubinemia in full term newborn infants following administration of Pregnane-3α,20β-diol, Nature **203**:1292, 1964.
2. Arias, I. M., et al.: Prolonged neonatal unconjugated hyperbilirubinemia associated with breast feeding and steroid Pregnane-3α,20β-diol in maternal milk that inhibits glucuronide formation in vitro, J. Clin. Invest. **43**:2037, 1964.
3. Atkinson, S. A., Bryan, M. H., and Anderson, G. H.: Human milk: differences in nitrogen concentration in milk from mothers of term and premature infants, J. Pediatr. **93**:67, 1978.
4. Auerbach, K. G., et al.: A symposium: breast feeding the premature infant, Keeping Abreast J. **2**:98, 1977.
5. Beck, F.: Breast feeding the baby with a cleft lip, Keeping Abreast, J. Hum. Nurturing **3**:122, 1978.
6. Bode, H. H., Vanjonack, W. J., and Crawford, J. D.: Mitigation of cretinism by breast feeding, Pediatr. Res. **11**:423, 1977.
6a. Brown, E. G., Ainbender, E., and Sweet, A. Y.: Effect of feeding stool endotoxins: possible relationship to necrotizing enterocolitis, Pediatr. Res. **10**:352, 1976.
7. Dahms, B. B., et al.: Breast feeding and serum bilirubin values during the first 4 days of life, J. Pediatr. **83**:1049, 1973.
8. Drew, J. H.: Breast feeding and jaundice, II. Infant feeding and jaundice, Keeping Abreast, J. Hum. Nurt. **3**:53, 1978.

9. Eckhert, C. D., et al.: Zinc binding: a difference between human and bovine milk, Science **195**:789, 1977.
10. Evans, G. W., and Johnson, P. E.: Defective prostaglandin synthesis in acrodermatitis enteropathica, Lancet **1**:52, 1977.
11. Filer, L. J., Steglink, L. D., and Chandramouli, B.: Effect of diet on plasma aminograms of low birth weight infants, Am. J. Clin. Nutr. **30**:1036, 1977.
12. Foliot, A., et al.: Breast milk jaundice: in vitro inhibition of rat liver bilirubin-uridine diphosphate glucuronyltransferase activity and Z protein-bromosulfophthalein binding by human breast milk, Pediatr. Res. **10**:594, 1976.
13. Fomon, S. J., and Ziegler, E. E.: Protein intake of premature infants: interpretation of data, editor's column, J. Pediatr. **90**:504, 1977.
14. Fomon, S. J., and Ziegler, E. E.: Milk of the premature infant's mother: interpretation of data, editorial, J. Pediatr. **93**:164, 1978.
15. Fomon, S. J., Ziegler, E. E., and Vazquez, H. D.: Human milk and the small premature infant, Am. J. Dis. Child. **131**:463, 1977.
16. Forbes, G. B.: Is human milk the best food for low birth weight babies? Abstracted, Pediatr. Res. **12**:434, 1978.
17. Gartner, L. M., and Arias, I. M.: Temporary discontinuation of breast feeding in infants with jaundice, J.A.M.A. **225**:532, 1973.
18. Gartner, L. M., and Lee, K.-S.: Jaundice and liver disease. In Behrman, R. E., Driscoll, J. M., Jr., and Seeds, A. E., editors: Neonatal-perinatal medicine diseases of the fetus and infant, ed. 2, St. Louis, 1977, The C. V. Mosby Co.
19. Gaull, G. E., Rassin, D. K., and Räihä, N. C. R.: Protein intake of premature infants: a reply, J. Pediatr. **90**:507, 1977.
20. Gaull, G. E., et al.: Milk protein quantity and quality in low–birth-weight infants, III. Effects on sulfur amino acids in plasma and urine, J. Pediatr. **90**:348, 1977.
21. Grady, E.: Breastfeeding the baby with a cleft of the soft palate: success and its benefits, Clin. Pediatr. **16**:978, 1977.
22. Grady, E.: Breast feeding the baby with a cleft of the soft palate, Keeping Abreast, J. Hum. Nurturing **3**:126, 1978.
23. Greenberg, J., Nazarian, L., and Green, J.: Personal communications, 1976 to 1978.
24. Heird, W. C., and Anderson, T. L.: Nutritional requirements and methods of feeding low birth weight infants. In Gluck, L., editor: Current problems in pediatrics, vol. VII, no. 8, Chicago, 1977, Year Book Medical Publishers, Inc., p. 1.
25. Hemmingway, L.: Breastfeeding a cleft-palate baby, Med. J. Aust. **2**:626, Sept. 9, 1972.
26. Jelliffe, D. B., and Jelliffe, E. F. P.: Human milk in the modern world, Oxford, 1976, Oxford University Press.
27. Jelliffe, E. F. P.: Infant feeding practices: associated diseases. In Neumann, C. G., and Jelliffe, D. B., editors: Symposium on nutrition in pediatrics, Pediatr. Clin. North Am. **24**:1, 1977.
28. Jelliffe, E. F. P.: Infant feeding practices: associated iatrogenic and commerciogenic diseases. In Neumann, C. G., and Jelliffe, D. B., editors: Symposium on nutrition in pediatrics, Pediatr. Clin. North Am. **24**:49, 1977.
28a. Johnson, P., and Salisbury, D. M.: Breathing and sucking during feeding in the newborn. In Hofer, M. A., editor: Ciba Foundation Symposium no. 33, parent-infant interaction, Amsterdam, 1975, Elsevier Scientific Publ. Co.
29. Kennell, J. H., et al.: Early neonatal contact: effect on growth, breast feeding and infection in the first year of life, Pediatr. Res. **10**:426, 1976.
30. Lubit, E. C.: Cleft palate orthodontics: why, when, how, Am. J. Orthod. **69**:562, 1976.
31. Luzeau, R., et al.: Demonstration of a lipolytic activity in human milk that inhibits the glucurono-conjugation of bilirubin, Biomedicine **21**:258, 1974.
32. Luzeau, R., et al.: Activity of lipoprotein lipase in human milk: inhibition of glucuro-conjugation of bilirubin, Clin. Chim. Acta **59**:133, 1975.
33. Mata, L. J., and Urrutia, J. J.: Intestinal colonization of breast fed children in a rural area of low socio-economic level, Ann. N.Y. Acad. Sci. **93**:1976, 1971.
34. Nau, J.: When a baby has surgery—an interview, Keeping Abreast J. **1**:38, 1976.
35. Office for Maternal and Child Health, HEW, sponsor: Human milk in premature infant feeding: summary of a workshop, Pediatrics **57**:741, 1976.

36. Räihä, N. C. R., et al.: Milk protein quantity and quality in low–birth-weight infants, I. Metabolic responses and effects on growth, Pediatrics **57**:659, 1976.

37. Rassin, D. K., et al.: Milk protein quantity and quality in low–birth-weight infants, II. Effects on aliphatic amino acids in plasma and urine, Pediatrics **59**:407, 1977.

38. Rassin, D. K., et al.: Milk protein quantity and quality in low–birth-weight infants. IV. Effects on tyrosine and phenylalanine in plasma and urine, J. Pediatr. **90**:356, 1977.

39. Russell, G., and Feather, E. A.: Effects of feeding on respiratory mechanics of healthy newborn infants, Arch. Dis. Child. **45**:325, 1970.

40. Sack, J., Amado, O., and Lunenfeld, B.: Thyroxine concentration in human milk, J. Clin. Endocrinol. Metab. **45**:171, 1977.

41. Simkins, T.: Feeding the premature infant: more questions than answers, Perinatol. Neonatol. **2**:30, 1978.

42. Snyderman, S. E.: The protein and amino acid requirements of the premature infant. In Jonxis, J. H. P., Visser, H. K. A., and Troelstra, J. A., editors: Nutricia Symposium, metabolic process in the foetus and newborn infant, Rotterdam, 1971, Stenfort, Kroesse, Leider, p. 128.

43. Sturman, J. A., Rassin, D. K., and Gaull, G. E.: A mini review: taurine in development, Life Sci. **21**:1, 1977.

44. Varma, S. K., et al.: Thyroxine, tri-iodothyronine, and reverse tri-iodothyronine concentrations in human milk, J. Pediatr. **93**:803, 1978.

45. Weatherly-White, R. C. A.: Guest comment: Breastfeeding the baby with a cleft lip, Keeping Abreast, J. Hum. Nurturing **3**:125, 1978.

46. Wong, P. W. K., Lambert, A. M., and Komrowe, G. M.: Tyrosinaemia and tyrosluria in infancy, Dev. Med. Child. Neurol. **9**:551, 1967.

47. Wong, Y. K., and Wood, B. S. B.: Breast milk jaundice and oral contraceptives, Br. Med. J. **4**:403, 1971.

CHAPTER 14

Medical complications of the mother

OBSTETRICAL COMPLICATIONS
Cesarean section

When delivery takes place by cesarean section, the mother becomes a surgical patient with all the inherent risks and problems. If the section is anticipated because of a previous section, cephalopelvic disproportion, or some other identifiable reason, a mother can prepare herself psychologically for the event and usually tolerates the process better. When the section is unplanned and done during the process of labor, it is psychologically more traumatic, and the mother tends to feel as if she has failed in her female role. In addition to this unexpected disappointment, there may be medical emergencies that also have an impact on the mother's well-being, such as a long hard labor, abruptio placentae, blood loss, toxemia, or infection.

The mother who plans to breast-feed following a cesarean section should be able to do so provided the infant is well enough. Depending on the type of anesthesia and the associated circumstances, the mother may feel alert enough to put the infant to breast within the first 12 hr. Mothers have nursed in the first hour after the surgery is over. Regional anesthesia permits the mother to remain awake, and she may be ready to nurse as soon as the intravenous lines and urinary catheter are all stabilized. The mother will need considerable help from the nursing staff. She should remain flat if she has had a spinal anesthetic to prevent developing a spinal headache. She can turn to one side and the infant can be placed on his side and offered the nipple by stroking the infant's perioral area with the nipple. If he is a normal full-term infant and has not been depressed by maternal medication, he should do well. If the mother can be turned to the other side, the infant should nurse on both sides. The bedside rails will help the mother turn as well as provide safety for her.

Fluids and medications in the first 48 hr postoperatively should not affect the infant adversely. Pain medication is required subsequently, usually for 72 hr or so. It is best given immediately after breast-feeding to permit the level to peak before the next feeding. The medication used should be limited to short-acting drugs that the adult eliminates quickly (i.e., within 4 hr) and that the newborn is able to excrete also. Aspirin, for instance, is in that category despite the theoretical risk of decreased platelet aggregation because it is readily excreted by both adult and infant. Codeine is also acceptable (Chapter 11).

There are some very positive factors associated with breast-feeding for the mother who has had a cesarean section. Lactation is advantageous to the postoperative uterus in that the oxytocin production stimulated by suckling will assist in the involution of the uterus. In addition, the traumatized psyche of a mother whose delivery did not occur naturally as planned is more quickly healed when she can demonstrate her maternal capabilities by breast-feeding.

Whether nursing can be introduced early or must await stabilization of medical problems in the mother or infant, it is a reasonable goal for the mother to seek, in most cases. Supportive nursing care will be critical to establishing successful lactation. But none of this can take place unless the physician has carefully assessed the condition of the mother and the infant in light of the advantages and disadvantages of breast-feeding to both.

The management should include the following:

1. A postoperative care plan must include sufficient rest. Most postpartum wards are not scheduled to include adequate rest for postoperative patients.
2. The family must be instructed on the needs for rest at home and assistance with the household chores.
3. The infant should be considered, when possible, in writing medication orders.

Toxemia

Toxemia presents a problem in management anytime it occurs. The clinical onset is insidious and may be accompanied by a variety of subtle symptoms but the diagnosis depends on the presence of hypertension and proteinuria.[5] It usually begins after the thirty-second week of gestation and has been observed to occur 24 to 48 hr or later postpartum. Convulsions, renal disease, and cerebral hemorrhage in the mother are all complications to be prevented by careful management. Because serious toxicity in the mother may necessitate delivery of a premature infant or an infant compromised by a poorly profused placenta or maternal medications, there are a number of contraindications to breast-feeding in the immediate postpartum period. Initial treatment of the preeclamptic patient includes bed rest, preferably lying on her side in a room that is darkened to prevent photic stimuli. Blood pressure and proteinuria are to be carefully watched. Sedation with phenobarbital, 60 mg every 6 hr, or diazepam (Valium), 10 mg intramuscularly, salt restriction, and possibly diuretics such as thiazide or furosemide are used. Hydralazine (Apresoline) and methyldopa (Aldomet) may be indicated as well, to bring down the blood pressure. Many patients recover quickly once the infant and placenta are delivered, requiring only 24 to 48 hr of postpartum sedation. Often the infant is small for gestational age or premature and may require special or intensive care; therefore the decision to breast-feed depends on the infant's condition. If the infant is full-term and well, then the breast-feeding is initiated when toxemia precautions are discontinued and when the mother's phenobarbital intake has been tapered off to about 180 mg/day or less, calculating that initially the amount of milk obtained is not so great as to provide a large dose of drug to the infant. Careful observation should be made to be sure the infant is not depressed by the accumulation of phenobarbital, however. Phenobarbital is a drug that can be and is given to newborns for several indications and therefore is of low risk. It is preferable to wait until the other medications can be discontinued, especially the diuretics, hydralazine, and methyldopa. Once the risk of convulsions is past, some attention can be given to manual expression or pumping even if the infant cannot be nursed yet. If medications are a problem temporarily, the milk will have to be discarded, but the expression of milk will serve to stimulate the breast and initiate lactation. Diminution of stress is a critical factor in toxemia therapy so the anxiety of the mother about being able to nurse must be managed with open discussion of the overall plan and where nursing fits in. On the other hand, the stress of early feedings that do not go well because the infant has been confused by initial bottle-feedings may also present a hazard in the course of management of toxemia. The single most important element in every case is communication with the patient about her expectations or needs regarding breast-feeding. The physician's therapeutic management design can put this in appropriate perspective.

Venous thrombosis and pulmonary embolism

Venous thrombosis and pulmonary embolism are the most common serious vascular diseases associated with pregnancy and the postpartum period.[5] Pulmonary embolism has assumed relatively greater importance because of the decline in morbidity and mortality from sepsis and eclampsia. Varicose veins also present more problems during pregnancy than at any other time. These diseases all represent common features in vein physiology as associated with the perinatal period.

The major concerns during lactation, in addition to the well-being of the mother, include the diagnostic procedures that might be necessary to establish the diagnosis and the systemic medications necessary for treatment that could have an impact on the nursing infant via the milk. Accurate diagnosis is urgent and is far more complex than therapy. Besides the health of the mother in this life-threatening state, any program of contraception after childbirth is fundamentally affected by the established diagnosis of thromboembolism. Thus the diagnosis must be accurate.

Diagnosis. Laboratory procedures such as evaluation of arterial blood gases, liver function studies, and fibrin/fibrinogen derivatives are not a problem to nursing. It might be noted that the absence of fibrin split products in plasma and serum virtually excludes the diagnosis of embolism, although their presence does not confirm it. The most definitive diagnosis is made with radioactive scanning procedures and angiography. At present, computer-assisted tomography and ultrasound are effective in major arterial aneurysms only. Radioactive materials vary in their half-lives and disappearance time from breast milk. They all appear in breast milk (Chapter 11).

Treatment. Anticogulant therapy is the treatment of choice for established venous thrombosis with or without embolism. Heparin can be given parenterally, since this large molecule does not cross the placenta or appear in breast milk. This therapy is adequate for the hospitalized patient, in whom constant monitoring of coagulation is possible. An alternative, self-administered subcutaneous heparin, has been reported by Kakkar and colleagues.[13] The cost of heparin and the patient's ability to learn self-administration are considerations. Warfarin has been considered the best replacement for heparin but it is secreted in the breast milk (Chapter 11 and Appendix F).

MATERNAL INFECTIONS
Bacterial infections

Urinary tract infection. Urinary tract infections are the most common of the postpartum bacterial infection. Any apparent infection is of concern because of the risk to the infant. Urinary tract infections, however, are "closed infections" and do not constitute a hazard except when the infection is due to β-hemolytic streptococci. The mother should be reminded to wash her hands thoroughly before handling the infant. The choice of medication is important when the mother is breast-feeding, since the majority of antibiotics reach the milk in some concentration. The medication should be one that could also be given to the infant, such as penicillin, ampicillin, and gentamycin. Under 1 month postpartum, sulfadiazine and sulfa-containing medications should not be given, since the hazard of interfering with bilirubin binding to albumin is significant. Beyond 1 month of age sulfa drugs are actually given to infants directly. Tetracycline and chloramphenicol should not be used. Forcing fluids and acidifying the urine via the diet are always helpful.

Breast abscesses in staphylococcal epidemics. Breast abscesses can occur in both mothers and infants in nursery epidemics with a virulent staphylococcus. Maternal abscesses may occur anytime from 2 weeks to 2 months postpartum. Transmission does not always go from infant to mother, since breast abscess has been seen in women who have delivered stillborn infants.

According to recent reports,[29] during a nursery epidemic, the colonized mothers who were nursing developed abscesses, whereas the ones not nursing did not. Both groups of infants were free of the disease but had positive nasal cultures for *S. aureus,* phage type 80/81. Shinefeld[29] states that, in his view, in times of epidemics with virulent strains of staphylocci, infants colonized with the epidemic organism should not be breast-fed. Breast abscesses should be looked for carefully in the mother and diagnosed by culturing the secretion from the nipple, since the skin and external nipple may well be colonized with the epidemic organism. The treatment is systemic antibiotics, careful drainage of the breast by massage or pump at intervals, and drainage of the abscess when surgically indicated.

Bacterial infections due to streptococcus, staphylococcus, or other transmissible organisms may cause skin lesions, pharyngitis, pneumonia, or endometritis. These should be treated promptly with antibiotics, and the infant permitted to breast-feed as soon as a therapeutic level of medications has been established for at least 12 hr. Usually infants who are bottle-fed are separated from their mothers longer, but they will not receive the valuable anti-infective properties of human milk. Often the question of isolation from the mother and interruption of feeding at the breast comes when symptoms of fever, pain, or malaise first develop in the mother and the diagnosis is still in question. A clinical judgment must be made as to the organ infected, whether bacteria are being actively extruded from the infected source, and the estimated virulence of the organism. A draining incision that appears to show that the infection is streptococcal in origin suggests early isolation and a conservative approach, whereas a low-grade fever within 24 hr of delivery with no localizing signs might warrant continuing active breast-feeding.*

Staphylococcal infections may be passed back and forth between the mother and infant. Identification of the infection and the etiological agent is important so that appropriate treatment may be initiated. Not all staphylococci are patholog-

---

*It should be pointed out that engorgement may be associated with a low-grade fever. The patient should be evaluated as to other possible causes, but if none are identified the probable diagnosis is engorgement. The best treatment is to nurse the infant as often as possible and see that the breasts are gently expressed to assure proper drainage of all alveoli.

ical, and removing this flora may permit growth of real pathogens. A mother and nursing infant with staphylococcal disease under medication need not be separated from each other. They should be isolated from other mothers and infants. Sometimes the best plan when the symptoms are mild is to discharge the nursing couple to prevent spread in the hospital and permit freedom of contact at home, with reasonable precautions (Table 14-7).

Gonorrhea. When gonorrhea is specifically diagnosed by identification of bacteria in the cervical smear or culture prior to delivery, antibiotics should be started immediately; the mother may handle and/or feed her infant 24 hr after the initiation of therapy. Because of the occasional occurrence of established infection in the neonate despite use of silver nitrate in the eyes at birth, it is appropriate to isolate the infant from the rest of the nursery population, although the infant need not be isolated from his mother once her treatment has been established. The Credé method of eye prophylaxis may fail because it is improperly done or the infection was established prior to birth because of prematurely ruptured membranes or the development of inclusion conjunctivitis.

Syphilis. A mother with positive syphilis serum reaction, which indicates a primary infection, should be treated immediately. If there are primary or secondary lesions that could contain the treponeme, the infant should be isolated from the mother as well as from other infants. The infant should have a diagnostic work-up for congenital syphilis and treatment instituted when appropriate. If there are lesions around the breast and nipple, nursing is contraindicated until treatment is complete and the lesions are clear. Following is an outline of the therapeutic decisions in relation to the syphilis VDRL antigen status of the infant[10]:

  I. Negative VDRL
      A. No disease: no treatment required
      B. Early disease
          1. Symptomatic: treat
          2. Asymptomatic: follow and repeat VDRL
 II. Positive VDRL
      A. Symptomatic
          1. Hydrops fetalis: treat
          2. Hepatosplenomegaly, jaundice: treat
          3. Mucocutaneous manifestations: treat
          4. Hematological manifestations: treat
          5. Nephrotic syndrome: treat
      B. Asymptomatic
          1. Perform quantitative VDRL on mother and infant
              a. If infant titer is fourfold higher: treat
          2. Perform quantitative immunoglobulin test
              a. If cord IgM is elevated ($\geq$ 21 mg/100 ml): treat
          3. Perform hematological studies (hemoglobin, hematocrit, reticulocyte count, platelet count, smear)
              a. If abnormal: treat
          4. Perform bone radiography
              a. If abnormal: treat
          5. Perform lumbar puncture
              a. If abnormal: treat
          6. If mother unreliable: treat

Tuberculosis. Controversy exists around the management of tuberculosis during pregnancy and lactation. All mothers with a positive tuberculin test reaction but no radiological evidence of tuberculosis are considered by Huber[9] to be infected but not diseased. Recent tuberculin conversion, which represents a state of undetermined activity, should be distinguished from well-contained tuberculosis. Dates and results of previous skin tests and recent exposure to active cases are important parts of the history. Because of the hazard that tuberculosis presents to the newborn, careful family studies, including tuberculin skin testing and chest x-ray examinations should be performed on contacts of both the mother and the infant. Huber[9] states that all mothers with a newly positive skin test and negative chest film should be started on a course of isoniazid at the beginning of the third trimester of pregnancy. Dosage is 5 mg/kg of body weight each day as a single dose. Therapy is continued for a year postpartum. If no active cases are identified in the household, no special precautions are indicated to protect the newborn. At one time, however, approximately half the neonates born to tuberculin-positive but bacteriological-negative mothers later became infected with tuberculosis. Since the advent of antituberculous drugs in recent years, however, breast-feeding has been permitted without difficulty in these cases.

When the mother has a positive tuberculin test and a positive chest film, considerable effort should be made to identify the organism in the sputum or gastric washings. If the mother is bacteriologically positive, she should receive triple therapy of isoniazid (INH), 300 mg/day, para-aminosalicylic acid, 12 g/day, and pyridoxine, 50 mg/day, regardless of the time in pregnancy. If she is bacteriologically negative, she should receive isoniazid in the third trimester. Minimum active tuberculosis is defined as parenchymal involvement without cavities. The pregnant woman with minimum active tuberculosis should be hospitalized for evaluation. Sputum sampling and gastric washings should be done and triple treatment begun immediately. It has been shown these patients are no longer infective to others as soon as therapy is initiated. Therapy should continue for 2 years. It is important to reassure the mother that if she is given triple treatment, there is no reason to believe the newborn will have the disease at birth. The controversy arises on postpartum management and separation of mother and infant.

When maternal pulmonary tuberculosis has been treated for at least a week, and if compliance with regard to maternal therapy is assured, infant and maternal contact can be permitted, provided the infant is receiving isoniazid prophylaxis. The isoniazid prophylaxis (30 mg/kg/day in two doses) is always indicated when the mother has any disease requiring triple therapy, even without any contact. If the mother has been treated during pregnancy and cultures are negative, 10 mg of isoniazid/kg/day is indicated for the infant, and no period of separation is necessary.

If it is safe for the mother to be in contact with her infant, then it is safe to breast-feed except for consideration regarding the medications. Since both mother and infant will be taking isoniazid it would be a matter of assuring that the accumulation in the infant is not excessive because isoniazid does pass into the breast milk. Dosages for infants range from 10 to 30 mg/kg/day. Hepatotoxicity is possible in either the mother or infant, which can be monitored with serial serum glutamic-oxaloacetic transaminase (SGOT) tests. Para-aminosalicylic acid (PAS) readily crosses the placenta, yet is reported by O'Brien[24] not to cross into breast milk; this is conflicting information. A drug that readily crosses the placenta is usually found in breast milk. PAS is not recommended nor is it used to treat newborns. Streptomycin or kanamycin is used instead as the second drug. Jelliffe and Jelliffe[11] point out that in technically undeveloped countries, maternal pulmonary tuberculosis is not a contraindication to breast-feeding. Active treatment is given the mother, while the infant receives isoniazid or BCG vaccine with an isoniazid-resistant strain. In these countries the risk to the infant of not being breast-fed far outweighs any risk of drug-related toxicity. That risk/benefit ratio is different in the Western world. In some populations, however, in which infant death from various infections is a major consideration, breast-feeding may be significant to survival. The isolated populations of the American Indian are such a group. Meticulous care must be given to assure that both mother and infant receive proper medication and vaccination against tuberculosis. Newborns and young infants are the most vulnerable group with the highest rate of complication.

Leprosy. Leprosy is not a contraindication to breast-feeding, according to Jelliffe and Jelliffe.[11] The urgency of breast-feeding is recognized in leprosariums, where the infant and mother are treated with diaminodiphenylsulfone by mouth. No mother-infant contact is permitted except to breast-feed.

Listeriosis. Listeriosis has been identified as the infecting organism in neonatal sepsis and meningitis in recent years and can result in neonatal death. *Listeria,* causing abortion, stillbirth, prematurity, and neonatal death, was described in the 1930s under various titles, including argyrophilic septicemia and pseudotuberculosis of the newborn. The early infection frequently is not recognized and is confused with aspiration pneumonia because of the respiratory symptoms. Examination of the meconium, placenta, and maternal lochia may locate the chief sources of the bacteria, since the symptom complex is not pathognomonic. Symptoms in the mother may be flulike or similar to infectious mononucleosis. The manifestations in the adult are protean and in the pregnant woman may lead to an early delivery of an infected infant. Otherwise the infection in adults may be mild and unrecognized, except in retrospect.

The outcome of listeriosis in the neonate depends on early and effective antibiotic therapy, since untreated infants usually do not survive over 4 days. Both mother and infant should be treated. At present, ampicillin is the treatment of choice and should be maintained in the newborn through the fourth week of life. Treatment in the mother should be maintained 6 to 8 days after symptoms have cleared or cultures are negative. If the mother's symptoms were mild and/or brief, and she is well postpartum, she can breast-feed as soon as the infant is well enough to be fed. Usually such infants require intravenous fluids and nutrition, at least briefly. Once the mother has had adequate medication to show negative cultures, her colostrum or milk can be expressed and given to the infant. The management of lactation and feeding in listeriosis is conducted supportively as it is in any situation in which the infant is extremely ill. Hospitalization is usually required for 4 weeks.

Because of the risk to the neonate it has been suggested that cultures for *Listeria* be done in the third trimester for all women when cultures are being done for gonococcus and herpes. It is certainly important to do such cultures when there is a flulike syndrome in the mother during the second half of pregnancy.

Bacterial diarrhea. Neonatal diarrhea due to various bacteria, but especially *E. coli,* is best managed by breast-feeding. Diarrhea in the mother due to infection is not a contraindication. Although infections of the gastrointestinal tract are among the principal causes of illness and death in infants in more than 85% of the world, death usually does not occur until after 4 months of age because of the incidence of early breast-feeding in other countries. Even when a diagnosis of infectious diarrhea is made in the mother, it is appropriate to treat with antibiotics that are also safe for the neonate and to start or continue breast-feeding. One should also obtain a culture from the infant without symptoms and treat accordingly. If this is a hospital-acquired disease, then the rigors of establishing the source of the outbreak are to be instituted. Epidemiological investigation and management of cases and contacts should be initiated. A surveillance system should be established for those in the cohort who are at home.

Viral infections

Rubella. Rubella can produce a variety of effects on the newborn in intrauterine infections from a classic constellation of defects to no apparent effect. Silent infections in the young infant are much more common than symptomatic ones. Schiff and co-workers[26] prospectively examined over 4000 infants born after the 1964 rubella epidemic using virological and serological techniques for the detection of infections in the newborn. The overall rate of congenital rubella was in excess of 2% during the epidemic, whereas it is usually 0.1 percent in endemic years. During the neonatal period 68% of the infected newborns in that study had subclinical infection; 71% of this group of neonates developed evidence of disease in the first 5 years of life. The infant who is shedding virus is contagious; he should be isolated until the presence or absence of infection can be established. The mother is not considered contagious once the placenta is delivered. The infant can be breast-fed. Isolation of the infant should not interfere with breast-feeding except for its inherent inconveniences. If the infant is clinically well the mother and infant can be discharged, even without all the laboratory results reported. At home they can nurse without restriction. Regardless of method of feeding, the family should protect pregnant women from contact with the infant until the rubella status is determined.

Rubella infection in the mother postpartum will be spread to the neonate long before it is identified. If breast-feeding, it should be continued. A sick breast-fed infant does better when breast-feeding is maintained.

Herpesvirus

CYTOMEGALOVIRUS. Cytomegalovirus is one of four known herpesviruses in the human. In addition to herpesvirus hominis (herpes simplex) and herpesvirus varicellae (varicella-zoster, V-Z) and Epstein-Barr virus (EBV), CMV has also been found to have ultrastructure and physiochemical properties of a herpesvirus.[7] CMV, EBV, and herpesvirus varicellae are believed to be antigenically related on the basis of crossreactions observed in indirect fluorescent antibody tests. Herpesvirus hominis and herpesvirus varicellae have antigenic similarities in crossneutralization tests. Two or more subgroups are believed to exist in the CMV group.

The significance for the newborn who does or does not have the virus, is whether or not it can be obtained by contact with his infected mother. If it can be picked up from extrauterine maternal contact, what are the risks of infection?

Table 14-1. Incidence of CMV in human milk of seropositive women*

Postpartum day	Number tested	Number positive	Percent positive
1-6 days	37	4	10.8
1-13 wk	26	13	50.0

*From Hayes, K.: N. Engl. J. Med. **287:**177, 1972, reprinted, by permission.

Seroepidemiological studies suggest that usually the infection is acquired in early infancy. A second rise in seroconversion rates occurs after puberty, suggesting venereal transmission at that time. CMV has been demonstrated in semen and cervical swabs. CMV cervicitis increases with gestational time during pregnancy. CMV has been isolated from the saliva and may well be transmitted by kissing.

Various studies[7,21] have detected that 3% to 28% of pregnant women have CMV in cervical cultures; 4% to 5% have CMV in their urine. CMV was found in the milk of seropositive women by Hayes and associates.[8] The data on these women with CMV-complement fixing (CF) antibody are shown in Table 14-1.

The time at which the virus gains access to the fetus may be an important determinant in the prognosis. Women who seroconvert early in pregnancy are more apt to have symptomatic infants, whereas infants born to mothers who seroconvert late in pregnancy are born with silent infections. It has been suggested that patients with periventricular calcifications acquire CMV encephalitis in the third or fourth month of gestation because this is the time that the subependymal matrix is most susceptible to damage by viruses. It has been observed that many infants are exposed to CMV during the descent through the birth canal because infections of the cervix at birth are not uncommon. This type of exposure is not associated with disease. Numazaki and co-workers[23] found 60% of Japanese infants to excrete virus in the urine or upper respiratory tract at 5 to 6 months of age. Some of the infections presumably occurred during passage through the birth canal, whereas others could have been transmitted through ingestion of the virus in mother's milk. In both instances, IgG antibody should have been present in the maternal serum, according to Hanshaw,[7] and have been transferred to the fetus prior to birth. It may well be that specific IgA is also transmitted. The newborn infant may be exposed to the virus at a time when he has received the passive transfer of antibodies from his mother. The lack of infection in the neonatal period may well be due to this passive and active transfer protection. These data provide evidence that infected mothers who are seropositive can breast-feed their infants safely.

HERPES SIMPLEX. Herpes simplex virus (HSV) infection in the neonatal period is often fatal or severely debilitating. Reviews spanning a 39-year period, including 276 patients, have been reported by Nahmias and colleagues.[22] The mode of transmission has been a critical question in management. Transplacental infections have been diagnosed because of the presence of HSV lesions at birth, recovery of the virus from the placenta or cord blood, demonstration of histological changes or the virus itself in the placenta, detection of elevated IgM levels in the cord blood, presence of typical congenital malformations, or presence of HSV viremia. Because the risk of exposure of the newborn to indivduals has not been fully determined, the question of removing personnel with herpetic lesions or subclinical infections from the nursery is still unsettled. No instances have been recorded of neonatal infection acquired from the mother after delivery, according to Nahmias and Visintine.[21] No information is available on transmission to the newborn of HSV by means of the breast milk. These authors recommended, therefore, that the possibility of mother-to-infant transmission of infection postpartum suggests that such infection might be prevented if the newborn does not have contact with his mother until her active infection is resolved.

CHICKENPOX. Chickenpox ranks as one of the most communicable diseases in a class with measles and smallpox. The incidence is reported at 5 cases/10,000 pregnancies.[36] There is no known reservoir of V-Z virus. Transfer is believed to be by respiratory droplet; contact infection from the lesions is also possible. In pregnancy, V-Z virus may be transmitted across the placenta, resulting in congenital or neonatal chickenpox. Most mothers and hospital personnel have had the disease and are not at risk. When chickenpox occurs in pregnancy, it is a highly lethal disease for the mother with death, when it occurs, usually resulting from varicella pneumonia, although there may be a bias of selective reporting (Table 14-2).

Perinatal chickenpox. Postnatally acquired chickenpox usually begins at 10 to 28 days of age and is more common than the congenitally acquired form but generally mild. Transmission in neonates is of a low order. Congenital chickenpox by definition occurs in infants less than 10 days of age. The attack rate is about 24% when the mother has the disease within 17 days of delivery. V-Z does not readily cross the placenta. Congenital chickenpox is associated with significant mortality. The case/fatality ratio is only 5%, that is 95% will either not get the disease or will not die. When the disease occurs more than a week before delivery,

Table 14-2. Fetal deaths in relation to gestational age following selected virus infections during pregnancy*

Infection	Weeks of gestation	Number of cases	Number of fetal deaths	Percent
Mumps	0-11	33	9	27.3
	12-27	51	1	2.0
	>28	43	0	—
Measles	0-11	19	3	15.8
	12-27	29	1	3.4
	>28	17	1	5.9
Chickenpox	0-11	32	5	15.6
	12-27	60	4	4.7
	>28	52	0	—
Controls	0-11	1010†	131	13.0
	12-27	392‡	15	3.8
	>28	152‡	1	0.7

*Modified from Siegel, M., Fuerst, H. T., and Peress, N. S.: N. Engl. J. Med. **274:**768, 1966; from Young, N. A.: Chickenpox, measles, and mumps. In Remington, J. S., and Klein, J. O., editors: Infectious disease of the fetus and newborn infant, Philadelphia, 1976, W. B. Saunders Co.
†Subjects attending prenatal clinic in first trimester without virus infections.
‡Controls matched for age, race, and parity of the mother and type of obstetrical service.

antibody titers in maternal and cord blood are the same. When the disease occurs within 4 days of delivery, maternal titers are positive and cord blood tests are negative. The greatest risk of nosocomial chickenpox exists when the mother develops lesions with 6 days of delivery. If the infant has lesions, he should be isolated with his mother and discharged as soon as condition permits. This infant should be allowed to breast-feed if the mother is well enough (Table 14-3).

When maternal chickenpox occurs within 6 days of delivery or immediately postpartum and no lesions are present in the neonate, mother and infant should be isolated separately. Only half the infants born to mothers who developed the disease 7 to 15 days before delivery will develop the disease. They should receive

Table 14-3. Guidelines for preventive measures after exposure to chickenpox in the nursery or maternity ward*

Type of exposure or disease	Locale of chickenpox lesions		Disposition
	Mother	**Neonate**	
A. Siblings at home have chickenpox when neonate and mother are ready for discharge from hospital	No	No	1. Neonate: protective isolation indicated. 2. Mother: with history of previous chickenpox, she may either remain with neonate or return to older children. Without previous history, she should remain with neonate until older siblings are no longer infectious.
B. Mother with no history of chickenpox exposed during period 6-20 days antepartum†	No	No	1. Exposed mother and infant: send home at earliest date unless siblings at home have communicable chickenpox. 2. Other mothers and infants: no special management indicated. 3. Physicians, nurses in delivery room and nursery: no precautions indicated if there is a history of previous chickenpox or zoster. In absence of history, immediate serologic testing‡ is indicated to determine immune status. Nonimmune personnel should be excluded from patient contact for 20 days.

*From Young, N. A.: Chickenpox, measles, and mumps. In Remington, J. S., and Klein, J. O., editors: Infectious disease of fetus and newborn infant, Philadelphia, 1976, W. B. Saunders Co.
†If exposure occurred less than 6 days antepartum, mother would not be potentially infectious until at least 72 hours postpartum.
‡Send serum to virus diagnostic laboratory for determination of complement-fixing (CF) antibodies or, preferably, indirect fluorescent antibodies. Personnel may continue to work for period of 9 days after exposure pending serologic results, since they are not potentially infectious during this period. CF antibodies to V-Z virus > 1:2 probably are indicative of immunity in the absence of recent infection caused by herpes simplex virus.
§Considered noninfectious when no new vesicles have appeared for 72 hours, and all lesions have progressed to the stage of crusts.
‖ZIG (zoster immune globulin) is available from Center for Disease Control. Atlanta, Georgia, or from regional consultants.

Continued.

Table 14-3. Guidelines for preventive measures after exposure to chickenpox in the nursery or maternity ward—cont'd

Type of exposure or disease	Locale of chickenpox lesions		Disposition
	Mother	Neonate	
C. Onset of maternal chickenpox ante-partum§ or post-partum	Yes	Yes	1. Infected mother and infant: isolate together until clinically stable, then send home. 2. Other mothers and infants: send home at earlier date. ZIG‖ or immune serum globulin may be given to exposed neonates. 3. Hospital personnel: same as B-3.
D. Onset of maternal chickenpox ante-partum§ or post-partum	Yes	No	1. Infected mother: isolate until no longer infectious.§ 2. Infected mother's infant: administer ZIG and isolate separately from mother. Send home with mother if no lesions develop by the time mother is noninfectious. 3. Other mothers and infants: same as C-2. 4. Hospital personnel: same as B-3.
E. Congenital chickenpox	No	Yes	1. Infected infant and its mother: same as C-1. 2. Other mothers and infants: same as C-2. 3. Hospital personnel: same as B-3.

zoster-immune globulin (ZIG) if available. If no lesions develop by the time the mother is noninfectious, they may be sent home together. When the mother and infant can be together, the child can be breast-fed (Table 14-7).

Measles. Measles is a highly communicable childhood disease, which is more severe in adult life or in the neonatal period. Measles is also a disease that can be prevented by immunization. The disease is contagious from the onset of the rash. Incidence of the disease in pregnancy prior to immunization is low, 0.4/10,000 pregnancies because most adults are immune.[36] Perinatal measles includes trans-placental infection as well as disease acquired postnatally by the respiratory route. Measles acquired in the first 10 days of life may be considered transplacental. When measles occurs after 14 days it is due to extrauterine exposure. The course of extrauterine exposure is mild. A case is described in which an infant developed the disease on the fourteenth day of age, and it had a very benign course. The infant had been nursed at the breast by his mother in whom the prodromata of measles occurred on the first day postpartum. Since secretory antibodies occur within 48 hr of onset, it is possible that the disease was mitigated by the presence of measles-specific IgA in the mother's milk.

As with chickenpox, the incidence of disease postpartum is minimal. The same precautions noted in the discussion of varicella are appropriate. If the mother is exposed just before delivery, mother and infant should be isolated separately, since only half the infants will acquire the disease. If the mother and infant can be isolated together because the infant has the disease, he can be breast-fed. Since specific antibodies are present in the milk in 48 hr, the value of the antibodies after that time would outweigh any theoretical risk (Tables 14-2 and 14-7).

Mumps. Mumps is also an acute generalized communicable disease. It is characterized by parotid gland swelling and involvement of other glands. It is also preventable by immunization. It is less contagious, thus more adults are still susceptible. Incidence in pregnancy is from 0.8 to 10 cases/10,000 pregnancies.[36] Mumps in pregnancy, however, is generally benign. Mumps virus has been isolated on the third postpartum day from the milk of a woman who developed parotitis 2 days antepartum. She did not breast-feed, and her infant did not develop clinical mumps (Table 14-2).

Mumps is not a major hazard in newborn nurseries. A mother with the disease should be isolated from the other patients but need not be separated from her infant. Clinically apparent mumps with parotitis during the first year of life tends to be very mild. Although mastitis is a rare complication of mumps in any mature female, no data are available to suggest that the incidence is greater in lactating women. Should it occur, breast-feeding should continue because the exposure has already occurred during the prodromata and the IgA in the breast milk may help to mitigate the symptoms in the infant.

Hepatitis. The two major types of hepatitis are hepatitis A and hepatitis B. Hepatitis A is defined as the virus that causes the short incubation form of viral hepatitis; it has also been referred to as infectious hepatitis. Its virus has not yet been isolated, although electron-microscopy has identified probable virus particles. Hepatitis B (HBV) is the virus that causes the long-incubation form of viral hepatitis. This form has also been called serum hepatitis and Australian antigen hepatitis. Most of the information available on epidemiology, immunology, mode of transmission, pathogenesis, and clinical disease is about hepatitis B, mainly because its virus has been isolated. Hepatitis A virus and the immune reactions to it are considered distinct from those of hepatitis B.[6]

TRANSMISSION

Carrier state in mothers. The chief concern here is the mode of transmission of the virus from mother to infant. The transmission of hepatitis B virus from mothers whose blood contains HB$_s$Ag to their infants has been described. This is called vertical transmission. It may occur transplacentally in utero, at the time of delivery, or shortly after delivery. The transmission between any two individuals who may be close contacts is termed horizontal transmission. Work in Taiwan where hepatitis occurs in 5% to 20% of the cases (one of the highest rates in the world), showed that 51 infants of 158 carrier mothers developed antigenemia within 6 months of life. This high frequency has not been observed in other populations. When the mother had a prenatal complement-fixation titer in her serum of 1:64 for HB$_s$Ag, over 90% of the infants were positive. This appears to be vertical transmission. The high incidence of transmission of hepatitis B virus in Taiwan and Japan from carrier mothers to infants suggests that the virus passes the placental barrier easily. In other countries, there has been almost no evidence (0% to 8.3%) of transplacental transmission carrier mothers with infants remaining negative (Table 14-4).

Table 14-4. Transmission of HBV from HB$_s$Ag-carrier mothers to neonates in various geographic areas*

Investigator	Location	Patients studied	Number infants HB$_s$ Ag-positive	Vertical transmission† (%)
Stevens (1975)	Taiwan	158	63	40
Okada (1975)	Japan	11‡	8	73
Schweitzer (1973)	United States	21	1	4.8
Schweitzer (1975)	United States	36	3	8.3
Skinhoj (1972)	Denmark	36	0	0
Papaevangelou (1973)	Greece	12	1	8.3
Punyagupata (1973)	Thailand	14	0	0
Ariz (1973)	Pakistan	26	1	3.8

*From Crumpacker, C. S.: Hepatitis. In Remington, J. S., and Klein, J. O., editors: Infectious disease of fetus and newborn infant, Philadelphia, 1976, W. B. Saunders Co.
†Vertical transmission means transmission from mother to infant and may occur in utero, at the time of delivery, or shortly after delivery.
‡One hundred thirty-nine HB$_s$Ag-positive carrier mothers were studied, but only eleven infants participated in follow-up.

Table 14-5. Transmission of HBV from mothers with acute hepatitis B during or after pregnancy*

	Investigator		
	Cossart (1974)	Merrill (1972)	Schweitzer (1973)
Acute hepatitis B during 1st and 2nd trimester			
Number of mothers	1	1	10
Number of infants	0	0	1
Transmission (%)	0	0	10
Acute hepatitis B during 3rd trimester or within 2 months postpartum			
Number of mothers	4	4	21
Number of infants	2	4	16
Transmission (%)	50	100	76

*From Crumpacker, C. S.: Hepatitis. In Remington, J. S., and Klein, J. O., editors: Infectious disease of fetus and newborn infant, Philadelphia, 1976, W. B. Saunders Co.

Mothers with acute hepatitis B in pregnancy. Infants born to mothers who have acute HB$_s$Ag-positive hepatitis during the perinatal period are at greater risk for transmission (Table 14-5). Studies in the United States by Schweitzer and co-workers[27,28] on a series of mothers who developed hepatitis within 2 months of delivery suggested that three newborns developed disease transplacentally (they had positive cord bloods), but the majority were infected at birth (eight infants of seventeen mothers). None of the HB$_s$Ag-positive infants were breast-fed; this excluded mother's milk as a mode of transmission in these cases. Schweitzer and colleagues[28] further demonstrated that the frequency of HBV transmission from mother to infant is high (76%) when the disease occurs in the third trimester or early in the postpartum period. Transmission is only 10% when the disease occurs in the first two trimesters. These data and other studies suggest that the neonate becomes infected primarily during the birth process itself. Antibody levels in the mother and cord blood are comparable. Thus it appears that the antibody crosses the placenta more easily than the virus.

Transmission via postpartum fecal-oral route. Transmission via the fecal-oral route can occur. Hepatitis is highly contagious. HB_sAg has been isolated from saliva, stool, urine, prostatic fluid, and seminal fluid. The incidence by this route, however, is small, as is demonstrated by the fact that few infants have a positive reaction when the mothers have the disease at delivery and the cord blood is negative.

Transmission via colostrum or breast milk. HB_sAg is found in breast milk, therefore transmission via the milk is possible. As noted earlier, infants of mothers with the virus in their milk but who did not breast-feed them developed virus and antibodies anyway.

CLINICAL MANAGEMENT. There is a high incidence of prematurity (35%) in infants born to mothers with hepatitis, regardless of the infection in the infant. The long-term effects of chronic neonatal HBV infections are not known. Fatal cases of neonatal hepatitis are rare (only five cases reported in the literature, all occurring in infants of carriers, with two in each of two families). Specific-antibody prophylaxis of infants born to mothers with acute HG_sAg-postive hepatitis at the time of delivery appears to be effective in preventing neonatal HBV infection. Both infants of carriers and those with acute hepatitis should receive high-titer hepatitis B–immune globulin (0.25 ml of a 16% solution) or standard immune globulin (2.0 ml) given immediately after delivery.

Because it is highly contagious, an HB_sAg-positive infant should be isolated and all secretion, excretions, and instruments handled with adequate precautions. Although there are no data to suggest that mother and infant should be isolated from each other, Crumpacker[6] and others are firm in their recommendation that mothers should be discouraged from breast-feeding (Table 14-7).

Toxoplasmosis

Toxoplasmosis is one of the most common infections of humans throughout the world.[25] The protozoan organism is ubiquitous in nature and is the cause of a variety of illnesses that were previously thought to be due to other agents or unknown causes. The normal host is the cat. In humans, prevalence of positive serological test titers increases with age, indicating past exposure, and there is equal distribution in males and females in the United States, but not in Norway, El Salvador, or Poland. The risk to the fetus is related to the time when the maternal infection occurs. In the last months of pregnancy, the protozoa are most frequently transmitted to the fetus but the infection is subclinical in the newborn. Early in pregnancy, the transmission to the fetus occurs less often but does result in severe disease. Once the placenta has been infected, it remains so throughout pregnancy. *Toxoplasma gondii* have been isolated from the milk, menstrual fluid, placenta, lochia, amniotic fluid, embryo, and fetal brain in 33% of the subjects in one series.

Table 14-6. Outcome of 180 pregnancies in which maternal toxoplasmosis was acquired during gestation: incidence of symptomatic congenital toxoplasmosis among offspring surviving the early newborn period*

Newborn	Number (%)	Percentage of total newborns
Not infected	110	61
Infected	64	36
Clinically normal	46† (72)	26
Clinically abnormal	18 (28)	10
Mild disease	11‡ (17)	6
Severe disease	7§ (11)	4
Neonatal deaths	6‖	3

*Adapted from Desmonts, G., and Couvreur, J.: Bull. N.Y. Acad. Med. **50**:146, 1974; from Remington, J. S., and Desmonts, G.: Toxoplasmosis. In Remington, J. S., and Klein, J. O., editors: Infectious disease of fetus and newborn infant, Philadelphia, 1976, W. B. Saunders Co.
†Seven not examined until 14 to 45 months postpartum.
‡Ten with isolated ocular lesions discovered during systematic fundus examinations; one had isolated intracranial calcifications.
§Five with involvement of eye and central nervous system present at birth; two with delayed onset of disease.
‖Two had generalized toxoplasmosis; four fetuses were lost to examination.

In various animal models, the toxoplasmas have been transmitted via the milk to the suckling young. They have been isolated from colostrum as well. The newborn animals became asymptomatically infected when nursed by an infected mother when her colostrum contained *Toxoplasma gondii*. Three of eighteen women were reported by Langer[16] to have *Toxoplasma gondii* in their milk. Two of these mothers had negative dye tests and complement. His results have been questioned because of the inadvertent presence of pollen grains in the preparation and the confusion between specimens.

Transmission during breast-feeding in humans has not been demonstrated, however. It is possible that unpasteurized cow's milk could be a vehicle of transmission. The human mother, however, would provide appropriate antibodies via her milk. From this information it appears there is no evidence to support depriving the neonate of his mother's milk when the mother is known to be infected with *Toxoplasma gondii*[25] (Tables 14-6 and 14-7).

Vulvovaginitis

Normally during pregnancy there is an increase in cervical and vaginal secretions. Only about 1% of women have symptomatic vulvovaginitis.[5] The normal flora of the vagina at a pH of 4.5 includes predominantly Döderlein's bacilli with some bacteroides, enterococci, group B β-hemolytic streptococci, diphtheroid organisms, or coliform bacteria. Vaginitis is identified when there is inflammation and discharge associated with an alkaline pH and absence of Döderlein's bacilli. The usual pathogens are *Trichomonas vaginalis* and *Candida albicans*.

Monilial vulvovaginitis. Monilial vulvovaginitis is usually benign, but bothersome except during pregnancy and lactation, when it is difficult to treat. The infant may become infected coming through the birth canal. It is manifest in the newborn as an oral infection, or thrush. The breast-fed infant may transmit the oral infection to the breast and then the infection is passed back and forth unless both mother and infant are adequately treated. *Candida albicans,* the causative organism, is a fungus, which thrives on milk in the breast or in the mouth. Early lesions in a newborn who is bottle-fed can be treated by rinsing the mouth with water after each feeding so there are no curds for the fungi to thrive on. When the infant is breast-fed, however, it is important to be vigorous with treatment immediately in an effort to avoid a chronic *Candida* infection of the breast.

The recommended treatment for the infant is rinsing his mouth with water after each feeding and giving 1 ml of nystatin (Mycostatin) suspension carefully by dropper onto the oral lesions. This treatment should be used for 2 weeks even though the mouth appears to have cleared prior to the fourteenth day. The major reason for apparent relapse is that therapy is terminated as soon as the caseous plaque seem to disappear. Simultaneous treatment of the mother should include the use of nystatin ointment to both nipple and areola areas after each feeding and appropriate washing each day. The absorbent pads the mother uses in her nursing brassiere should be changed with each feeding and be of the disposable variety.

If this infant also is given a rubber nipple or uses a pacifier, these should be boiled daily for 20 min and discarded after a week of therapy and new ones used. Reseeding can occur from other articles that are placed in the mouth. Properly treated, thrush should not be a cause for weaning from the breast.

Trichomonas vaginalis infection. A common cause of vaginitis is the parasite, *Trichomonas vaginalis,* which usually causes an asymptomatic infection in both male and female. The parasite is found in 10% to 25% of women in the childbearing years. It is transmitted predominantly by sexual intercourse. Symptoms are common in pregnancy when the infection is more difficult to cure. There is some evidence that growth of the parasite is enhanced by estrogens. It is more difficult to treat in women taking oral contraceptives. The difficulty encountered in lactation stems from the fact that the drugs of choice are contraindicated for the infant during lactation. The organism has not been identified as a particular threat to the neonate who is otherwise healthy. The treatment of choice is metronidazole (Flagyl). Metronidazole, however, does appear in the breast milk with milk levels parallelling serum levels.[1,2] Severe systemic reactions occur including headache, nausea, vomiting, and diarrhea when taken in conjunction with alcohol. Leukopenia and neurological symptoms have been described in adults who take metronidazole. Concern has been expressed because of the tumorgenicity in laboratory animals. On the other hand, metronidazole is given to children with serious infections with sensitive parasites such as amebas. It is recommended therefore that the use of metronidazole be limited to those patients in whom local palliative treatment has been inadequate. The peak serum levels occur about 1 hour after oral ingestion; therefore therapy, which is usually given three times a day, should be timed so that the peak serum levels occur between nursings. Roughly, three times a day would be after alternate feedings. An alternative approach would be to pump the breasts for the week of therapy. It should be pointed out again that the infant who is solely breast-fed is at greater risk than the older infant who is getting other nourishment (Chapter 11). Thus the older infant (over 6 months of age) may not get much drug when doses are carefully timed.

Table 14-7. Management of infectious disease

Organism	Condition	Isolate from mother	Mother can visit nursery	Mother can breast-feed	Immediate treatment	Contact with pregnant women allowed
Bacteria	Premature rupture of membranes; longer than 24 hr without fever					
	Full-term infant	No	Yes	Yes	Observe	Yes
	Premature infant	No	Yes	Yes	Treat with ampicillin and kanamycin	Yes
	Maternal fever greater than 38° C twice, 4 hr apart, 24 hr before to 24 hr after delivery, or endometriosis; full-term or premature infant	Yes, until mother afebrile 24 hr	No, until mother afebrile 24 hr	No, until mother afebrile 24 hr	Treat with ampicillin and kanamycin	Yes
Salmonella, Shigella		No	Yes, if culture negative	Yes, if culture negative	In most cases	Yes
Staphylococcus		No	Yes	Yes	Yes	Yes
Group B β-streptococcus	Mother with possible cervical culture but otherwise negative obstetrical history	No	Yes	Yes	Yes	Yes
	Mother with possible cervical culture and obstetrical history of fever, premature rupture of membranes >24 hr, fetal distress, meconium, low Apgar score, any symptoms of prematurity	No	Yes	Yes, after treatment	Treat with ampicillin and kanamycin	Yes
	Infant with surface colonizing					
	Negative history and PE	No	Yes	Yes	Observe	Yes
	With premature rupture of membrane or maternal infection	No	Yes	Yes	Treat with penicillin	Yes
Group A streptococcus	Mother with infection	Yes	Not in acute stage	Not in acute stage; after 24 hr treatment	Prophylactic penicillin for 10 days	Yes

Gonorrhea					
Mother with positive smear or culture; infant well	No	Yes, after treatment	Yes, after treatment	AgNO₃ to the eyes, once in delivery room and one in nursery	Yes
Infant with conjunctivitis	No	Yes, after treatment	Yes, after treatment	Penicillin IM or IV, plus chloramphenicol drops topically	Yes
Syphilis					
Mother with positive VDRL or clinical disease not treated	Only if mother with second-degree disease or with skin lesions	No, if skin lesions; yes, otherwise	Yes	Penicillin IM or IV after work-up done; follow-up after discharge	Yes
Mother treated	No	Yes	Yes		Yes
Tuberculosis					
Mother with inactive disease	No	Yes	Yes	Consider BCG if follow-up in doubt	Yes
Hepatitis					
Mother had in first trimester, well at delivery	No	Yes	Yes		Yes
Mother with active hepatitis at delivery or in third trimester	No, may room-in after good handwash technique followed	No	No	Pooled globulin or hyperimmune if available	Yes
Mother is chronic carrier	No	Yes, not kiss other infants	Ask for infectious disease opinion		Yes
Protozoa					
Toxoplasma					
Toxoplasmosis	No	Yes	Yes		No

$AgNO_3$

MATERNAL DIABETES

Pregnancy has become a more common event in the well-controlled diabetic and fertility rates compare with those of nondiabetics. Much has been said about labor and delivery in the diabetic and almost nothing about lactation in these mothers. Textbooks on diabetes often do not mention lactation except those written prior to 1960, perhaps reflecting the national trends away from breast-feeding. A mother, although diabetic, should be offered the same opportunity to breast-feed that is offered to all patients unless her disease has so incapacitated her that any stress is out of the question.

Brudenell and Beard[4] indicate that when the diabetic infant's progress is uneventful and he can be treated normally, there is no contraindication to breast-feeding. They believe that lactation is more difficult in diabetic mothers, perhaps as a result of operative delivery or the need to keep the infant in a special care unit for the first few days of life.

During the last stages of pregnancy in normal women, there is a more or less constant excretion of lactose in the urine. During the last few days before delivery there is a marked rise in the level of lactose in the urine with the height reached on the day of delivery. Following delivery, the lactose excretion immediately drops to a low level where it remains for from 2 to 5 days, followed by a sudden large excretion of lactose in the normal woman. Lactosuria in the diabetic may lead to diagnostic confusion. It occurs normally late in pregnancy and in the postpartum period before the infant takes much milk, if the mother does not nurse, or if the supply of milk exceeds the requirement of the infant. Lactose reabsorbed from the breasts is excreted in the urine.

In the diabetic lactating woman, the concentration of lactose in the breast milk remained remarkably constant despite very marked elevations or depressions of the blood glucose concentration, according to Joselin and associates.[12] During lactation, lactosuria occurs physiologically and must be distinguished from glucosuria. Lactation is recorded by Wilder[35] as decreasing the blood sugar level. The sparing effect of lactation on the insulin requirement has been observed by many, including Joselin and co-workers.[12] The depression of the level of the blood sugar in normal nursing diabetic women may lead to hypoglycemic symptoms. The simultaneous lactosuria may be misdiagnosed as glucosuria and excessive insulin be taken. The improved tolerance has been explained by the transference of sugar from the blood to the breast for conversion to galactose and lactose. Joselin and colleagues[12] report that the majority of patients at the Joselin Clinic, as well as those at Johns Hopkins Hospital, breast-feed in whole or in part. They recommend the increased administration of the B vitamins for the diabetic during lactation, based on work by Tarr and McNeile.[30]

Diet for the lactating diabetic

Although it is clearly demonstrated that all lactating mothers have an increased energy requirement, it is critical to the diabetic to identify this need and provide for it in dietary adjustments. The 300 kcal required by the infant initially means at least 500 to 800 additional kcal in the mother's diet. Since the milk is synthesized from maternal stores and substrates, the plasma glucose levels in the lactating diabetic will be lower. The daily maternal insulin requirement is usually much less. The balance is a significant one between the needs of the infant and the energy and nutrition production in the mother. Most postpartum women, including the diabetic, have fat stores developed during pregnancy in preparation by the body for lactation. The diabetic, when balancing diet and insulin, needs to consider that the course of lactation mobilizes these fat stores as substrate for the mammary gland. It has been recommended by Tyson[31] that the diet include no less than 100 g of carbohydrate and 20 g of protein. This will permit the continued mobilization of fat stores to produce the glucose needed for mother and milk. When a diabetic increases fat metabolism there is always the risk of ketonemia and ketonuria. This indicates a need for increased kilocalories in both the diabetic and the nondiabetic. With some careful observations of blood and urine sugar levels and anticipatory guidance, lactation can be managed without hypoglycemia or hyperglycemia.

Adjustments to lactation for the diabetic

The literature is singularly devoid of any specific discussion of the management of lactation for the diabetic with the notable exception of a personal experience recorded by Miller.[18] Miller points out that management depends on the classification of the diabetes.

The mild, or class A, diabetic whose condition can be controlled by diet alone will have to modify her diet to include the increased caloric needs, taking adequate protein, in particular. It has been stated by O'Brien[24] and Vorherr[33] that little or no tolbutamide or other antidiabetic agents appear in breast milk. It should be noted, however, that most diabetic specialists believe there is no place for these oral medications in females in the childbearing years. The mother with insulin-dependent diabetes will usually be able to increase her diet and maintain her insulin level, although some may find insulin requirements will be reduced also. Monitoring blood sugars and acetone will be necessary at first to achieve the correct balance.

Although hypoglycemia does not cause a reduction in lactose in the milk, the phenomenon of hypoglycemia itself will cause increased secretion of epinephrine in insulin shock. The epinephrine will inhibit milk production and the ejection reflex. Miller[18] points out the necessity of using a method of testing the urine that measures only glucose, such as Tes-Tape.* Otherwise the physiologic lacturia may cause inappropriate conclusions as to insulin requirements. Acetone signals a need for increased calories and carbohydrate. In addition, elevated acetone can cause increased acetone in the milk itself, which is a stress to the newborn liver. If one merely increases insulin to clear the acetone, it may predispose to hypoglycemia. Each individual mother will identify the point below which she can not reduce her insulin dosage without producing acetonuria.

Usually the insulin requirements are proportional to needs during pregnancy. One who takes large doses may even have to drop the dose by 50% and increase her dietary intake 100%. While the infant is nursing exclusively at the breast, adjustment is usually smooth. Weaning may present some need for day-to-day adjustment, since the amount of milk taken by the infant varies. Many infants take more 1 day and less the next, and it is less pedictable. If blood sugars cannot be controlled by diet during this time, then insulin will have to be decreased. If the weaning is gradual and continuous, the adjustment will be similar.

---

*Tes-Tape is manufactured by the Lilly Co.

Special features of lactation for the diabetic

Some diabetics enjoy a postpartum remission of their diabetes that may be minimal or complete. The remission may last through lactation; it may last several years. This remission has been attributed to the hormone interactions that affect the hypothalamus and pituitary gland during pregnancy, labor, delivery, and lactation. Many diabetics report a feeling of well-being during lactation.

Diabetics are prone to infection, and therefore mastitis presents a particular problem. With careful anticipatory care, avoidance of fatigue, and antibiotics for at least 10 days when indicated, mastitis should not pose a threat. Monilial infections are more common because of the glucose-rich vaginal secretions, and most diabetic women are alert to the early signs of a fungal vaginitis. Infection of the nipples can also occur due to *Candida albicans* even though the infant does not have obvious thrush. Early specific treatment with nystatin ointment to the breast and nystatin suspension for the infant whenever sore nipples do not respond to the usual nonspecific treatment is recommended. Treatment of both mother and infant simultaneously is necessary or they will reseed each other.

The advantages of breast-feeding to the diabetic beyond the experience of nurturing and nourishing include the advantages of transient amenorrhea. The decreased or absence of menstrual bleeding preserved iron stores. In addition, it keeps chances of pregnancy minimal as the postpartum infertility of the lactating diabetic is thought to be more consistent and predictable than in the nondiabetic. Miller concludes, "The diabetic mother who chooses to nurse her baby presents a situation about which little is known. In addition to the usual advantages which nursing affords the baby, it is highly beneficial to the mother because lactation is an anti-diabetogenic factor. The metabolic process of milk production and lactose supply added to the hormone balance during lactation serves to improve the health of the diabetic mother on both the clinical and physical levels. The chief problem to overcome is adjusting the diet and insulin to correspond with the mother's requirements during this remission."[18]

Infants of diabetics present a special problem in breast-feeding as noted by Lubchenco[17] because they are often premature, frequently have respiratory distress syndrome and hyperbilirubinemia, and may be poor feeders at first. Hypoglycemia is the immediate problem and its management may initially preclude dependency on breast milk as the sole source of nourishment. Since less than half do develop problems, many need not be separated from their mothers. For those requiring special or intensive care, lactation may have to be postponed briefly, depending on the infant's status.

THYROID DISEASE

The thyroid gland is intimately involved with hormone activity of pregnancy. The metabolic and hormonal demands of pregnancy alter the thyroid gland. Conversely, the outcome of pregnancy may be altered by changes in the thyroid gland. The thyroxine-binding globulin increases secondary to the increased estrogens. The normal pregnant woman may be euthyroid yet there are changes in the basal metabolic rate, radioactive iodine uptake, and thyroid size.

Thyroid disease is four times more common in women then men and thyroid abnormality is common in pregnancy. The diagnosis is more difficult to make during pregnancy because of problems with the interpretation of thyroid function tests. Treatment must take into account the presence of the fetus once the management decision is made.

Maternal hypothyroidism

It has long been held that hypothyroidism is associated with infertility. There is a low incidence of hypothyroidism during pregnancy. Because of the difficulty in maintaining pregnancy in hypothyroid individuals, the number of women who are truly hypothyroid at delivery is also low. There are women who are maintained on thyroid treatment for one reason or another who do have children. If hypothyroidism is diagnosed, it should be treated with full replacement therapy equivalent to 3 grains of desiccated thyroid daily. The medication should be continued after delivery. The mother should be permitted to breast-feed without question. Previous reports have indicated that thyroid does not appear in human milk. Data from Bode and co-workers[3] indicate there is measurable thyroid in milk of normal women. In any event breast-feeding is not contraindicated. If the mother is truly hypothyroid, particular care should be used to rule out hypothyroidism in the infant, using neonatal screening with T_4 and TSH if necessary. Diagnosis can be performed by evaluating blood values and is not a hazard to the nursling.

Hyperthyroidism. The diagnostic procedures and therapeutic management of the mother with possible hyperthyroidism presents some hazards to the breast-fed infant. The diagnosis can be made without radioactive material. The combination of an elevated serum T_4 and a normal resin triiodothyronine uptake is helpful. These two determinations can be combined to obtain a free tyroxine index, which reflects these determinations in a single value. Whether the patient is operated on eventually or not, her thyrotoxicosis must first be medically stabilized.

The treatment includes antithyroid medication with thiourea compounds, which inhibit the synthesis of thyroid hormone by blocking iodination of the tyrosine molecule. Propylthiouracil (PTU) and methimazole (Tapazole) are the treatments of choice for the mother. The major difficulty in their use in pregnancy is that PTU may cause fetal goiter and possibly hypothyroidism. The goiter is thought to be the result of inhibition of fetal thyroid hormone production by PTU with resulting increase in fetal TSH and thyroid gland enlargement. In forty-one pregnancies in thirty patients receiving antithyroid medication, five infants developed goiters. Goiter development was not dose related. It has been recommended that the maternal therapy also include dessicated thyroid on the basis that the various components of thyroid metabolism cross the placenta at different rates.[5]

The lactating mother presents a somewhat similar problem. Vorherr[33] reports 4.5% to 6% of PTU appears in breast milk, which could become an undesirable cumulative dose when the infant is nursed six to eight times per day. It has been suggested that the infant can be breast-fed and monitored biochemically. Now that microtechniques are available for determining T_3, T_4, and TSH levels, monitoring should not be a technical problem. Physical examination would reveal bradycardia or other signs of hypothryroidism and goiter. It has also been suggested that the infant may be given 0.125 to 0.25 grain of thyroid daily. Certainly this situation should be under close medical surveillance and continually monitored by microanalysis. The clinical judgment rests with the physician as to whether sufficient medication is reaching the infant. The older infant (over 6 months of age) who is getting other diet such as solids would be at less risk than the newborn, who depends solely on breast milk.

MALIGNANCY AND OTHER SITUATIONS REQUIRING RADIOACTIVE EXPOSURE

The treatment of a lactating woman with malignancy may well necessitate the use of radioactive compounds for diagnosis and treatment or the use of anti-metabolites. Since the breast is a minor route of excretion for most of these compounds, it is probably inappropriate to continue nursing during such exposure. Although the dose of the material in a single aliquot of milk may be small, the effects are cumulative (Appendix F). There are no long-range studies to indicate the outcome of offspring exposed in utero. In addition, a mother with malignancy should be encouraged to spare all her resources to overcome the disease. Lactation is as draining in such a situation as pregnancy.

Diagnostic or therapeutic measures using radioactive materials are contraindicated in pregnancy and lactation, since they tend to accumulate in the fetoneonatal thyroid and the maternal breast. If radioactive testing is deemed essential before treatment can be carried out, a test dose of ^{131}I can be given and breast-feeding discontinued for 48 hr. The validity of the test during lactation has been questioned because the mammary gland may divert a disproportionate amount of ^{131}I to the milk. The milk should be expressed during the 48 hr period and discarded.[34]

SMOKING

The pharmacological effects of nicotine have been studied in the fetuses of experimental animals. The active components of cigarette smoke, nicotine and carbon monoxide, have been implicated in the birth-weight reduction seen in infants of mothers who are heavy smokers. Nicotine has acetylcholine-like actions on the CNS, skeletal muscle, and upper sympathetic and parasympathetic ganglia. Nicotine initially stimulates and then depresses. Nicotine has been shown to interfere with the let-down reflex, but it does not appear to disrupt lactation once it has been initiated. Smoking has been associated with a poor milk supply. It has been reported by Arena[2] that women who smoke ten to twenty cigarettes a day have 0.4 to 0.5 mg of nicotine/L in their milk. He further calculated by Clark's law of dosage calculation that this is equivalent to a dose of 6 to 7.5 mg of nicotine in an adult. In an adult, 4 mg of nicotine has produced symptoms, and the lethal dosage is in the range of 40 to 60 mg for adults. On the basis of gradual intake over a day's time the neonate would metabolize it in the liver and excrete the chemical through the kidney. Low-grade responses to nicotine would be subtle in the neonate and require specific monitoring to detect. The effects of smoking need further study and clarification in lactation. Recent evidence has pointed to the effect on nutrition as being related to the low birth weight associated with infants of heavy smokers. The effect of chronic elevation of blood carbon monoxide levels on milk is unknown.

In counseling the nursing mother who smokes, consideration should be given to the data. The data suggest that mothers not smoke while nursing, or at least until they have initiated let-down, that they not blow smoke in the infant's face, and that they be cautious about the hot ashes. If it is not possible to stop, they should cut down and also consider low-nicotine cigarettes.

If the mother smokes marijuana an entirely different risk is created. Animal studies have shown that structural changes occur in the brain cells of newborn animals nursed by mothers whose milk contained cannabis. Nahas and co-workers[19,20] describe impairment of DNA and RNA formation and of proteins essential for proper growth and development. Results seen in some humans suggest that serious and long-lasting effects can occur. Impairment of judgment and behavioral changes may actually interfere with an individual's ability to care for the infant or adequately breast-feed. If the mother smokes while nursing there is not only the drug in her milk but the effect of the smoke that the infant inhales from the environment. Since brain cell development is still taking place in the first months of life, any remote chance that DNA and RNA metabolism is altered should be viewed with concern.

THE MOTHER WHO REQUIRES HOSPITALIZATION
Emergency admission

The mother who suddenly develops an emergency condition that requires hospitalization presents a unique problem in management. It is patently obvious that the emergency condition must be dealt with appropriately medically, surgically, or psychiatrically. It is equally important in all three situations to deal with her as a lactating mother, since failure to do so may have an impact on the successful outcome of the primary condition.

Medical admission. Medical problems such as acute infection or metabolic disturbances should be analyzed in relationship to lactation and to the infant and, in addition, to any other children at home. Is it contagious? In the case of lactation, will the drugs pass into the breast milk? If so, are there alternative treatments? What is the prognosis for recovery? Is the recovery phase less than 2 weeks and is maintaining lactation justified? This decision should not be made in the abstract without an understanding of the mother's commitment to further breast-feeding. If the prognosis is poor for recovery or the drugs involved are contraindicated for the infant but necessary for the mother, provision should be made for the mother's adjusting. It should be kept in mind that abrupt cessation of lactation can cause a flulike syndrome, which will confuse the management picture. It may be advisable to include the mother's obstetrician or pediatrician in the discussion to provide the mother with the necessary support to accept alternatives (Chapter 11).

Surgical admission. Surgical emergencies such as trauma, appendicitis, or chylocystitis will require immediate attention, including anesthesia and surgery. If it is a self-limited disease with a short postoperative course, as in appendicitis, the mother can go back to breast-feeding on return home. If the hospitalization will be more prolonged, as in trauma with immobilizing fractures, different considerations are important. It is possible to have the infant brought to the hospital several times a day for nursing. Unless the mother is mobile enough to provide some of the infant's bedside care, rooming-in is too taxing on the recovering patient. It is also stressful to other patients and staff who are not equipped for neonates. The mother would require a single room. If she has provision for her own nursing care or if the nursing staff is agreeable, an arrangement could be worked out. The only contraindication would be whether it would interfere with recovery. When bone healing is important, dietary demands of bone healing and lactation, especially in calcium, phosphorus, and vitamin intakes should be accounted for. If the mother is to be cared for but immobilized at home, nursing is easier but provision for ample assistance would be mandatory. The needs for assistance would not differ for the breast- or bottle-fed infant of the same age.

Psychiatric admission. The onset of a psychiatric crisis in a lactating mother is rarely a problem unless the mother has already been identified as having a psychiatric problem. The role of the mother in lactation will be a part of her psychiatric care, and the decision to breast-feed or not should be worked out with her psychiatrist. Most psychiatric wards can accommodate young infants whether breast- or bottle-fed, so it is less of a novelty than on the medical and surgical wards. The management of postpartum psychosis includes the concerns of the mother caring for the infant as part of recovery. The drugs used when the mother is nursing should be appropriate.

Elective maternal admission to the hospital

There are occasions when a lactating mother may have to plan for hospitalization. The urgency will be determined by the underlying disease. If the admission date can be made for over a month away, there is time for gradual weaning of the infant, if this is necessary. If weaning is appropriate and/or necessary the impact will largely be determined by the age of the infant. A very young infant who would profit greatly by continued breast-feeding is one type of problem. If the child is a year old, it may be less traumatic for him to be weaned when the separation time is going to be greater than 48 to 72 hours. A child who is also receiving solids and some other liquids from a cup can sustain himself during the separation without much more than sadness. If the caretaker and the surroundings are familiar, the support of this infant is easier. For the mother of the older child the impact of forced separation during hospitalization is also easier and less likely to produce "milk fever."

The young infant can be sustained by bottle-feedings or "wet nursing" by another lactating mother until he can be breast-fed by his own mother again. The mother in the first few months of lactation will have more problems with engorgement, discomfort, and even malaise. Provision should be made to express or pump milk to maintain supply if she will be nursing again or pumping minimally for comfort if lactation is to be discontinued. Milk can be collected in sterile bottles and sent home for the infant. When the admission is elective, plans can be made in advance to have a pump available, renting one if the hospital is not equipped. Methods for collecting, refrigerating, and getting milk home to the infant can be planned along with her other needs, such as a babysitter.

During an elective admission for a self-limited disease, rooming-in for the infant may be possible if the circumstances of the illness permit. It should be pointed out that the prime purpose of the hospitalization is to treat an illness. If surgery is involved, rooming-in should not be a stress to the mother when she is in the operating room, recovery room, or heavily medicated.

The purpose of this section is to point out that it is possible to maintain lactation when hospitalization is necessary for the mother. It is possible to have the infant accompany the mother or vice versa in a rooming-in arrangement. The theoretical threat of infection in the hospital setting is outweighed by the advantages of human milk in most cases. On the other hand, the decision rests with the physician in charge of the case who will have the responsibility of looking at the total picture, including the medical problem in question, the necessary treatment, and the short-range prognosis for resuming normal breast-feeding. Here again the expertise of the mother's obstetrician and the infant's pediatrician may be invaluable.

REFERENCES

1. American Academy of Clinical Toxicology: Breast feeding and drugs in milk, Vet. Hum. Toxicol. **20**:346, Oct., 1978.
2. Arena, J. M.: Contamination of the ideal food, Nutr. Today **5**:2, 1970.
3. Bode, H. H., Vonjonack, K., and Crawford, J. T.: Mitigation of cretinism by breast feeding, Pediatr. Res. **11**:423, 1977.
4. Brudenell, M., and Beard, R.: Diabetes in pregnancy, Clin. Endocrinol. Metabol. **1**:691, 1973.
5. Burrow, G. N., and Ferris, T. F.: Medical complications during pregnancy, Philadelphia, 1975, W. B. Saunders Co.
6. Crumpacker, C. S.: Hepatitis. In Remington, J. S., and Klein, J. O., editors: Infectious disease of fetus and newborn infant, Philadephia, 1976, W. B. Saunders Co.
7. Hanshaw, J. B.: Cytomegalovirus. In Remington, J. S., and Klein, J. O., editors: Infectious disease of fetus and newborn infant, Philadephia, 1976, W. B. Saunders Co.
8. Hayes, K., et al.: Cytomegalovirus in human milk, N. Engl. J. Med. **287**:177, 1972.
9. Huber, G. L.: Tuberculosis. In Remington, J. S., and Klein, J. O., editors: Infectious disease of fetus and newborn infant, Philadelphia, 1976, W. B. Saunders Co.
10. Ingall, D., and Norins, L.: Syphilis. In Remington, J. S., and Klein, J. O., editors: Infectious disease of fetus and newborn infant, Philadelphia, 1976, W. B. Saunders Co.
11. Jelliffe, D. B., and Jelliffe, E. F. P.: Human milk in the modern world, Oxford, 1978, Oxford University Press.
12. Joslin, E. P., et al.: The treatment of diabetes mellitus, Philadelphia, 1959, Lea & Febiger.
13. Kakkar, V. V., et al.: Low doses of heparin in prevention of deep vein thrombosis, Lancet **2**:669, 1971.
14. Kilham, L.: Mumps virus in human milk and in milk of infected monkey, J.A.M.A. **146**:1231, 1951.
15. Kohn, J. L.: Measles in newborn infants (maternal infection), J. Pediatr. **3**:176, 1933.
16. Langer, H.: Repeated congenital infection with toxoplasma gondii, Obstet. Gynecol. **21**:318, 1963.
17. Lubchenco, C. O.: Infants of diabetic mothers, an editorial, Keeping Abreast J. **1**:107, 1976.
18. Miller, D. L.: The diabetic nursing mother, Keeping Abreast J. **1**:102, 1976.
19. Nahas, G. G.: Marijuana, J.A.M.A. **233**:79, 1975.
20. Nahas, G. G., et al.: Inhibition of cellular mediated immunity in marijuana smokers, Science **183**:419, 1974.
21. Nahmias, A. J., and Visintine, A. M.: Herpes simplex. In Remington, J. S., and Klein, J. O., editors: Infectious disease of fetus and newborn infant, Philadelphia, 1976, W. B. Saunders Co.
22. Nahmias, A. J., Alford, C., and Korones, S.: Infection of the newborn with Herpesvirus hominis. In Schulman, I., editor: Advances in pediatrics, Chicago, 1970, Year Book Medical Publishers.
23. Numazaki, Y., et al.: Primary infection with human cytomegalovirus: virus isolation from healthy infants and pregnant women, Am. J. Epidemiol. **91**:410, 1970.
24. O'Brien, T. E.: Excretion of drugs in human milk, Am. J. Hosp. Pharm. **31**:844, 1974.
25. Remington, J. S., and Desmonts, G.: Toxoplasmosis. In Remington, J. S., and Klein, J. O., editors: Infectious disease of fetus and newborn infant, Philadelphia, 1976, W. B. Saunders Co.
26. Schiff, G. M., Sutherland, J., and Light, I.: Congenital rubella. In Thalhammer, O., editor: Prenatal infections. International Symposium of Vienna, Sept. 2-3, 1970, Stuttgart, 1971, George Thieme Verlag.
27. Schweitzer, I. L., et al.: Factors influencing neonatal infection by hepatitis B virus, Gastroenterology **65**:227, 1973.
28. Schweitzer, I. L., et al.: Viral hepatitis B in neonates and infants, Am. J. Med. **55**:762, 1973.

29. Shinefeld, H. R.: Staphylococcal infections. In Remington, J. S., and Klein, J. O., editors: Infectious disease of fetus and newborn infant, Philadelphia, 1976, W. B. Saunders Co.
30. Tarr, E. M., and McNeile, O.: Relation of vitamin B deficiency to metabolic disturbances during pregnancy and lactation, Am. J. Obstet. Gynecol. **29:**811, 1935.
31. Tyson, J. E.: The diabetic nursing mother, an editorial, Keeping Abreast J. **1:**106, 1976.
32. Varma, S. K., et al.: Thyroxine, tri-iodothyronine, and reverse tri-iodothyronine concentrations in human milk, J. Pediatr. **93:**803, 1978.
33. Vorherr, H.: Drug excretion in breast milk, Postgrad. Med. **56:**97, 1974.
34. Weaver, J. C., Kamm, M. L., and Dobson, R. L.: Excretion of radioiodine in human milk, J.A.M.A. **172:**872, 1960.
35. Wilder, R. M.: Clinical diabetes mellitus and hyperinsulinism, Philadelphia, 1940, W. B. Saunders Co.
36. Young, N. A.: Chickenpox, measles, and mumps. In Remington, J. S., and Klein, J. O., editors: Infectious disease of fetus and newborn infant, Philadelphia, 1976, W. B. Saunders Co.

CHAPTER 15

Human milk as a prophylaxis in allergy

The association of allergy with cow's milk has been documented in the literature for decades. The incidence of allergy has been noted to progressively increase since the original comments on the subject by Rowe[17a] in 1931. The incidence has been said to have increased ten times in 20 years. This apparent increase has been attributed to increased recognition, increased incidence of allergy, and a gradual decrease in infection as a source of morbidity due to the use of antibiotics and immunization. Glaser[3] attributes this apparent rapid increase in the development of allergic diseases in the past 30 to 40 years to the abandonment of breast-feeding when safe pasteurized milk became available about 50 years ago. It has been noted that 20% of all children were allergic by 20 years of age. Studies of office pediatrics have shown a third of the visits are a question of allergy. A third of all chronic conditions under age 17 are due to allergy, and a third of the days lost from school are due to asthma. In the evaluation of 2000 consecutive unselected newborns in pediatric practice, it was found that 50% had allergic family histories. Grulee and co-workers[7] observed in 1934 that eczema was seven times more common in infants fed cow's milk than in those who were breast-fed.

There is no question that heredity plays a part in the development of allergic disease. Kern[10a] has noted that the outstanding etiological factor in human hypersensitiveness is hereditary. He states that there are few diseases in which heredity is so clearly identified and which are so commonplace. Glaser speculated years ago that if a child was at high risk for developing allergy, prophylaxis should be able to change the outcome. The original work on prophylaxis was done by Glaser and Johnstone[5] and reported in 1953. Only 15% of a group of children whose mothers controlled their own diet in pregnancy and controlled the infant's diet and environment at birth did develop eczema, whereas 65% of the sibling controls and 52% of nonrelated controls receiving cow's milk developed similar allergic illnesses. Although as a retrospective study it was open to some criticism, it did begin to look at a very significant issue, that is, reducing the incidence of allergic manifestations in high-risk individuals by a new type of preventive measure.

A second study was designed in 1953 and carried out prospectively by Johnstone and Dutton[9] to investigate dietary prophylaxis of allergic disease. They observed a difference over 10 years in the incidence of asthma and perennial allergic rhinitis in those fed soybean milk (18%) and those fed evaporated milk (50%). No infant in this study of 283 children was breast-fed, however. Halpern[8] reported the study of 1753 children fed breast milk, soy milk, and cow's milk from birth to 6 months of age who were followed until they were 7 years or older. The children included those with high-risk, low-risk, and no-risk family histories for allergy. They reported in 1973 no difference in outcome related to early diet. There was a relationship to the family history, however.

In a prospective study to identify the development of reaginic allergy, infants of allergic parents were placed in a study or control group. The study group followed an allergen-avoidance regimen, including breast-feeding. At 6 months and 1 year there was less eczema than the controls had had at 6 months. Lower serum total IgE levels were also reported[15] (Table 15-2).

Interest in identifying the immunological aspects of clinical allergy led to a number of studies. Kletter and associates[12] reported that hemagglutinating antibodies to cow's milk were present in the sera of some newborns but usually at levels lower than those of the mother. The earliest rise in titer was detected at 1 month and a peak was seen at 3 months in infants given cow's milk from birth. Antibodies belonged mainly to the IgG group with their rise and fall paralleling hemagglutinating antibodies. IgA antibodies were in low titer and IgM rarely detected. The delayed exposure to cow's milk in breast-fed infants resulted in lower mean values of milk antibodies, and peak values were attained more slowly. An inverse relationship exists between duration of breast-feeding and levels of titers of humoral antibodies.

Antibody-facilitated digestion and its implications for infant nutrition have been presented by Freed and Green.[1] They suggest a model of digestion in which oligopeptides in the small bowel are bound to secretory antibodies, which hold

Table 15-1. Some diseases possibly preventable by protecting relatively immunodeficient infants from adverse antigen experience*

Disease	Status
Eczema	Established
Asthma	Probable
Hay fever	Probable
Infantile gut and respiratory infection	Probable
Intestinal allergy	Probable
Septicemia and renal *E. coli* infection	Probable
Sudden death	Probable
Ulcerative colitis	Possible

*From Soothill, J. T.: Proc. R. Soc. Med. **69**:439, 1976.

Table 15-2. Preliminary analysis of a prospective study of the development of allergy by offspring of allergic parents*†‡

Treatment	Cases with eczema	Cases with no eczema
Breast-feeding regimen	2	24
Conventional management	10	17

*From Matthew, D. J., et al.: Lancet **1**:321, 1977.
†p < 0.05.
‡All avoided *Dermatophogoides*, pets, and allergenic bedding.

them in contact with proteases. This facilitates the breakdown and utilization of the oligopeptides. They consider immunity and digestion to be closely related. Breast-feeding, they point out, with colostrum and then mature human milk provides the immature gut of the infant with both immunity and "digestivity."

Eighteen patients with documented malabsorption of cow's milk, which improved by feeding them human milk, were studied by Savilahti[18] after challenge with powdered milk. Eight patients had clinical reactions; the number of IgA- and IgM-containing cells increased by almost two and a half times in the intestinal mucosa. When breast milk resumed, the findings returned to normal. There was a rise in serum antibodies of both hemagglutination and IgA. There was no change in IgE antibodies or serum complement. Multiple other findings, including villous atrophy and round cell infiltration, were noted. After the age of 2, all the infants became tolerant of milk, which the researchers suggest indicates immunological immaturity is part of the pathogenesis. Walker presented similar arguments and conclusions in a symposium discussion.[20]

The role of heredity in allergy was studied by Kaufman and Frick.[10] They described unilateral family history as allergy in one parent, bilateral as involving both parents. They followed ninety-four infants from birth for 24 months. Significantly more infants developed allergy if they were from a bilaterally allergic family. In the first 3 months there was less atopic dermatitis in the breast-fed infants with unilateral history than with bilateral history. Kimball[11] presents similar relationships to family history in a study of breast-fed infants (Table 15-3).

These data are augmented by findings by Murray[16] examining nasal-secretion eosinophilia in relationship to respiratory allergy, associated with a screening procedure for hearing loss. In a group of children with a history of allergy in the immediate family, an association between early introduction of solid food and the presence of a nasal-secretion eosinophilia was significantly positive.

Although modern processing of cow's milk has diminished the problem, it has not eliminated it, and it would appear that given high-risk factors or strong family history of allergy, an effort to avoid unnecessary exposure to known allergens is an easy way to avoid some medical problems.

Intrauterine sensitization and allergy in the newborn breast-fed infant were described by Matsumura[14] and his colleagues in Japan. Glaser[4] also identified the fact that under certain conditions an infant with a predisposition for allergy may become actively sensitized in utero because of the mother's overindulgence in

Table 15-3. A study of 1378 children*†

Number of babies	Duration of breast-feeding	Allergy	Allergy without family history
268	0-4 days	11.6% (31)	35.5% (11)
136	less than a month	10.3% (14)	29.0% (4)
123	1-2 months	9.7% (12)	25.0% (3)
323	2-6 months	6.5% (21)	19.0% (4)
528	6 months plus	4.0% (21)	0% (0)

*From Kimball, E. R.: La Leche League International information sheet no. 203, 1964, p. 5.
†Numbers in parentheses indicate number of infants with allergy.

certain foods in pregnancy. The infant will then respond to reexposure with allergic symptoms on first contact with that same food. Kuroume and associates[13] showed in intrauterine sensitization that hemagglutinating antibody titers against lactalbumin and soybean in the amniotic fluid were high. They suggest this measurement of amniotic fluid as an instrument to predict future allergy.

It has been suggested that for the first 6 weeks or so of life, the intestinal tract is immature anatomically and immunologically. The early absorption of protein macromolecules in young animals is well recognized. The subepithelial plasma cells of the lamina propria mucosae and lymph nodes do not make IgA initially. Gradually the levels increase until they reach adult values at 2 years of age. Children with a strong family history of allergy have a more prolonged deficiency of IgA, lasting 3 months or longer. The early introduction of foods other than human milk has been associated with a rise in antibodies in the blood and eosinophilia, as noted earlier. Providing the infant with breast milk to which he will not become sensitized is the most direct way of dealing with the problem.

The total approach to the potentially allergic individual should include diet in pregnancy to exclude known common food allergens plus any known to cause problems in the members of that family. From birth until 6 months the infant should receive no cow's milk formula. In addition, the diet of the mother should be restricted as in pregnancy and the environment made as allergen free as possible. If the infant is not breast-fed, he should receive a cow's milk–free formula. Even though this regimen will not totally prevent all the potentials for allergy, it will help to minimize the insults by foreign protein (Appendix K).

Walker[20] summarizes by saying that it has been shown that antigens cross the intestinal barrier in physiological and pathological states. He states it is most important to prevent excessive penetration of antigens in patients that are susceptible to the disease via the following steps:

1. Identify the population at risk
2. Encourage breast-feeding in infancy
3. Decrease antigen load with elemental formulas
4. Conduct direct research at identification and prevention

REFERENCES

1. Freed, D. L. J., and Green, F. H. Y.: Hypothesis antibody-facilitated digestion and its implications for infant nutrition, Early Hum. Develop. **1:**107, 1977.
2. Gerrard, J. W.: Allergy in infancy, Pediatr. Ann. **3:**9, Oct., 1974.
3. Glaser, J.: Prophylaxis of allergic disease in infancy and childhood. In Speer, F., and Dockhorn, R. J., editors: Allergy and immunology in children, Springfield, Ill., 1973, Charles C Thomas, Publishers.
4. Glaser, J.: Intrauterine sensitization and allergy in the newborn breast fed infant, editorial, Ann. Allergy **35:**256, 1975.
5. Glaser, J., and Johnstone, D. E.: Prophylaxis of allergic disease in newborn, J.A.M.A. **153:**620, 1953.
6. Glaser, J., Daeyfuss, E. M., and Logan, J.: Dietary prophylaxis of atopic disease. In Kelley, V. C., editor: Brennemann's practice of pediatics, vol. II, Hagerstown, Md., 1976, Harper & Row, Publishers.
7. Grulee, G. G., Sanford, H. N., and Herron, P. H.: Breast and artificial feeding, J.A.M.A. **103:**735, 1934.
8. Halpern, S. R., et al: Development of childhood allergy in infants fed breast, soy, or cow milk, J. Allergy Clin. Immunol. **51:**139, 1973.

9. Johnstone, D. E., and Dutton, A. M.: Dietary prophylaxis of allergic disease in children, N. Engl. J. Med. **274:**715, 1966.

10. Kaufman, H. S., and Frick, O. L.: The development of allergy in infants of allergic parents: a prospective study concerning the role of heredity, Ann. Allergy **37:**410, 1976.

10a. Kern, R. A.: Prophylaxis in allergy, Ann. Intern. Med. **12:**1175, 1939.

11. Kimball, E. R.: La Leche League International information sheet no. 203, p. 5, 1964.

12. Kletter, B., et al.: Immune response of normal infants to cow milk, I. Antibody type and kinetics of production, Int. Arch. Allergy **40:**656, 1971.

13. Kuroume, T., et al.: Milk sensitivity and soybean sensitivity in the production of eczematous manifestations in breast-fed infants with particular reference to intrauterine sensitization, Ann. Allergy **37:**41, 1976.

14. Matsumura, T., et al.: Congenital sensitization to food in humans, Jpn. J. Allergy **16:**858, 1967.

15. Matthew, D. J., et al.: Prevention of eczema, Lancet **1:**321, 1977.

16. Murry, A. B.: Infant feeding and respiratory allergy, Lancet, **1:**497, 1971.

17. Ratner, B.: A possible causal factor of food allergy in certain infants, Am. J. Dis. Child. **36:**277, 1928.

17a. Rowe, A. H.: Food allergy, Philadelphia, 1931, Lea & Febiger, p. 20.

18. Savilahti, E.: Intestinal immunoglobulins in children with coeliac disease, Gut **13:**958, 1972.

19. Soothill, J. T.: Some intrinsic and extrinsic factors predisposing to allergy, Proc. R. Soc. Med. **69:**439, 1976.

20. Walker, W. A.: Antigen absorption from the small intestine and gastrointestinal disease, symposium on gastrointestinal and liver disease, Pediatr. Clin. North Am. **22:**731, 1975.

CHAPTER 16

Induced lactation and relactation (including nursing the adopted baby)

Induced lactation is the process by which a nonpuerperal woman is stimulated to lactate, in other words, breast-feeding without pregnancy. Relactation is the process by which a woman who has given birth but did not initially breast-feed is stimulated to lactate. This may also apply to the situation in which a mother may have initially breast-fed her infant, weaned him, and then wishes to reinstitute lactation. Induced lactation and relactation are not new concepts but rather are well known to history and to other cultures. The motivation historically has been to provide nourishment for an infant whose mother has died in childbirth or is unable to nurse him for some reason. A friend or relative would take on the care of the child and with it the responsibility to nourish the infant at the breast, since there were no other alternatives. Relactation has been used in times of disaster or disease to provide safe nutrition to weaned or motherless infants. Numerous accounts of induced lactation are recorded in medical literature and reviewed in the writings of Foss and Short[8] as well as Brown.[2] Mead[15] recorded the phenomenon in her writings about New Guinea in 1935. Other anthropologists have made similar observations in other preindustrialized societies of women who have not borne children who, after a few weeks of placing the suckling infant to the breast, produce milk adequate to nourish the infant. Until recently, Western world literature reported the phenomenon as an anecdotal report as part of the discussion of aberrant lactation. Cohen[6] reported in 1971 a patient who had been nursing an adopted child very successfully for weeks when first seen in his pediatric office.

Today the interest in induced lactation in the industrialized world stems from a desire on the part of some adopting mothers to nurture the adopted child at the breast even if she was unable to carry the infant in utero. The interest in relactation comes from mothers of sick or premature infants who wish to breast-feed their infants after the days and weeks of neonatal intensive care are over. These mothers, although postpartum, have not been lactating.

The process of induced lactation is separate from galactorrhea, or inappropriate lactation, which has been described in the medical literature for over 100 years.[22] Abnormal lactation has been observed in a number of circumstances in nulliparous and parous women and even in males. There are many eponyms for these conditions, usually based on the name of the physician who first described the syndrome, such as Chiari-Frommel and Ahumada-del Castillo-Argonz. Normally in the absence of suckling, lactation ceases 14 to 21 days after delivery. Milk flow that continues beyond 3 to 6 months after abortion or any termination or pregnancy is termed abnormal or inappropriate lactation, or galactorrhea. Also included in this group of galactorrhea is lactation in a woman 3 months after weaning or the secretion of milk in a nulliparous woman in association with hyperprolactinemia and amenorrhea. Although these cases are pathological in nature and therefore different from the groups under discussion, it is noteworthy that some knowledge of the initiation and maintenance of lactation has been gained from the study of these syndromes.

Lactation has been induced in nonpregnant and nonparturient animals by the continual systematic application to the mammary gland of the suckling animal or mechanical milking apparatus. The response is effected through the release of mammotrophic hormone from the anterior pituitary gland. This effect is abolished if the pituitary stalk is transected. Ruminants respond to the addition of estrogen or estrogen-progesterone combinations, which facilitate mammary growth. Again in ruminants, growth hormone and thyroid hormone have been shown to increase milk yield, although prolactin does not. This suggests that prolactin is not deficient in ruminants. Selye and McKeown[18] showed in 1934 that suckling stimulus inhibits sexual cyclicity in rats. They further showed that when the main milk ducts to all the nipples are cut and the escape of milk has been rendered impossible, the mechanical stimulation of the nipples by nursing would also inhibit the sexual cyclicity of the normal estric, nonlactating adult rat. These studies demonstrate the significance of suckling in triggering the lactation cycle.

Because the motivation, goals, and physiological problems may be slightly different, induced lactation and relactation shall be considered separately.

INDUCED LACTATION

When a mother wishes to nurse her adopted infant, the goal is usually to achieve a mother-infant relationship that may also have the benefit of some nutrition. Put in that perspective then, success can be evaluated on the basis of whether or not the infant will suckle the breast and achieve some comfort and security from this opportunity and close relationship with his new mother. As has been well described by Avery,[1] this is nurturing with the emphasis on nursing, not on "breast-feeding" or nutrition. She further notes that "breast-feed" is not an actual word whereas nurse is defined as nourish or nurture. A mother who is interested in inducing lactation to nurse an adopted infant may need to understand that she may never be able to completely sustain the infant by her milk alone without supplementation. Neither the physician nor the mother should be disappointed. The nurturing goal is still achieved.

Preparation for induced lactation

Normally the breast is prepared through pregnancy for the time when lactation will begin by the proliferation of the ductal and alveolar system. Thus it is not inappropriate to assume that a period of similar preparation should take place in induced lactation. It has been suggested that the woman should begin systematically to manually express the breasts and stimulate the nipples for up to 2 months prior to the arrival of the infant, if time permits. A hand pump or other pumping devices can be used, but manual expression may work as well or better. Sometimes some secretion can be produced in this manner if it is carried out systemically on a uniform schedule throughout the day. The schedule should be practical, that is, include times when a mother could take a moment for this activity, such as morning and night plus any times she uses the bathroom.

In other cultures in which lactation is induced as a survival tactic for the infant, no period of preparation is available. The infant is put to the adoptive mother's breast and allowed to suckle. Stress has been placed on herbal teas and good nourishment for the mother, while the infant is also given prechewed food, gruel, or animal milk. Mead attributes much of the success of induced lactation in New Guinea to the ingestion of ample supplies of coconut milk by the new mother.

Adoption is not an easy process, and in fact, it can be quite stressful to become an instant parent. In assisting such a mother, consideration should be given to the infant's age, previous feeding experience, and any medical problems that may exist. Provision for additional nourishment during the process of establishing some milk secretion is most important. Some infants are easily confused by switching back and forth between breast and bottle because the sucking technique is slightly different. Other nourishment can be offered by dropper or as solid foods. There is, however, a unique system for providing nourishment for the infant while suckling at the breast. It is called Lact-Aid and is described on pp. 262 to 264.

Drugs to induce lactation

As described in Chapter 1, estrogen and progesterone stimulate the proliferation of the alveolar and ductal systems. These hormones work in association with an increase in prolactin production. Although the prolactin level is high during pregnancy, milk secretion is inhibited by the presence of the estrogen and progesterone. After delivery has occurred and the placenta is removed, there is a marked fall in estrogen and progesterone, and prolactin initiates milk production. Efforts to simulate this hormonal stimulation have had variable success and are not recommended in this situation because of the possible effect on the infant via the milk. Women taking birth control pills have been noted in some cases to have breast enlargement. In addition, although estrogen and progesterone may enhance proliferation, they may inhibit lactation per se. The dosage recommended by Waletzky and Herman[24] of conjugated estrogens is 2.5 mg twice a day for 14 days beginning on the fourth day of a regular menstrual cycle. Giving 0.35 mg norethindrone once daily with the morning dose of estrogen prevents breakthrough bleeding. Medication is given for 2 weeks and is comparable in dosage to 2 weeks of birth control pills. This may be accompanied by some side effects. This regimen has been followed in concert with other efforts to stimulate lactation.

Oxytocin, on the other hand, is a critical component in the milk ejection reflex and may be helpful in the early initiation of ejection. Physiologically stimulation of the nipple in the lactating woman results in the release of oxytocin by the hypothalamus, which then triggers the release of milk by stimulating the contraction of the myoepithelial cells and the ejection of milk (Fig. 8-9). The effect of intranasal administration of oxytocin on the let-down reflex in lactating women was well described by Newton and Egli.[16] (Oral administration by tablet has not been as effective.) Since that time oxytocin nasal spray has been utilized in nonpuerperal lactation with some success in enhancing let-down but not necessarily altering the volume produced. Continued use of oxytocin over weeks has been associated with diminished effect or even suppression of lactation. The chief benefit of oxytocin is often to break the cycle of failure and instill a feeling of confidence once it has been demonstrated that some secretion can be produced.

Chlorpromazine has been observed to act as a galactogogue as well as a tranquilizer when given to patients in large doses (up to 1000 mg or more). The effect has been observed in both male and female patients in mental institutions. The drug has been reported to increase pituitary prolactin secretion severalfold. It acts via the hypothalamus, probably by reducing prolactin inhibitory factor levels. Using this information, women well motivated to lactate who have attempted induced lactation by suckling a normal infant have had the process enhanced by small doses of chlorpromazine, according to Brown.[4] In a program to induce lactation in refugee camps in India and in Vietnam, nonlactating women were given 25 to 100 mg of chlorpromazine three times a day for a week to 10 days while infants were initially put to breast. Brown reports apparent enhancement of lactation with this treatment. Chlorpromazine has the added pharmacological effect of acting as a tranquilizer. The program of management in these women was supportive in other ways and also included the usual herbal medicines associated with lactation in these Eastern cultures. There was no control group. It is possible that the drug contributed to both the physiological and psychological well-being of the women wishing to lactate. It has been suggested that the wish to lactate is a strong component of success, since woman whose breasts are frequently stimulated sexually do not begin to lactate. Theophylline can also increase pituitary prolactin secretions, according to Vorherr[17]; therefore both tea and coffee should enhance prolactin secretion and thus lactation. However, excessive amounts may inhibit let-down.

Since the role of prolactin is the initiation and maintenance of lactation, whereas oxytocin regulates the glandular empting via the milk-ejection reflex, it is reasonable to speculate that enhancing prolactin release would be productive in inducing lactation. The exact activating mechanism of the neuronal reflex arc from breast to brain has not been deciphered. Secretion of prolactin appears to be influenced, if not controlled, by changes in hypothalamic dopamine turnover. Correspondingly, suckling has been observed to deplete dopamine stores.

Investigation of other drugs that are known to stimulate prolactin release has identified some possible therapeutic materials. McNeilly and colleagues[4] have reported metoclopramide induces prolactin release regardless of the route of administration. Prolactin levels are increased three to eight times normal levels within 5 min when a 10 mg dose is given either intravenously or intramuscularly. The effect is achieved within an hour when metoclopramide is given orally. The effect persists for 8 hr. No reports are available for its use in nonpuerperal women at this time, although metoclopramide has been used to enhance lactation and for relactation (p. 262).

The regulation of prolactin secretion in humans has been studied to further the understanding of abnormal lactation as well as provide information on the regulation of pituitary function of the brain. It has been shown experimentally that the hypothalamus secretes PIF, which acts on the mammotropin-releasing cells of the pituitary to inhibit release of the hormone prolactin. The hypothalamus can also regulate prolactin secretion by a stimulatory mechanism, the secretion of thyrotropin-releasing hormone (TRH). When human volunteers (nonpregnant, nonlactating) are given infusions of TRH, increases in thyrotropin and prolactin are observed within minutes of injection with values peaking in 20 min. The level of thyroid hormone in the volunteers initially influences the results. Hypothryoid patients have been observed to secrete excessive amounts of prolactin, whereas

Table 16-1. Influence of drugs on prolactin secretion*

Pharmacological agents	Plasma prolactin concentration	Mechanism of drug action
L-Dopa	Decrease	Increase in hypothalamic dopamine–catecholamine levels, leading to enhanced activity of prolactin-inhibiting factor (PIF)
Ergot alkaloids (ergocornine, ergocryptine)	Decrease	Direct inhibition of adenohypophyseal prolactin secretion; possible increase of hypothalamic PIF activity (continued PIF function)
Thyrotropin-releasing hormone (TRH; pyroglutamyl-histidylprolin-amide) Theophylline	Increase	Direct stimulation of adenohypophyseal lactotrophs for increased prolactin secretion
Phenothiazines (chlorpromazine) Amphetamine α-Methyldopa	Increase	Decrease in hypothalamic dopamine–catecholamine levels, leading to diminution of PIF activity
Metoclopramide	Increase	Inhibition of hypothalamic PIF secretion through dopamine antagonism
Sulpiride	Increase	Increase in hypothalamic prolactin-releasing hormone

*From Vorherr, H.: Human lactation and breast feeding. In Larson, B. L., editor: Lactation, New York, 1978, Academic Press, Inc., p. 182.

hyperthyroid patients are relatively insensitive to TRH. This may explain some of the variable results obtained with prolactin-stimulating drugs used in the practical application to stimulate lactation. Studies of relactation have been done using TRH but not of de novo induced lactation.

Table 16-1 summarizes the influence of drugs on prolactin secretion.

Jelliffe[11] points out that the most important factor for continued production of milk is not drugs or hormones but "mulging." He explains that mulging (stimulation) is a word created in 1975 by N. W. Pirie to mitigate the confusion between the words sucking and suckling. The word comes from the Latin mulgere, to milk.

Composition of milk in induced lactation

Concern has been expressed that the composition of the milk produced by stimulation of suckling rather than as a result of pregnancy might indeed differ from "normal human milk." Such induced milk is not different in other species that have been studied extensively, including bovine and rat. In developing countries the fact that the infants showed normal growth and weight gain was taken as evidence that the milk is adequate. Vorherr[22,23] reported the analysis of the galactorrheal secretion produced by the breast following hyperstimulation. The comparative analysis is shown in Table 16-2. The induced lactational milk did not differ from puerperal milk. Brown[2] reported higher values of fat, protein, and lactose in

Table 16-2. Composition of normal breast milk and "galactorrhea milk"*

Milk components and properties	Normal breast milk	"Galactorrhea milk"
Components		
Fat (g/100 ml)	3.7	3–8
Lactose (g/100 ml)	7.0	3–5
Total protein (g/100 ml)	1.2	2–7
Sodium (mg/100 ml)	15	70
Potassium (mg /100 ml)	50	5
Calcium (mg/100 ml)	35	38
Chlorine (mg/100 ml)	45	50
Phosphorus (mg/100 ml)	15	2
Ash (mg/100 ml)	20	40–70
Properties		
Specific gravity	1030–1033	1031
Milk pH	6.8–7.3	7.3
Daily volume	400–800 ml	1–120 ml

*From Vorherr, H.: The breast: morphology, physiology and lactation, New York, 1974, Academic Press, Inc.

galactorrheal milk, but the volume of secretion was small in these subjects. It is probably of little value to try to analyze a given mother's secretions, since there is no evidence to question the composition. In tandem nursing where a mother continues to nurse an older child and puts an adopted newborn on the breast simultaneously, the composition of the milk might be in question.

Management of the mother and infant when lactation is induced

The collected experience of counseling women in the Western world who wish to induce lactation has been reported by Hormann[10] and Avery[1]; the latter author has now had contact with several thousand such women. Others have had experience with smaller series. The request for information and advice is increasing and becoming widespread throughout the United States and other Western countries.

Because there are simple means of supplementing the nutritional needs of the infant, the counseling should center on the relationship and the nurturing aspects. When the process is undertaken in preindustrialized nations, the anti-infective properties become important even though total nourishment may not be possible. Success is measured by having the infant content to nurse at the breast.

The woman should be encouraged to come to the physician's office for a counseling visit prior to the arrival of the adoptive infant to discuss the process of induced lactation. Actually, parents who are planning to adopt an infant should have a preliminary visit with their pediatrican so that some understanding of parenting can be discussed, just as any couple should do prior to the birth of their first child. At this visit to discuss lactation with the couple, it is helpful to explore their motives and general concepts of what is involved. It has been pointed out by all authors on the subject that the husband's interest in and support of lactation is critical to success. His participation in the preparation of the breasts may be a means by which the father can share intimately and constructively in the process. Instruction of the mother in preparation of the breast for suckling is also critical in induced lactation, whereas with puerperal lactation it may not be necessary at all. Exercises to stimulate the nipple should be undertaken several times a day and will be most successful if they are scheduled for times when and situations in which it is easy, feasible, and readily remembered. A few minutes multiple times a day is more successful and less likely to *overemphasize* milk versus mothering than rigid excessive exercises once or twice a day. Manual manipulation with gentle traction or horizontal and vertical stretching can be suggested. Avery[1] suggests that the father be encouraged to assist in breast massage and other techniques. She notes that "many adoptive parents felt that this technique (fondling and suckling of the breasts by the husband) added to the mutual sharing in preparation for adoptive nursing similar to the closeness many couples experience in preparing for natural childbirth." Raphael[17] reports that among forty adoptive nursing mothers there were dozens of variations on the theme of preparation. A positive attitude seemed to be the only consistent factor.

The need for dietary counseling is obvious. Lip service in behalf of well-balanced nutritious meals is not enough. Discussion should center around the absolute needs in kilocalories, fluids, and nutrients to produce milk (Chapter 9).

The physician should point out that stimulation of the nipples may well cause amenorrhea. Although the variation in menses is not uniform, it should be explained that decreased flow, irregular cycles, or total cessation of menstrual flow is possible. On the other hand, the menstrual cycle may be maintained and the flow of milk may seem to vary during menses. Changes in breast size, heaviness, and feeling of fullness may accompany the induced lactation. There may be an associated weight gain of 10 to 12 lb, on the average, according to Avery,[1] attributed to the response of the body to developing stores for lactation, just as in pregnancy (i.e., increased fluid retention and appetite increase). The weight gain may be a simple phenomenon of excessive intake. However, there is no need to gain excessive weight during this experience. Mothers (who may be nutritionally depleted) in non-Western countries who induce lactation are given added diet, nourishment, and herbal teas but do not usually gain weight. Failure to experience change in breast size, menstrual regularity, or weight should not be construed as a failed response.

Rigid conformity to a system of feeding may be a symptom of a more serious problem. Women who are rigid and compulsive may have trouble lactating because of the inability to have a good ejection reflex, which can be inhibited by stress and emotional conflict. Mothers who demonstrate an inordinate attention to volume of production of milk over and above the value of the relationship may feel as if they have failed.

Nutritional supplementation. The need to supplement the infant's intake while the milk supply is being developed should be discussed. The older infant who has already been receiving solid foods can be continued on solids by spoon with careful attention to nutritional content so that the diet includes a balance of protein and other nutrients. Supplements with milk or formula should be appropriate to the age of the infant. The infant under 6 months should receive infant formula rather than whole milk, if donor breast milk is not available. The milk supplements should be full strength, 20 kcal/oz and provided during the feeding by dropper or Lact-Aid or after the nursing by dropper, spoon, or cup in preference to a rubber nipple, which may confuse the infant in his adaption to nursing at the breast.

The process of induced lactation requires considerable commitment and determination. It is far more arduous a task than initiating postpartum lactation, but it is possible and worth the effort, according to the many mothers who have attempted it. The situation is better managed if a doula is available. It is appropriate for the physician to suggest that in addition to medical support the mother seek counseling from a lactation counselor experienced in induced lactation. Day-by-day contact for verbal support may be helpful, and these needs may be beyond the scope of a busy office practice. The nurse practitioner may be invaluable in this situation, particularly if home visits are made.

Appendix J includes reading material on induced lactation for the parents.

RELACTATION

The need to relactate exists in a number of circumstances, including the following:

1. A sick or premature infant cannot be fed initially or even until he is several weeks or months old.
2. An infant is weaned prematurely because of illness in the infant or in the mother.
3. An infant who was not previously breast-fed develops an allergy or food intolerance.
4. A mother who has lactated weeks, months, or years before is nursing an adopted infant.

Historical reviews provide many examples of infants suckled in times of crisis by women who have not lactated for years. The process of reestablishing lactation under these circumstances is generally easier than that of nonpuerperal lactation. Investigations have shown that a breast that has been previously primed by pregnancy to respond to prolactin will produce milk more readily.

Although the general process of nipple stimulation, having the infant suckle the breast, and setting the stage for lactation is similar, the woman who has experienced successful lactation previously may have not only the physiological but also the psychological edge.

Drugs to induce relactation

Some medications that have been tried in relactation seem only to work when the breast has been primed by mammogenesis, that is, by pregnancy.

Pyroglutamyl-histidyl-prolinamide, or TRH (Thyroliberin), has been used by Tyson and others to induce lactation. Each woman in their study was primed with estrogens beforehand. TRH stimulates the pituitary to release both TSH and prolactin. Drugs that produce a decrease in hypothalamic catecholamines, such as phenothiazines, reserpine, meprobamate, amphetamines, and α-methyldopa, cause an increase in prolactin secretion by blocking hypothalamic PIF.

The feasibility of pharmacologically manipulating puerperal lactation was demonstrated by Canales and co-workers[5] using bromocriptine and TRH sequentially. They suppressed lactation using bromocriptine orally for 8 days in four mothers whose infants were premature and/or ill and could not be nursed. These mothers did not lactate during this time. On the eighth day they were given TRH intravenously and then daily orally for 4 days (eighth to twelfth postpartum day). On the fourteenth day they initiated breast-feeding by putting the infant to the breast. Prolactin levels were measured from the day of birth. Levels were de-

Table 16-3. Data regarding mothers taking metoclopramide*

Num-ber	Age of mother (yr)	Age of infant (mo)	Daily dose (mg)	Length of treatment (days)	Side effects	Result	Education level of mother
1	27	2	30	6	None	Increase in milk volume; infant not weaned	University
2	25	10	30	10	None	Same as above	University
3	29	1	20	7	None	Same as above	High school
4	35	3	30	7	None	Same as above	University
5	20	2	20	7	None	Same as above	High school

*From Sousa, P. L. R., et al.: J. Trop. Pediatr. **21**:214, 1975.

pressed by bromocriptine and noted to rise when the TRH was given. The mothers subsequently nursed successfully.

Lactation can be reestablished with metoclopramide, according to Sousa and associates.[19] Metoclopramide is a derivative of procainamide, as is sulpiride. Studies done by McNeilly and colleagues[14] showed that metoclopramide and sulpiride are potent stimulators of prolactin release. These authors demonstrated marked increase in prolactin when metoclopramide is given, as noted earlier in this chapter. Sousa and co-workers[19] used metoclopramide to reestablish lactation in women who had experienced diminished milk supply. All five mothers experienced increased production of milk when 10 mg was given orally every 8 hr for 7 to 10 days. No side effects were noted, although this drug is known to cause cardiac arrhythmias and extrapyramidal signs in some adults. No side effects were noted in the infants either, but the level of drug was not measured in the milk. The results were encouraging, but further study is needed to determine the minimum dosage necessary to produce the effect and the amount passed into the milk. The summation of the data on patients treated by Sousa and associates[19] is recorded in Table 16-3.

LACT-AID NURSING SUPPLEMENTER AND OTHER DEVICES

Although many mechanical devices have been developed since Roman times to augment lactation and give other feeding opportunities, the Lact-Aid nursing supplementer provides a unique ability to nourish an infant adequately while he suckles at the inadequately lactating breast (Fig. 16-1). The suckling stimulates the mother's own supply. On the other hand, the infant continues to suckle the breast because there is milk available. The device has been carefully engineered to provide a source of milk that is obtained by suckling, not by gravity. The capillary tube through which the milk flows can be placed along the human nipple without interfering with suckling. The plastic bags that serve as reservoirs for the supplemental milk are sterile and disposable. The milk is naturally warmed by hanging the bag beside the mother's breast, as shown in Fig. 16-1. See Appendix H for a full description.

Gradual weaning from the Lact-Aid can be provided by putting less and less in the bag each day so that the infant can obtain milk from the breast in increasing amounts as the nipple stimulation effects milk production.

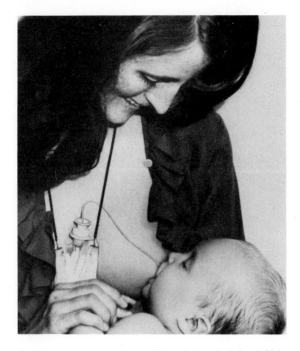

Fig. 16-1. Lact-Aid nursing supplementer in use. (From Avery, J. J.: Lact-Aid nursing supplementer instruction book, Denver, 1977, Resources in Human Nurturing, International.)

Experience in Rochester was initially obtained using Lact-Aid for adoptive induced lactation when the infant was 2 months old or older and needed instant supplementation. An increasing number of mothers wish to nurse their sick premature infants, however. It is often not possible to put the infant to breast for weeks. Meanwhile the mother may pump but only obtains minimal volume. When the infant is finally ready for discharge, it is mandatory that he continue to receive reliable nourishment every day. Starving the infant into submission is inappropriate and dangerous. Lact-Aid is an excellent alternative.

For years mothers of premature and sick infants have been assisted in breast-feeding their infants in preparation for discharge from the hospital and during early weeks at home by using dropper feeding, complementary feeds by bottle after each breast-feeding, or solids. The success rate was low and the aggravation for the mother often insurmountable.

Experience has now been gained in Rochester with twenty infants who have thrived with the assistance of supplements from Lact-Aid in these circumstances. Weaning from the Lact-Aid was not a problem for the infants. It was a problem, however, for one mother who could not nurse without the Lact-Aid even though it contained less than an ounce of formula per feeding and the breast was supplying the rest. She seemed to use the Lact-Aid as a "crutch." Careful anticipatory counseling should avoid this.

Lact-Aid should be started with a full understanding of its role in nourishment of the infant as well as with a plan for weaning from it that begins the first day. Weaning should be appropriate to the age of the infant and his nutritional needs.

The nourishment provided should be regular-strength formula, 20 kcal/oz and not just water, sugar water, or diluted formula. Starvation, even for a day or so, in a premature infant compromises the growth, especially of the brain. An infant who has been in the intensive care nursery is in special jeopardy (Fig. 13-13).

Other devices, such as hand pumps, the Egnell electric pump, and the Whittlestone psychological breast milker, which are useful in initiating relactation or induced lactation as well as puerperal nursing, are illustrated in Appendix G.

SUMMARY

Careful medical management of the adopted infant who is breast-fed is important. Many times the prenatal care of this infant as a fetus in utero has not been optimal. Any failure in growth should be identified quickly so that appropriate supplementation can be provided. In cases of relactation to provide for sick or premature infants, close follow-up is mandatory. A child who does not have a powerful suck may well appear to be very content yet be underfed. This situation was clearly described by Gilmore and Rowland,[9] who reported three cases of malnutrition while breast-feeding, attributed to the failure of the mother to recognize signs of growth failure and dehydration.

Relactation and induced lactation are special events requiring the positive support of medical personnel. The physician can serve as a well-informed stable resource in a process that will require considerable effort and commitment by the participants.

REFERENCES

1. Avery, J. L.: Induced lactation: A guide for counseling and management, Denver, 1979, Resources in Human Nurturing, International.
2. Brown, R. E.: Some nutritional considerations in times of major catastrophe, Clin. Pediatr. **11:**334, 1972.
3. Brown, R. E.: Breast-feeding in modern times, Am. J. Clin. Nutr. **26:**556, 1973.
4. Brown, R. E.: Relactation: an overview, Pediatrics **60:**116, 1977.
5. Canales, E. S., et al.: Feasibility of suppressing and reinitiating lactation in women with premature infants, Am. J. Obstet. Gynecol. **128:**695, 1977.
6. Cohen, R.: Breast-feeding without pregnancy: letter to the editor, Pediatrics **48:**996, 1971.
7. Evans, T. J., and Davies, D. P.: Failure to thrive at the breast: an old problem revisited, Arch. Dis. Child. **52:**974, 1977.
8. Foss, G. L., and Short, D.: Abnormal lactation, J. Obstet. Gynecol. Br. Emp. **58:**35, 1951.
9. Gilmore, H. E., and Rowland, T. W.: Critical malnutrition in breast fed infants, Am. J. Dis. Child. **132:**885, 1978.
10. Hormann, E.: A study of induced lactation, La Leche League International bulletin, Franklin Park, Ill., 1976, La Leche League International.
11. Jelliffe, D. B.: Hormonal control of lactation. In Schams, D., editor: Ciba Foundation Symposium no. 45, breast feeding and the mother, Amsterdam, 1976, Elsevier Scientific Publ. Co.
12. Jelliffe, D. B., and Jelliffe, E. F. P.: Human milk in modern world, London, 1976, Oxford University Press.
13. Larson, B. L.: Lactation: a comprehensive treatise, IV. The mammary gland/human lactation/milk synthesis, New York, 1978, Academic Press, Inc.
14. McNeilly, A. S., et al.: Metoclopramide and prolactin, Br. Med. J. **2:**729, 1974.
15. Mead, M.: Sex and temperament in three primitive societies, New York, 1963, Dell Publishing Co., Inc., p. 186.
16. Newton, M., and Egli, G. E.: The effect of intranasal administration of oxytocin on the let-down of milk in lactating women, Am. J. Obstet. Gynecol. **76:**103, 1958.
17. Raphael, D.: Breast feeding the adopted baby. In Raphael, D.: The tender gift: breast feeding, New York, 1976, Schocken Books.

18. Selye, H., and McKeon, T.: The effect of mechanical stimulation of the nipples on the ovary and the sexual cycle, Surg. Gynecol. Obstet. **59:**886, 1934.
19. Sousa, P. L. R., et al.: Re-establishment of lactation with metoclopramide, J. Trop. Pediatr. **21:**214, 1975.
20. Turkington, R. W.: Human prolactin, Am. J. Med. **53:**389, 1972.
21. Tyson, J. E.: Mechanisms of puerperal lactation. In Tyson, J. E., editor: Symposium on pregnancy, Med. Clin. North Am. **61:**153, 1977.
22. Vorherr, H.: The breast; morphology, physiology and lactation, New York, 1974, Academic Press, Inc.
23. Vorherr, H.: Human lactation and breast feeding. In Larson, B. L., editor: Lactation, New York, 1978, Academic Press, Inc., p. 182.
24. Waletzky, L. R., and Herman, E. C.: Relactation, Am. Fam. Pract. **14:**69, 1976.

CHAPTER 17

Reproductive function during lactation

FERTILITY

Gonadotropic and ovarian function during lactation has been only minimally investigated. The major body of knowledge has been collected regarding the postpartum return of the menstrual cycle and ovulation in the woman who is lactating as compared to the nonlactating woman.

The amenorrhea of lactation has been attributed to an imperfect balance of hypothalamoanteropituitary function and gonadotropin secretion. Secretion of follicle-stimulating hormone (FSH) and luteinizing hormone (LH) is generally diminished whenever prolactin is released from the acidophilic cells of the hypothalamoanteropituitary axis. Although the inhibition of FSH and LH has been reported by some, other investigators found no difference between lactating and nonlactating postpartum women. It has been suggested[4] that the ovaries are refractory to gonadotropic stimulation during the early postpartum period and lactation. This has been attributed to the conditions in pregnancy in which high sex steroid plasma levels and large amounts of human chorionic gonadotropin (HCG) led to ovarian inactivity. The ovarian quiescence has been observed in the early postpartum period as well. The antigonadotropic activity of prolactin present during the early months of nursing augments this effect on the ovary. The levels of gonadotropin in all postpartum women for the first weeks of the postpartum period are decreased, which substantiates the theory that there is postpartum ovarian refractoriness. In the first 2 weeks postpartum low levels of FSH are found in urine and plasma. Beling and co-workers[1] report estrogen excretion to be low with a linear increase during the first 5 to 8 weeks. When lactating postpartum women are given intramuscular gonadotropins, there is no increase in urinary steroids, according to studies by Zarate and associates.[19] The prolactin cell predominance may be responsible for the decreased activity of the pituitary-ovarian axis postpartum. Myometrial and endometrial involution are also considered to reduce fertility. Animal studies have shown that the release of FSH and LH is inhibited by intense suckling. In addition, animals in which the nipple is stimulated while the milk ducts have been tied off still show a suppression of estrous and menstrual cycles. Selye and McKeown[15] concluded that interruption of sexual cyclicity during lactation is a result of the nursing and not due to the secretory activity of the mammary gland.

Clinically, the perceptible measurement of the return of fertility is the onset of

Table 17-1. Percentage of ovulatory first cycles by duration from birth and nursing status at time of first bleeding day postpartum* †

	Day of first bleeding			
Ovulatory first cycles	0-29	30-59	60 or more	Total
Fully nursing				
Number of patients	—	8	19	27
Ovulatory (%)	—	0	58	41
Partial nursing				
Number of patients	—	7	38	45
Ovulatory (%)	—	29	79	75
Nursing suspended				
Number of patients	—	18	80	98
Ovulatory (%)	—	83	93	91

*From Perez, A., et al.: Am. J. Obstet. Gynecol. **114**:1041, 1967.
†In the twelve patients who became pregnant during amenorrhea, first bleeding day is defined as ovulation day plus 9.

menstruation. Return of reproductive function varies, depending on the length and degree of lactation. Most studies do not, in fact, report the completeness of lactation, that is, whether the infant is totally breast-fed or is also receiving solid foods or supplemental bottles. By the end of the third month only 33% of lactating women have had a menstrual period, whereas 91% of nonlactating women have had their period. At 9 months, 65% of those women who are still lactating have had the return of menstruation. Vorherr[18] further reports that 30% become pregnant within 1 year after delivery; 40% of those who became pregnant at 1 year were still lactating. Of the lactating women not using contraception, more than half will become pregnant during the first 9 months of lactation. Another view of the statistics, however, indicates that lactation does exert an inhibitory effect on reproductive function. A mother who nurses at least 20 weeks will postpone menstruation 12 weeks and ovulation 18 weeks.

The period of lactational amenorrhea does offer a measure of conception protection for 3 months. The nonlactating woman has a return of her period at 25 days at the earliest, of ovulation at 25 to 35 days, and a 5% chance of regaining fertility prior to 6 weeks postpartum.

Perez and colleagues[12] diagnosed the first postpartum ovulation by endometrial biopsy, basal body temperature, vaginal cytology, and cervical mucus in a group of 200 women in a prospective study. The dates of first ovulation, first menses, and nursing status were analyzed. No woman ovulated before the thirty-sixth day, whether lactating or not. The intensity and length of nursing affected the date when ovulation occurred, according to the researchers. About 78% of the women ovulated prior to the first menses. Twelve pregnancies occurred with first ovulation. Of the 170 women who breast-fed, 24 ovulated while completely nursing, 49 while partially nursing, and 97 after weaning (Table 17-1).

Following is a general summation of available data on return of ovulation and menstruation[18]:

    I. Nursing mothers
        Earliest possible menstruation: 4 to 6 weeks postpartum (pp)

Most women menstruating: fourth month pp
Return of menstruation: 6 weeks pp—15%
                                12 weeks pp—45%
                                24 weeks pp—85%
Earliest possible ovulation: 6 weeks pp
Return of ovulation: 6 weeks pp—5%
                              12 weeks pp—25%
                              24 weeks pp—65%
First ovular cycle: preceded in about 80% by one or more anovular cycles
Early pp: mainly anovular cycles
Later pp: more often ovular cycles
Ovular cycles: in about 50% of regularly menstruating mothers

  II. Amenorrheic nursing mothers
Endometrium: state of undifferentiation or hypoproliferation
Return of ovulation: 6 weeks pp—2%
                              16 weeks pp—10%
                              After first menstruation—14%

 III. Nonnursing mothers
Earliest possible menstruation: 4 weeks pp
Most women menstruating: third month pp
Return of menstruation: 6 weeks pp—40%
                                12 weeks pp—65%
                                24 weeks pp—90%
Earliest possible ovulation: 3½–5 weeks pp
Ovular cycles: in about 50% with first menstrual period pp
Early pp ovulation: possible occurrence late in the menstrual cycle—shortening of secretory phase and greater tendency toward irregular menses
Return of ovulation: 6 weeks pp—15%
                              12 weeks pp—40%
                              24 weeks pp—75%

 IV. Amenorrheic nonnursing mothers
Return of ovulation: 12 weeks pp—20%
                              16 weeks pp—40%

Data collected in preindustrialized societies show more prolonged lactational amenorrhea, which is probably due to more prolonged total breast-feeding and, to a degree, the relative malnutrition of the mother. Peters and associates[13] indicate that the mean duration of breast-feeding in their study of women in India is 16½ months and of amenorrhea 12 months.

A significant distinction should be made between token breast-feeding with early solids and more rigid feeding schedules and the ad lib breast-feeding around the clock with no solids until the infant is 6 months old. The amount and frequency of sucking are closely related to the continued amenorrhea in most women. When a totally breast-fed infant sleeps through the night at an early age, requiring no suckling for 6 hours or so at night, the suppressive effect on menses diminishes. It has also been shown that if the infant uses a pacifier rather than receive his

Table 17-2. Distribution of natural mothering* sample by months of breast-feeding† ‡

Months of breast-feeding	Number of experiences	Percent of total experiences
12	1	3.5
13–16	5	17.2
17–20	7	24.2
21–24	4	13.7
25–28	6	20.7
29–32	3	10.3
33–36	2	6.9
37	1	3.5

*Natural mothering includes, among other things, no pacifiers used, no bottles used, no solids or liquids for 5 months, no feeding schedules other than infant's, presence of night feedings, and presence of lying-down nursing (naps, night feedings).
†From Kippley, S.: Breast feeding and natural child spacing, New York, 1974, Harper & Row, Publishers, copyright © 1974 by Sheila K. Kippley, reprinted by permission of Harper & Row, Publishers.
‡N = 29 experiences (22 mothers). Mean months of breast-feeding = 22.8; median months of breast-feeding = 23.0.

Table 17-3. Distribution of natural mothering* sample by months of amenorrhea† ‡

Months of amenorrhea	Number of experiences	Percent of total experiences
1–4	2	6.9
5–8	2	6.9
9–12	7	24.1
13–16	9	31.0
17–20	5	17.2
21–24	2	6.9
25–28	1	3.5
29–30	1	3.5

*Natural mothering includes, among other things, no pacifiers used, no bottles used, no solids or liquids for 5 months, no feeding schedules other than infant's, presence of night feedings, and presence of lying-down nursing (naps, night feedings).
†From Kippley, S.: Breast feeding and natural child spacing, New York, 1974, Harper & Row, Publishers, copyright © 1974 by Sheila K. Kippley, reprinted by permission of Harper & Row, Publishers.
‡N = 29 experiences (22 mothers). Mean months of amenorrhea = 14.6; median months of amenorrhea = 14.0.

nonnutritive sucking at the breast, the suppression of ovulation is diminished (Tables 17-2 and 17-3).

CONTRACEPTION DURING LACTATION
Natural child spacing

Although lactation provides some degree of protection early in the postpartum period, a woman who is seriously concerned about avoiding conception should be informed of her options. If she does not wish to use contraceptives, medications, or devices, she should be instructed in the external signs of ovulation. In most studies of lactation, the initial menses occur prior to the onset of ovulation. The risk of pregnancy during lactational amenorrhea, however, is about 5% unless some effort is made to identify ovulation by basal temperature or cervical secretions.

Oral contraceptives and lactation

The significant issues related to lactation and the use of oral contraceptives are the potentially adverse effects of oral contraceptives on milk production, uterine involution, and growth and development of the breast-fed infant. A case is reported by Curtis[5] of breast enlargement in a breast-fed male infant whose mother began taking norethynodrel with ethynylestradiol 3-methyl ether (Enovid) on the third day postpartum. Breast enlargement began on the third week of life. The mother had noted her milk was not as "rich" and started supplements the second week. Nursing was discontinued at about 4 weeks of age and the breasts of the infant returned to normal in 2 to 3 weeks. The additional risks to the mother of thromboembolism, hypertension, and cancer have also been discussed extensively in the literature.

The data available have been well reviewed by Vorherr.[17,18] He summarizes the information by noting that preparations containing 2.5 mg or less of a 19-norprogestogen and 50 μg or less of ethinylestradiol or 100 μg or less of mestranol present no hazard to mother or infant. He further points out that milk yield can be decreased with larger doses of oral combination contraceptives containing estrogen and 5 to 10 mg of progestogen/dose. Only two studies of many suggest any variation in the content of the milk (protein, fat, and calcium) (Table 17-4) due to oral contraceptives.

Toddywalla and colleagues[16] reported the effect of injectable contraceptives as well as oral combinations on milk production. They found an increase in the protein content of the milk and slight increase in quantity from the group given injection of 150 mg of medroxyprogesterone (Depo-Provera) every 3 months. The group receiving 300 mg of medroxyprogesterone every 6 months showed a significant increase in quantity but a decrease in protein, fat, and calcium as compared to controls (who used mechanical means of contraception).

It is the concern of many that use of any hormone combination to suppress ovulation during lactation is contraindicated because of the potential risk to the infant, not only immediately but also in the long-range view. As discussed earlier, there have been reports of enlargement of the breasts in male and female infants when nursed by mothers taking oral contraceptives with higher dosages of estrogen and/or progesterone than are presently used.

No adverse effects on the infant during the ensuing years in bone maturation, genital development, or impaired fertility have been substantiated. Vorherr responds to the reports of such effects in animal studies by pointing out that (1) only small amounts of progesterone reach the infant and the androgenic capabilities are a fraction of those of testosterone, (2) long-range follow-up from the middle 1950s of nursing mothers given up to 20 mg of progestogen/day showed no bone maturation acceleration in infancy nor impairment of ovarian function and fertility in the infants' reproductive years, and (3) the dosages given the animals in the studies reporting abnormalities were excessive on a comparable weight basis (1 mg in a 6 g newborn rat).

Table 17-4. Effect of contraceptive steroids on lactation*

Agents	Milk yield	Comments
Estrogens		
Ethinylestradiol (50 μg)	No change	Placebo controls
Mestranol (80 μg)	No change	Placebo controls
Progestins		
Depo-Provera†	No change	No placebo controls
(150–250 mg medroxy-progesterone acetate)	No change	No placebo controls
Ethinylestrenol (0.5 mg)	No change	Placebo controls; no adverse effects on infants' weight gain
Lynestrenol (0.5 mg)	No change	No change in infant's growth curve
Norethindrone (10 mg)	No change	No placebo controls
Norethisterone (200 mg)	No change	No placebo controls
Estrogen–progestin combinations		
Anovlar (4 mg norethindrone + 50 μg ethinylestradiol)	Decrease by 40%	No placebo controls
C-Quens†	No change	No placebo controls
(2 mg chlormadinone acetate + 80 μg mestranol, sequential)	Decrease by 32%	No placebo controls; infants' weight gain 10% less than controls
Deladroxate (150 mg dihydroxy-progesterone + 10 mg estradiol enanthate)	Slight decrease	No change in infants' weight
Enovid† (2.5, 5, 10, 20 mg nor-ethynodrel + 100 μg mestranol)		
Enovid 2.5	No change	No placebo controls
	No change	No placebo controls; "patient's acceptance was excellent"
Enovid 5	No change	No placebo controls
Enovid 5, 10, 20	Decrease by 40% to 80%	Textbook information, no details regarding data evaluation
Ovulen† (1 mg ethynodiol diacetate + 100 μg mestranol)	No change	No placebo controls
	"Nursing function occasionally impaired"	No placebo controls
	Decrease by 30%	No placebo controls
	Decrease by 32% to 55%	No placebo controls; infants' weight gain 27% less than controls

*From Vorherr, H.: Human lactation and breast feeding. In Larson, B. L., editor: Lactation: a comprehensive treatise, New York, 1978, Academic Press, Inc.
†Consideration of results of various publications.

It is too early in the history of oral contraceptives to be entirely sure that there is no long-range increase in risk of cancer in the infants so nursed.

Intrauterine devices and other contraceptive methods

Various alternatives to oral contraceptives do exist and have been observed to have different degrees of reliability. The intrauterine devices (95% to 98% effective), cervical caps and diaphragms (85% to 88% effective), condoms (80% to 85% effective), vaginal suppositories, jellies, or creams (80% effective) have no known contraindication during breast-feeding, since no chemicals are absorbed. The only contraceptive that is 100% effective is abstinence. Many cultures and societies place taboos on sexual intercourse for the nursing mother as an effective means of spacing children. Usually there are no medical contraindications to sexual relationships during lactation.

SEX AND THE NURSING MOTHER
Sexual arousal associated with suckling

If one examines the normal adult female in regard to the menstrual cycle, sexual intercourse, pregnancy, childbirth, and lactation, one observes that these events are all influenced by the interaction of the same hormones. Not only the presence of estrogen, progesterone, testosterone, FSH, LH but oxytocin and prolactin as well. The breast is known to respond during all these phases, enlarging before menstruation, during pregnancy, before orgasm, and during lactation.[6] The nipples also respond during these phases. Furthermore, it is noted that the uterus contracts during childbirth, orgasm, and lactation. Body temperature rises during ovulation, childbirth, orgasm, and lactation. As pointed out in Chapter 3, oxytocin is a critical element in the let-down reflex during lactation. Oxytocin levels also rise during orgasms and labor, and oxytocin causes the uterus to contract and the nipples to become erect. Newton and Newton[11] report other similarities in women during these events, including sensory perception and emotional reactions. Following are the psychophysiological similarities between lactation and coitus[11]:

1. The uterus contracts.
2. The nipples become erect.
3. Breast stroking and nipple stimulation occur.
4. The emotions experienced involve skin changes (vascular dilation and raised temperature).
5. Milk let-down (or ejection) reflex can be triggered.
6. The emotions experienced may be closely allied.
7. An accepting attitude towards sexuality may be related to an accepting attitude to breast-feeding (and vice versa).

Given the biological and hormonal similarities of lactation to the other events in the sexual cycle of the adult female, it is not surprising that some women experience some form of sexual gratification during suckling on certain occasions. It has been reported by Masters and Johnson[10] in a study of 111 parturient women, only twenty-four of whom breast-fed, that there was sexual arousal experienced during suckling on some occasions. The exact incidence of this response is unknown, but it is believed to be uncommon. Nursing mothers may have an element of guilt surrounding these experiences and thus it is underreported. It has been suggested that guilt leads to early weaning in some cases. For some women the breasts are highly erogenous. The handling and manipulation of the breast necessary during lactation by both mother and infant can, in the right circumstances and mood, be stimulating. Clearly the majority of women who enjoy breast-feeding have no feelings or responses to the stimulation of the breast that could be construed as sexual arousal, although they enjoy breast-feeding and the intimacy with their infant that it provides. The erotic response to nursing the infant has no significance in terms of being normal or abnormal compared to a woman who has not had the experience of lactational arousal. The decline of breast-feeding because of feelings of shame, modesty, embarrassment, and distaste has been reported by Bentovim[2] and interpreted as indicating that breast-feeding is viewed as a forbidden sexual activity. For such women any sexual allusions and excitement accompanying breast-feeding are not permissible and cause shame. Such attitudes are more common in lower social groups and need to be considered in counseling mothers about breast-feeding prepartum or when premature weaning takes place. Major changes in the number of women who breast-feed may not be possible until society can accept the breast in its relationship to nurturing the infant and also as an object of less sexual ambivalence.

The sexual activity of the nursing mother

A review of the limited data available on lactating women in the Masters and Johnson study does indicate that in their group of 111 postpartum women, the nursing mothers were more eager to resume sexual relations postpartum than nonnursing mothers. The data were independent of the fear of pregnancy. They report that this interest was apparent 2 to 3 weeks postpartum. Individual reports through a questionnaire reported by Ladas[9] indicated that 30% of nursing mothers believed their sexual relationships were improved and 2.5% believed they were worse postpartum. The individual testimonies of nursing mothers reported by Ladas indicated they had a better feeling about themselves as well as their relationships with their husbands and family in general.

More general observations indicate that although some women may have increased interest in sexual relations while nursing, others may experience no interest at all for 6 months or so. Whether this is due to the saturation of the mother's needs for intimate relationship and stimulus through nursing, general fatigue, or fear of pregnancy is debatable. Sexual stimulus may trigger the ejection reflex, and milk ejection may have a negative effect on some men. The total knowledge of nursing and suckling as a biological phenomenon will help couples to understand such reactions and thus avoid inappropriate response psychologically. The conflict in some adult men over their role in regard to the nursing mother's breasts is usually a result of guilt or upbringing. There is no need to advise against fondling the lactating breast during lovemaking, although physicians have often imposed rigid restrictions on sexual activity in the lactating woman. There is no scientific basis for such restriction and no difference in the incidence of infection and mastitis associated with such activity. Unusually restrictive protocols are often imposed on patients without medical indication. Bradley[3] recommends, in fact, oral and manual manipulation of the breasts by the husband during both pregnancy and lactation to prevent sore nipples.

NURSING WHILE PREGNANT

Pregnancy can and does occur while lactating. When it does occur it produces a number of questions. There is no need to hastily wean the first infant from the breast, which is often ordered by the physician. It is possible to lactate throughout pregnancy and to then have two infants at the breast postpartum. It is now a sufficiently common event to be called tandem nursing. Obviously the amount of nourishment provided the first infant at the breast depends on his age and other supplements. When the infant at the breast is only a few months old when pregnancy occurs, there is some rationale to continued breast-feeding for the benefit of the infant until it is time to wean to solids and other liquids at 6 months of age or so. This child will be about a year old when the new infant arrives and if still at the breast may have demands in excess of the mother's ability to provide. Concern had been expressed that the older infant will take much of the nourishment needed by the new infant. In some societies it is believed that a suckling infant will "take the spirit" from the newly conceived fetus; thus weaning is mandated once pregnancy is confirmed. The milk produced immediately postpartum by the mother who never stopped nursing appears to be colostrum. The kangaroo has been observed to have a teat for the older offspring with mature milk and a teat for the new offspring who requires significantly different nourishment. Such a provision does not exist for the human. It has been shown by mothers who wish to maintain both infants at the breast that it can be done without any apparent effect on the nourishment of the new infant. Counseling of such a mother should take into account the mother's resource to get adequate rest, nourishment, and psychological support to withstand the added demand on her, physically and mentally.

If the first child is older and will be well beyond a year of age when the new infant arrives, the need for physical nourishment is minimal and continuation at the breast is more for the security and psychological benefits. Abrupt weaning should be avoided and the consideration be given to the impact of separation when the mother is confined during the birth of the new infant. (Perhaps this is an argument for 12 hr hospitalizations for delivery.) The first few days of colostrum are most vital for the new infant and the supply is not infinite; therefore priorities need to be set as far as the older child is concerned.

Many of the changes in child-rearing practices in recent years have increased the freedom and response to human needs. Carried to extremes, instant gratification becomes a right rather than a privilege. Sometimes a mother may need help in seeing that she need not feel guilty if she decides to wean the older child. If it is only an occasional feeding or suckling experience for added security, especially when security is threatened by the arrival of a new infant, it is tolerable in terms of endurance for the mother and she agrees willingly. When, however, continuing nursing becomes a strain or is painful or stressful, she should feel no guilt in stopping. When the mother feels real resentment toward the older child who is nursing, Pryor[14] points out that it is time to gently but firmly wean. If such a situation could be anticipated, it is probably easier for the older child to be weaned prior to delivery of the new infant. As with any such decisions to wean, it is best to work this decision out in frank discussion with the mother (and father, too, if he is available) so that any guilt, resentment, or feeling of failure can be dealt with openly. Many patients automatically suspect the physician of being antagonistic to breast-feeding if the physician suggests weaning. Even when the reason is purely but urgently medical, discussion should be open and include options and alternatives and their risks. Pryor[14] expresses it succinctly when she says, "Weaning is part of the baby's growing up, but it is sometimes part of the mother's growing up, too."

The dilemma of tandem nursing and weaning the older child has been dealt with in other societies with various manipulations such as painting the breast with pepper or bitter herbs to make it taste terrible. Having the mother leave the child with other caretakers is also done. The provision of love and affection during this difficult adaptation for the child is what makes the difference between a traumatic occasion and a step toward growing up. Equally important is the provision of some opportunity for the mother to express her concerns and doubts during the process to her physician, who should be neither judgmental or unduly rigid in his medical care plan.

REFERENCES

1. Beling, C. G., Frandsen, V. A., and Josimovich, J. B.: Pituitary and ovarian hormone levels during lactation, Acta Endocrinol. **155**(suppl.):40, 1971.
2. Bentovin, A.: Shame and other anxieties. In Ciba Foundation Symposium no. 45, breast feeding and the mother, Amsterdam, 1976, Elsevier Scientific Publ. Co., p. 159.
3. Bradley, R. A.: Husband-coached childbirth, New York, 1965, Harper & Row, Publishers.
4. Brambilla, F., and Sirtori, C. M.: Gonadotropin-inhibiting factor in pregnancy, lactation and menopause, Am. J. Obstet. Gynecol. **109**:599, 1971.
5. Curtis, E. M.: Oral-contraceptive feminization of a normal male infant, Obstet. Gynecol. **23**:295, 1964.
6. Eiger, M. S., and Olds, S. W.: The complete book of breastfeeding, New York, 1972, Bantam Books, Inc.
7. Gioiosa, R.: Incidence of pregnancy during lactation in 500 cases, Am. J. Obstet. Gynecol. **70**:162, 1955.
8. Kippley, S.: Breast feeding and natural child spacing, New York, 1976, Harper & Row, Publishers.
9. Ladas, A. K.: How to help mothers breast feed: deductions from a survery, Clin. Pediatr. **9**:702, 1970.
10. Masters, W. H., and Johnson, V. E.: Human sexual response, Boston, 1966, Little, Brown & Co.
11. Newton, N., and Newton, M.: Psychologic aspects of lactation, N. Engl. J. Med. **277**:1179, 1967.
12. Perez, A., et al.: First ovulation after child birth: the effect of breast feeding, Am. J. Obstet. Gynecol. **114**:1041, 1972.
13. Peters, H., Israel, S., and Purshottan, S.: Lactation period in Indian women—duration of amenorrea and vaginal and cervical cytology, Fertil. Steril. **9**:134, 1958.
14. Pryor, K.: Nursing your baby, New York, 1973, Pocket Books.
15. Selye, H., and McKeown, T.: The effect of mechanical stimulation of the nipples on the ovary and the sexual cycle, Surg. Gynecol. Obstet. **59**:856, 1934.
16. Toddywalla, V. S., Joshi, L., and Virkar, K.: Effect of contraceptive steroids on human lactation, Am. J. Obstet. Gynecol. **127**:245, 1977.
17. Vorherr, H.: The breast: morphology, physiology and lactation, New York, 1974, Academic Press, Inc.
18. Vorherr, H.: Human lactation and breast feeding. In Larson, B. L., editor: Lactation: a comprehensive treatise, New York, 1978, Academic Press, Inc.
19. Zarate, A., et al: Ovarian refractoriness during lactation in women: effect of gonadotropin stimulation, Am. J. Obstet. Gynecol. **112**:1130, 1972.

CHAPTER 18

Breast milk banks and wet nursing

BREAST MILK BANKS

Because of the renewed interest in providing human milk for the sick newborn and the premature infant, it is often necessary to store milk for infants, especially in the hospital. Milk banks have been in continuous operation for 50 years, according to Siimes and Hallman,[9] who report the collection of 5000 L/million members of the general population annually (24.4 L/donating mother). The indications for use of such milk have been alluded to in other chapters, but are briefly summarized as follows:

1. The mother plans to breast-feed the infant ultimately, but needs to provide pumped milk until he can go to breast.
2. The infant requires the special nutritional benefits of human milk, such as those infants who are recovering from intestinal surgery.
3. The infant weighs 1500 g or less and has difficulty digesting and absorbing other milks.
4. The infant is at risk of infection or necrotizing enterocolitis. Although effects are not clearly demonstrated with mature milk, fresh colostrum is held to be especially protective.
5. The physician believes the infant would benefit from the nourishment in human milk.
6. The mother is temporarily unable to completely nourish a breast-fed infant. It may be that the mother's supply is inadequate when she first puts the infant to breast after weeks of pumping or the mother has been ill or hospitalized. Usually these infants are already at home.

Structure of a milk bank

There has been a resurgence of interest in milk banks in recent years, paralleling the interest in breast milk in general. Banks have been reinstated after years of dormancy. The Mother's Milk Unit in California,[7] for instance, is part of a total transplant program. There are many hospitals, particularly those with intensive care nurseries, that are collecting and storing breast milk for use with hospitalized infants without the fanfare of being labeled a bank. In England and Wales, five large-scale human milk banks provide milk for infants in a large geographical area.

Whether a major project is launched and funds sought for its maintenance or a hospital merely wishes to provide a service for its patients, there are some ground rules that are helpful to follow. The hospital administration should be

THE UNIVERSITY OF ROCHESTER
SCHOOL OF MEDICINE AND DENTISTRY
AND
STRONG MEMORIAL HOSPITAL
601 ELMWOOD AVE.
ROCHESTER, NEW YORK 14642

DEPARTMENT OF PEDIATRICS

AGREEMENT WITH STRONG MEMORIAL HOSPITAL
AND MOTHERS DONATING BREAST MILK

I, _____, agree to contribute
my milk, which I carefully collect, taking the prescribed precautions
in its collection. I am in good health and not on medications. I
agree to discard milk collected if I am temporarily ill or temporarily
on medication. I understand that Strong Memorial Hospital will pay a
small stipend for my contribution. I understand they will provide me
with small sterile bottles to be used in refrigerating or freezing the
collected milk.

Signed_____ Date _____

Witnessed_____ Date _____

Fig. 18-1. Release form used at Strong Memorial Hospital for mothers who donate their milk to milk bank. (Courtesy Strong Memorial Hospital, Rochester, N.Y.)

informed so that proper permissions for donors and recipients can be provided. Establishment of the hospital's liability should also be investigated because a well-meaning donor or physician could be placed in jeopardy for their generous act if these seemingly stringent details are not identified and dealt with. A sample permission sheet is provided in Fig. 18-1.

Most hospitals find it convenient to receive and disburse the milk through a member of the nursery staff, such as the unit manager. The Louisville Breast Milk Program[2] has developed a system that involves the hospital pharmacy and a pharmacist as a part-time coordinator. The Mother's Milk Unit of the Northern California Transplant Bank affiliated with Stanford University School of Medicine uses a full-time coordinator and has a medical director.[4]

Operation of a milk bank

Experience with milk bank operation in Rochester spans almost 20 years. In the late 1950s and early 1960s, prior to intravenous alimentation, milk was provided for sick newborns postoperatively who could not tolerate other formulas, yet were gradually starving on intravenous fluids alone. Milk was collected fresh from volunteers, usually mothers on the postpartum floor who were not going to feed their own infants. Multiple donors were often used for a single infant; thus much colostrum was provided, which may, in retrospect, be why the infants did so well and infection was no problem. Mothers washed their hands and their breasts and used a sterile hand pump. Milk was refrigerated immediately in sterile bottles or given immediately to the infant. Mothers who were asked to donate had had a normal pregnancy and delivery, were serologically negative, had received no medications, and had no indications of infection. No infant had any infections while taking the milk.

In 1968 the demand for milk had become so frequent, particularly for small infants, that collections were begun from regular donors. These women were healthy and met all the criteria just mentioned but were also nursing their own infants. They continued to contribute as long as they nursed their own infants. It was also required that their infants were well and had not been jaundiced in the neonatal period. These mothers hand pumped or manually expressed milk and placed it in sterile bottles provided by the hospital. The milk was immediately placed in the deep freeze in the mother's home until she had collected daily samples for a week or two. The hospital provided transportation for picking up the milk. The milk was labeled with donor name, date, and time. The need for milk became so great that the hospital began to pay the donors by the ounce for milk and in turn they brought the frozen milk to the hospital and received another supply of sterile bottles. This provided a steady supply of easily digested nourishment for infants whose nutritional state was critical. An infant was always given milk from the same donor, and since there was a corps of regular donors, this did not present a problem. Milk was not pooled from multiple donors. If a mother was ill or taking medication she continued to pump to maintain her volume but did not save the milk. Most mothers pumped from one breast while their infant nursed on the other, although some mothers pumped first and fed their infant afterward. During the 9 years that the system was active there were no illnesses in any infant attributable to milk.

At present the infants whose mothers are willing to provide their own milk are permitted to have breast milk. Because of the expressed concern of some immunologists about host graft reaction in immature infants, no infant receives fresh milk from another mother. Frozen milk that has been thawed is used when milk is not available from an infant's own mother and before he is ready for gastric feedings of formula. Mothers also freeze their milk for their own infant if he is still unable to take cow's milk.

Qualification of donors

A mother who is willing to donate milk should be healthy and fulfill these qualifications:

1. Had normal pregnancy and delivery
2. Is serologically negative

3. Has no infection
4. Is taking no medications
5. Is capable of carrying out sterile technique
6. If donating for other infants, own child is healthy and without jaundice

Pregnancy and delivery should have been relatively uncomplicated. The mother should have a negative serologic reaction and negative chest x-ray results and be taking no medications, including birth control pills or any over-the-counter medications such as aspirin or acetaminophen. Her infant should be well and should not have had neonatal jaundice. Some banks obtain approvals from the mother's obstetrician and pediatrician (Figs. 18-2 and 18-3). If the mother is donating only for her own infant, the state of the infant's health obviously does not

---

(OBSTETRICIAN)

NORTHERN CALIFORNIA TRANSPLANT BANK
MOTHER'S MILK UNIT

Dear Doctor:

I have volunteered to be a donor to the Mother's Milk Unit of the Northern California Transplant Bank, Institute for Medical Research. If this meets with your approval, please provide them with the information listed below.

Thank you,

_____

_____

- -

TO: Mother's Milk Unit
    Northern California Transplant Bank
    751 S. Bascom Ave.
    San Jose, Calif. 95128

I recommend Mrs._____as a donor to the Mother's Milk Unit. To the best of my knowledge she had a normal pregnancy, is free of any condition that will impair the quality of mother's milk. Specifically, I believe her Wasserman and TBN and/or chest x-ray are negative. She has had no evidence of hepatitis, no tumors and is taking no medication. To my knowledge, she has no perinatal viral infection. HAA results:

_____
M.D.
_____
                                   M.D.
_____

Fig. 18-2. Communication to donor's obstetrician requesting pertinent medical information and approval of mother's participation in milk banking program of Northern California Transplant Bank. (Courtesy Northern California Transplant Bank, Mother's Milk Unit, San Jose, Calif.)

```
                                              (PEDIATRICIAN)

NORTHERN CALIFORNIA TRANSPLANT BANK
MOTHER'S MILK UNIT


Dear Doctor:


I have volunteered to be a donor to the Mother's Milk Unit of the

Northern California Transplant Bank, Institute for Medical Research.

If this meets with your approval, please so indicate below.

                                 Thank you,

                                 _____

                                 _____


──────────────────────────────────────────────────────────

TO: Mother's Milk Unit
    Northern California Transplant Bank
    751 S. Bascom Ave.
    San Jose, Calif. 95128



    I approve of_____donating milk to

    the Mother's Milk Unit.      _____
                                                    M.D.
                                 _____

                                 _____
```

Fig. 18-3. Communication to donor's pediatrician requesting pertinent medical information and approval of mother's participation in milk banking program of Northern California Transplant Bank. (Courtesy Northern California Transplant Bank, Mother's Milk Unit, San Jose, Calif.)

prevent her from donating. Anytime the mother becomes ill she should discard milk from the previous 24 hr period and not save milk until the illness is over and any medications stopped (Fig. 18-4).

Discarding milk during maternal illness is the hardest regulation for a mother to adhere to. The wish to contribute may overshadow the mother's understanding of the risk it poses for an infant receiving such milk. On the East coast in 1977 a mother developed diarrhea and continued to contribute for her own infant as well as others. This was the source of a serious outbreak of *Salmonella* in the nursery, resulting in unnecessary death and illness for many infants. This is one factor that has persuaded some banks not to pay donors for fear of developing a problem similar to that of blood banks, in which paid donors have more hepatitis and other problems than volunteers. The one limiting factor in donating milk, however, is that one has to be lactating. Becoming a professional donor of milk today is highly unlikely. The amount of protein has been noted to be lower after a year of lactation, thus it is advisable to limit a given mother's contributions to 10 months or, at most, 12 months postpartum.

Technique for collection

It is of prime importance to maintain cleanliness and minimize the bacteria in the process of collection. The mother should be instructed in washing her hands

NORTHERN CALIFORNIA TRANSPLANT BANK
MOTHER'S MILK UNIT

DONOR INFORMATION

Donor No.:_____

Date:_____

Name:_____ Age:_____ Blood type:_____

Address: _____City: _____

Cross streets:_____Phone No.:_____

Husband's name: _____No. of children:_____

Infant's name:_____ Birth date:_____

Hospital delivered: _____ City:_____

Obstetrician:_____

Address: _____Private:_____ Clinic:_____

Pediatrician: _____

Address: _____Private: _____Clinic:_____

Home visit:_____By: _____

Permission slip from obstetrician: _____

Permission slip from pediatrician:_____

Skin test (TBN):_____ Chest x-ray:_____

Do you smoke?_____ If yes, how many cigarettes a day?_____

Are you taking any medication?_____If yes, what kind and why?_____

_____

Storage facilities: _____Referred by: _____

Please draw a simple map, on back, of how we find your home.

_____
Donor signature

Fig. 18-4. Intake information sheet obtained on all donors of milk by Northern California Transplant Bank. (Courtesy Northern California Transplant Bank, Mother's Milk Unit, San Jose, Calif.)

and her breasts. Any equipment used such as hand pumps, tubing, and collecting bottles should be sterile. If an electric pump is used, the parts that come in contact with the milk should be sterile and/or disposable. The Egnell pump has the most advantages (Fig. 18-5). Many hospitals own an Egnell pump or one may be rented from a local rental company or may be available through the local La Leche League. The Louisville bank restricts milk collection to use of the Egnell pump, which they have available on a rental basis. They also suggest preping the breasts with pHisoHex and removing it with two gauze squares moistened with sterile water. It would be important to check milk samples for pHisoHex content if this were done daily. A simple soap may be preferable. Providing the mother with a preparatory kit has many advantages.

Many hospitals use the 4 oz sterile water-nursing bottles packaged by formula companies for collections by discarding the water at the time of collection and then

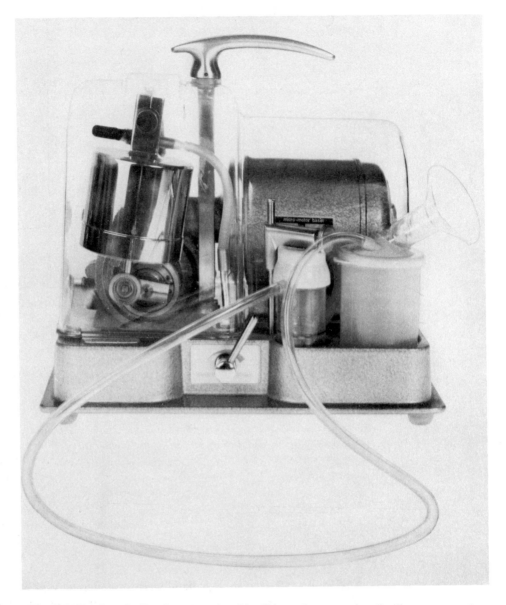

Fig. 18-5. Egnell pump. Egnell pump works with milking action on areola rather than vacuum extraction. Parts of pump that come in contact with milk can either be disposed of or sterilized. (Courtesy Egnell, Inc., Cary, Ill.)

filling them with milk. The Louisville program suggests the use of 50 ml plastic centrifuge tubes,* which are presterilized and have tight-fitting tops. These tubes have the advantage of more appropriate volume and easy measurability and sterility. Whether slightly acid human milk will leach plasticizers from plastic containers when stored in the freezer for weeks or months is unknown.

---

*No. 25330, manufactured by Corning Glass Works.

However, Paxson and Cress[8] have reported a significant difference in the survival of the leukocytes when the milk is collected and stored in plastic containers rather than glass, since the cells apparently stick to the glass. The phagocytosis of these cells, however, is not affected by the container. The researchers further demonstrated that varying the osmolarity or protein concentration does not alter the number or the phagocytosis of the cells. Because they believe the main reason for feeding preterm infants human milk is for the protection against infection, they suggest nasogastric feedings instead of nasojejunal feeding (to maintain pH in the acid range rather than placing in small bowel where pH is 6.5 to 8). They alternate feedings with formula to also provide increased kilocalories. The milk is collected in sterile plastic containers and maintained in the refrigerator until feeding it to the infant, thus avoiding heating, freezing, and alkaline solutions. It appears plastic containers may have a significant advantage in maintaining the stability of all constituents in human milk collections.

Storage and testing of milk samples

Fresh refrigerated unsterilized human milk can be used for 24 hr following collection. Donors are instructed to bring milk to the nursery within 3 hr if it is to be used fresh. If it is to be frozen, this should be done immediately at 0° F ($-18°$ C) (standard home freezer) or in top of a refrigerator freezer. The milk stored in the latter should be deep frozen within a week if it is to be stored any length of time. The milk kept at $-18°$ C can be kept for 6 months.

All samples should be labeled with name of donor, date, and time. Milk is stored in the freezer in such a way that the oldest milk is used first, and all milk of a single donor is kept together.

Monitoring for bacterial contamination is done on multiple samples before an individual is accepted as a donor. Studies are done on pooled samples; Siimes and Hallman[9] believe that pooling provides more stable nutritional content. To be accepted, the milk must contain less than 10,000 *Staphylococcus albus*/ml, less than 4000 *Staphylococcus aureus*/ml, and no gram-negative bacterial growth. Testing of milk samples from a given donor should also be done on a regular basis by a bacteriology laboratory approved for testing milk samples. Usually random samples taken every 2 weeks will suffice. When a hospitalized mother is contributing fresh milk to her own infant it is usually not cultured.

Testing milk for protein, fat, and carbohydrate is not necessary and is costly and time consuming. A new quick method of analysis has been suggested by Lucas and co-workers.[6] It involves standard hematocrit microtubes and a centrifuge. The percentage of cream or "creamatocrit" is read from the capillary tube. There is a linear relationship to fat and energy content.

$$\text{Fat(g/L)} = \frac{(\text{Creamatocrit [\%]} - 0.59)}{0.146}$$

$$\text{kcal/L} = (290 + 66.8) \times \text{Creamatocrit (\%)}$$

Accuracy is within 10%.

The effect of heating and freezing on the various constituents of human milk has been studied by a number of investigators. Their data should be considered before deciding how to store milk for special purposes.

Heat treatment. When human milk was pasteurized at 73° C for 30 min, there was little IgA, IgG, lactoferrin, lysozyme, and C_3 complement left, and when the temperature was kept at 62.5° C for 30 min there was a loss of 23.7% of the lysozyme, 56.8% of the lactoferrin, 34% of the IgG, but no loss of IgA, according to work done by Evans and associates.[1] Similar studies of heat treatments of graded severity were carried out by Ford and colleagues[3] (Tables 18-1 to 18-4).

Table 18-1. Immunoglobulin activity (mg/ml) in unheated and heat-treated human milk*

Heat treatment	IgA	IgM	IgG
None	0.50	0.10	None detected
56° C 30 min	0.48	0.10	None detected
62.5° C 30 min	0.39	0	None detected
70° C 15 min	0.24	0	None detected
80° C 15 min	0.10	0	None detected

*From Ford, J. E., et al.: J. Pediatr. **90**:29, 1977.

Table 18-2. Total lactoferrin and unsaturated iron-binding capacity in unheated and heat-treated human milk*

Heat treatment	Lactoferrin† (mg/ml)		Unsaturated iron-binding capacity‡ (μg of Fe/ml)		
None	3.4	3.7	3.4	3.1	3.1
56° C 30 min	—		3.0	—	—
Holder pasteurization (62.5° C 30 min)	1.2	1.5	1.3	0.7	0.8
65° C 15 min	1.0	1.0	0.6	0.4	0.4
70° C 15 min	0.2	0.1	0.1	0	0
75° C 15 min	0.2	0.2	0	0	0

*From Ford, J. E., et al.: J. Pediatr. **90**:29, 1977.
†Duplicate determinations were made on each test sample.
‡Each value represents a different preparation of milk.

Table 18-3. Influence of different heat treatments of human milk on its lysozyme activity*

Heat treatment	Lysozyme activity (μg of egg white lysozyme equivalent/ml milk)†	
None	98	99
HTST pasteurization	103	107
62.5° C 30 min	103	105
70° C 15 min	62	68
80° C 15 min	35	37
90° C 15 min	7	7
100° C 15 min	2	3

*From Ford, J. E., et al.: J. Pediatr. **90**:29, 1977.
†Each value represents a different preparation of milk.

The findings were similar. Pasteurization at 62.5° C for 30 min (Holder method) reduced IgA by 20% and destroyed IgM and lactoferrin. Lysozyme was stable at 62.5° C but destroyed at 100° C, as was lactoperoxidase and the ability to bind folic acid against bacterial uptake. Growth of *E. coli* increased in heated milk. B_{12}-binding capacity declined progressively with increasing temperature of the heat treatment. These data raise the question as to whether any heat treatment might not increase the risk of enteric infection in the infant. Some milk banks have advocated heating when the bacterial count is at a certain level, which may be too cumbersome to be practical. Ford and colleagues[3] suggest that for batch processing, 62.5° C for 30 min may be the method of choice.

The alterations of the lymphocyte and antibody content after processing were studied by Liebhaber and co-workers.[5] They, too, found significant changes with heat, including a decrease in total lymphocyte count and in specific antibody titer to *E. coli*.

Welsh and May[10] discuss anti-infective properties of breast milk and provide two tables (Tables 18-5 and 18-6) to demonstrate the stability of the antibacterial and antiviral properties of human milk. Siimes and Hallman[9] have relied on heat treatment of their milk samples, 60° C for 10 min. They do save fresh milk collected from donors who have been identified to consistently have no bacteria in their milk separately for immediate feeding to high-risk neonates.

Lyophilization and freezing. The impact of lyophilization was similar to heating, showing a decrease in total lymphocyte count and in immunoglobulin concentration and specific antibody titer to *E. coli*.

Freezing specimens up to 4 weeks showed no change in IgA or *E. coli* antibody titer, although the lymphocyte count was decreased. The technique involved freezing to −23° C and thawing at 1, 2, 3, and 4 weeks. Although there were cells present after freezing, they showed no viability when tested with the trypan blue stain exclusion method. The loss of cells may be desirable if the graft versus host reaction in a premature infant who is possibly immunodeficient is of concern. Evans and associates[1] reported their results with 3-month storage at −20° C and

Table 18-4. Influence of different heat treatments of human milk on its capacity to bind added [^{3}H] cyanocobalamin and [^{3}H] folic acid*

Heat treatment	Unsaturated binding capacity (ng/ml)	
	Cyanocobalamin	Folic acid
None	43.4	21.9
HTST pasteurization	26.2	—
62.5° C 30 min	22.6	19.7
65° C 15 min	18.4	16.4
70° C 15 min	14.4	14.2
75° C 15 min	14.0	11.5
80° C 15 min	15.0	10.2
85° C 15 min	18.4	4.2
90° C 15 min	21.6	2.4
95° C 15 min	22.8	1.5
100° C 15 min	18.6	1.5

*From Ford, J. E., et al.: J. Pediatr. **90:**29, 1977.

Table 18-5. Antibacterial factors in breast milk*

Factor	Shown in vitro to be active against	Effect of heat
L. bifidus growth factor	Enterobacteriaceae, enteric pathogens	Stable to boiling
Secretory IgA	E. coli; E. coli enterotoxin; C. tetani, C. diphtheriae, D. pneumoniae, Salmonella, Shigella	Stable at 56° C for 30 min; some loss (0% to 30%) at 62.5° C for 30 min; destroyed by boiling
C_1-C_9	Effect not known	Destroyed by heating at 56° C for 30 min
Lactoferrin	E. coli; C. albicans	Two thirds destroyed at 62.5° C for 30 min
Lactoperoxidase	Streptococcus; Pseudomonas, E. coli, S. typhimurium	Not known; presumably destroyed by boiling
Lysozyme	E. coli; Salmonella, M. lysodeikticus	Stable at 62.5° C for 30 min; activity reduced 97% by boiling for 15 min
Lipid (unsat'd fatty acid)	S. aureus	Stable to boiling
Milk cells	By phagocytosis; E. coli, C. albicans By sensitized lymphocytes: E. coli	Destroyed by 62.5° C for 30 min

*From Welsh, J. K., and May, J. T.: J. Pediatr. **93:**1, 1979.

Table 18-6. Antiviral factors in breast milk*

Factor	Shown in vitro to be active against	Effect of heat
Secretory IgA	Polio types 1, 2, 3, coxsackie types A9, B3, B5; ECHO types 6, 9; Semliki Forest virus, Ross River virus, rotavirus	Stable at 56° C for 30 min; some loss (0% to 30%) at 62.5° C for 30 min; destroyed by boiling
Lipid (unsat'd fatty acids and monoglycerides)	Herpes simplex; Semliki Forest virus, influenza, dengue, Ross River virus, Murine leukemia virus, Japanese B encephalitis virus	Stable to boiling for 30 min
Nonimmunoglobulin macromolecules	Herpes simplex; vesicular stomatitis virus	Destroyed at 60° C; stable at 56° C for 30 min; destroyed by boiling for 30 min
	Rotavirus	Unknown
Milk cells	Induced interferon active against Sendai virus; Sensitized lymphocytes? Phagocytosis?	Destroyed at 62.5° C for 30 min

*From Welsh, J. K., and May, J. T.: J. Pediatr. **93:**1, 1979.

of freeze-drying and reconstitution (lyophilization). They found no significant change in lactoferrin, lysozyme, IgA, IgG, and C_3 after 3-month freezing but a small loss of IgG after lyophilization (Table 18-7). These researchers propose that "human milk should be collected in as sterile a manner as possible and deep frozen shortly after collection. If a donor mother maintains a low bacterial count in her milk, then its use unheated should be considered. Pasteurization, if used, should be at minimum temperature capable of adequate bacterial killing (about 62° C for 30 min)."[1]

Table 18-7. Effect of deep freezing (3 m) at $-20°$ C and lyophilization of human milk proteins (mg/100 ml milk)*

	Raw milk (mean ± SE)	Deep frozen milk			Lyophilized milk		
		Mean ± SE	Mean as % raw	P	Mean ± SE	Mean as % raw	P
α_1-Antitrypsin (16 samples)	2.38 ± 0.3	1.98 ± 0.2	83.2	<0.05	2.22 ± 0.3	93.3	>0.1
IgA (8 samples)	9.55 ± 0.84	9.25 ± 0.83	96.9	>0.1	9.33 ± 0.74	97.7	>0.1
IgG (16 samples)	0.42 ± 0.05	0.42 ± 0.04	100	>0.1	0.33 ± 0.04	78.6	<0.05
Lactoferrin (11 samples)	332 ± 71.7	338 ± 57.4	102	>0.1	363 ± 79	109.3	>0.1
Lysozymes (11 samples)	5.1 ± 1.26	4.6 ± 0.67	90.2	>0.1	4.8 ± 1.19	94.1	>0.1
C_3 (16 samples)	1.35 ± 0.13	1.26 ± 0.11	93.3	>0.1	1.27 ± 0.13	94.1	>0.1

*From Evans, T. J., et al.: Arch. Dis. Child. **53:**239, 1978.

Financial aspects

Established milk banks have various financial structures. The Louisville bank has demonstrated that given a small amount of seed money, a viable self-sustaining program can be developed. Their income includes charges for equipment rental and for processing milk. Certainly the hospital should recover costs of collecting and processing. This should be a reimbursable item of hospital costs. Precedent for this has been set in the United States.

Siimes and Hallman[9] report that generally $4/L is paid to the donor, which, added to costs of equipment rental and milk processing, brings the costs of feeding an infant to $13/L.

WET NURSING

Although feeding an infant by one who is not his mother is an established means of sustaining life, it is uncommon in Western cultures. There are no medical contraindications provided the nursing woman is in good health and taking no medications. The chief obstacle is psychological or social. Actually women who are trying to develop a supply of milk when their own infant cannot nurse because of prematurity or illness would be greatly benefited by having a vigorous normal suckling infant nurse at their breasts. Perhaps as breast-feeding knowledge and understanding reach a greater number of professionals and women, such opportunities may be more common. At present it is significant to recognize this as a viable option.

REFERENCES

1. Evans, T. J., et al.: Effect of storage and heat on antimicrobial proteins in human milk, Arch. Dis. Child. **53:**239, 1978.
2. Fleischaker, J. W., Nowak, M. M., and Quinby, G. E.: The Louisville Breast Milk Program: the organization and operation of an in-hospital human milk bank, Keeping Abreast J. **2:**124, 1977.
3. Ford, J. E., et al.: Influence of heat treatment of human milk on some of its protective constituents, J. Pediatr. **90:**29, 1977.
4. Harrod, J. R.: Personal communication regarding Mother's Milk Unit, California Transplant Bank, July, 1978.

5. Liebhaber, M., et al.: Alterations of lymphocytes and of antibody content of human milk after processing, J. Pediatr, **91:**897, 1977.

6. Lucas, A., et al.: Creamatocrit: simple clinical technique for estimating fat concentration and energy value of human milk, Br. Med. J. **1:**1018, 1978.

7. Mother's Milk Unit, California Transplant Bank: A symposium on breast milk banking: procedures and protocols, San Jose, Calif., 1977.

8. Paxson, C. L., and Cress, C. C.: Survival of human milk leukocytes, J. Pediatr. **94:**61, 1979.

9. Siimes, M. A., and Hallman, N.: A perspective on human milk banking, 1979, J. Pediatr. **94:**173, 1979.

10. Welsh, J. K., and May, J. T.: Anti-infective properties of breast milk, J. Pediatr. **94:**1, 1979.

CHAPTER 19

The role of mother support groups and community resources

Certain changes in cultural aspects of Western civilization have contributed to the widespread use of artificial feedings for human infants as well as to the changing structure of the family. Urbanization has been associated not only with industrialization but also with the separation of generations from one another. This has produced the nuclear family. These are smaller, mobile, isolated families often stranded in a large urban population. The young couple and their new infant are totally without personal human resources. That is, there is no one who cares enough to give individual support to the family. There is no one to turn to, to share the experience with, and receive advice, encouragement and support from.

Rites de passage were described by the French author Van Gennep[14] as the ceremonies and rituals that mark special changes in people's lives. The list includes marriage, motherhood, birth, death, circumcision, graduation, ordination, and retirement. In our present culture there is support for most of these events except birth and motherhood. The most critical rite de passage in a woman's life, Raphael[10] points out, is when she becomes a mother. Raphael further distinguishes this period of transition with the term "matrescence," "to emphasize the mother and to focus on her new life-style." Traditional cultures herald a mother giving birth, whereas our culture announces the birth of an infant. The former highlights the mother, the latter the infant. Matrescence is a time of coddling. In preindustrial societies the mother is coddled for some time after birth, having only the responsibility of the infant's care while the mother's needs are met by doulas. Mothering the mother should be part of the postpartum support for a new mother.

A number of other forces added momentum to the bottle-feeding trend that began in the 1920s when manufacturers finally were able to mass-produce an inexpensive container and rubber nipple with which to feed infants cheaply. Pediatrics was a new specialty to guard the health of children. The stress was on measuring and calculating. Physicians seemed more secure when they could prescribe nutrition. The rise in the female labor force has also been credited with having an impact on the method of feeding infants. They were no longer brought everywhere with the mother to be nursed but left behind to be bottle-fed. The new technology of the infant food industry was a continuing influence on nutritional thinking of both medical and lay groups.

Breast-feeding was never totally abandoned. There was always a group of women who prepared themselves for childbirth and read and researched feeding and nutrition and chose to breast-feed. In the middle 1940s Dr. Edith Jackson began the Rooming-In Project in New Haven. Families in New Haven who sought "childbirth without fear" and an opportunity to room-in with their infants usually wished to breast-feed. In the rooming-in unit breast-feeding was often contagious because one mother successfully nursing would encourage others to try. Hospital stays averaged 5 to 7 days, during which time the mother-infant couple were cared for as a pair. About 70% of the patients left the hospital breast-feeding. Students and staff who were exposed to the philosophy of this unit went to many parts of the country taking with them tremendous commitment to prepared childbirth and nurturing through breast-feeding. The classic article on the management of breast-feeding by Barnes and associates[2] was published as a result of counseling hundreds of nursing mothers.

DEVELOPMENT OF MOTHER SUPPORT GROUPS

There still remained the need for nuclear families to have access to support and just friendly conversation about healthy infants, mothering, and breast-feeding. The La Leche League was developed to meet these needs in Franklin Park, Illinois in 1956. The original intent was to provide other nursing mothers with information, encouragement, and moral support. There are thousands of local chapters now and a network of state and regional coordinators who all synchronize their activities with the headquarters in Franklin Park. There is an excellent publication, *The Womanly Art of Breastfeeding,*[7] which was prepared by the original group of mothers. They continue to provide information and updated publications about common questions that arise during lactation. Local groups offer classes to prepare mothes to breast-feed. They help with suggestions about the nitty-gritty details of preparation, nutrition, clothing, and mothering in general. They also provide every mother with a telephone counselor. To be qualified to serve as a consultant to another mother, a member must demonstrate knowledge and expertise in breast-feeding as well as an understanding of how to counsel and render support. "Telephone mothers" do not give medical advice and are instructed to tell a troubled mother to call her own physician for such advice. Interested local physicians provide medical expertise for the group in situations in which a medical opinion is appropriate. The league provides support for mothers to reduce the time the physician needs to spend counseling on the nonmedical aspects of lactation. Most information needed by the new mother is not medical.

Similar programs have been developed in fifteen other countries. A well-established and respected program in Norway is Ammehjelpen, in Australia, the Nursing Mothers' Association of Australia, and The National Childbirth Trust in the United Kingdom.

The International Childbirth Education Association also provides resources for the new family. Their program makes preparation and training available for couples during pregnancy and afterward as parents. Their scope embraces the entire childbirth concept, of which breast-feeding is part.

Sociologist Alice Ladas[5] studied women who attended La Leche League preparation classes and compared them to a similar group who attempted to breast-feed but did not have this preparation. She was able to clearly demonstrate that the women who attended such programs had more confidence and seemed to profit by receiving accurate, up-to-date and relevant information as well as receiving individual and group support.

Silverman and Murrow[11] studied league activities and concluded that group dynamics are important, and feelings of normalcy are reinforced. The information and experience were shown to be important, but the support from the group had the greatest influence on success in breast-feeding. Meara[8] reports similar observations on league activities in a nonsupportive culture.

A follow-up study of breast-feeding in Oxford was carried out by Sloper and co-workers.[12] In this study they observed that significantly more mothers went home breast-feeding, mothers nursed longer, and solid foods were started later. They attribute this shift to the change in advice and support given in the hospital and at home visits.

COMMUNITY RESOURCES

Most hospitals provide training in preparation for childbirth. Part of the program should be about the new infant and how to plan for his care. These programs often serve as the initial stimulus to consider breast-feeding. Jelliffe and Jelliffe[4] suggest modifications of health services to promote breast-feeding (Table 19-1).

The YWCA in most communities provides preparation for childbirth. These classes usually provide programming that appeals to young and unwed women, a group in need of services rarely provided by other sources.

The Visiting Nurses Association and the public health nurses on the staff of the local county health department are special resources, particularly skilled at

Table 19-1. Possible modifications of the health services designed to promote breast-feeding in a community*

Health service	Modifications
Prenatal	Information on breast-feeding (preferably from breast-feeding mothers); breast preparation; maternal diet; emotional preparation for labor
Puerperal care	Avoid maternal fatigue/anxiety/pain (e.g., allow mothers to eat in early labor; avoid *unnecessary* episiotomy; relatives and visitors allowed; privacy and relaxed atmosphere; organization of day with breast-feeding in mind); separate mother and newborn as little as possible and stimulate lactation (e.g., no prelacteal feeds; first breast-feeding as soon as possible; avoid *unnecessary* maternal anaesthesia; permissive schedule; rooming-in); lactation "consultants" (advisers—preferably women who have breast-fed), adequate "lying-in-period"; in hot weather, extra water by dropper or spoon
Premature unit	Use of expressed breast milk (preferably fresh); contact between mother and infant with earliest return to direct breast-feeding
Children's wards	Accommodation in hospital (or nearby) for mothers of breast-fed infants
Home visiting	Encourage, motivate, support
Health center	Supplementary food distribution (e.g., formula and weaning foods) according to defined, locally relevant policy
General	Supportive atmosphere from all staff; avoid promotion of unwanted commercial infant foods (e.g., samples, posters, calendars, brochures, etc.); adopt minimal bottle-feeding policy and practical health education concerning "biological breast-feeding"

*From Jelliffe, D. B., and Jelliffe, E. F. P.: Human milk in the modern world, Oxford, 1978, Oxford University Press, copyright D. B. and E. F. P. Jelliffe 1978.

counseling new mothers with their infants. They can provide valuable information to the physician who is working with an infant who fails to thrive at the breast by witnessing the breast-feeding scene at home.

The Academy of Pediatrics[1] has made a statement in support of human milk in 1978.* They have summarized a lengthy presentation with the following:

1. Full-term newborn infants should be breast-fed, except if there are specific contraindications or when breast-feeding is unsuccessful.

2. Education about breast-feeding should be provided in schools for all children, and better education about breast-feeding and infant nutrition should be provided in the curriculum of physicians and nurses. Information about breast-feeding should also be presented in public communications media.

3. Prenatal instruction should include both theoretical and practical information about breast-feeding.

4. Attitudes and practices in prenatal clinics and in maternity wards should encourage a climate which favors breast-feeding. The staff should include nurses and other personnel who are not only favorably disposed toward breast-feeding but also knowledgeable and skilled in the art.

5. Consultation between maternity services and agencies committed to breast-feeding should be strengthened.

6. Studies should be conducted on the feasibility of breast-feeding infants at day nurseries adjacent to places of work subsequent to an appropriate leave of absence following the birth of an infant.

---

*Initiated by the Nutrition Committee of the Canadian Paediatric Society, this statement was prepared by both the Committee on Nutrition of the American Academy of Pediatrics and the Nutrition Committee of the Canadian Paediatric Society. Copyright American Academy of Pediatrics, 1978.

REFERENCES

1. American Academy of Pediatrics Committee on Nutrition: Pediatrics **62:**591, 1978.
2. Barnes, G. B., et al.: Management of breast feeding, J.A.M.A. **151:**192, 1953.
3. Ciba Foundation Symposium no. 45, breast feeding and the mother, Amsterdam, 1976, Elsevier Scientific Publ. Co.
4. Jelliffe, D. B., and Jelliffe, E. F. P.: Human milk in the modern world, Oxford, 1976, Oxford University Press.
5. Ladas, A. K.: How to help mothers breast feed, Clin. Pediatr. **9:**702, 1970.
6. Ladas, A. K.: The less viable option: breast feeding, J. Trop. Pediatr. **18:**318, 1972.
7. La Leche League: The womanly art of breastfeeding, ed. 2, Franklin Park, Ill., 1976, La Leche League International.
8. Meara, H.: A key to successful breast feeding in a nonsupportive culture, J. Nurse Midwife. **21:**20, 1976.
9. Pryor, K.: Nursing your baby, New York, 1973, Harper & Row, Publishers.
10. Raphael, D.: The tender gift: breast feeding, New York, 1976, Schocken Books.
11. Silverman, P. R., and Murrow, H. G.: Caregiver during critical role in the normal life cycle, unpublished report, Harvard Medical School.
12. Sloper, K. S., Elsden, E., and Baum, J. D.: Increasing breast feeding in a community, Arch. Dis. Child. **52:**700, 1977.
13. Thompson, M.: The effectiveness of mother to mother help, research on the La Leche League International program, Birth Fam. J. **3:**1, Winter, 1976-1977.
14. Van Gennep, A.: Rites of passage, Vizedom, M. B., and Caffee, G. L., translators, London, 1960, Rutledge & Kegan Paul, Publishers.

Growth and development

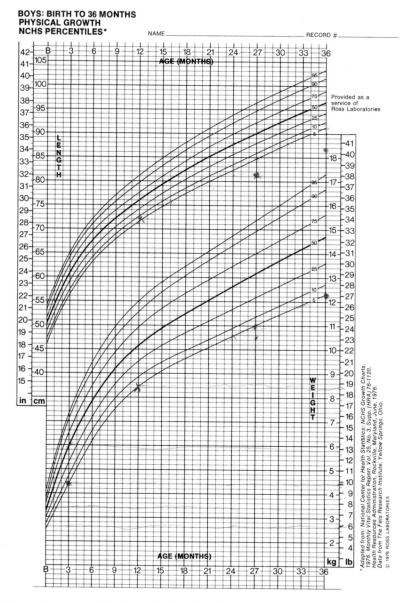

**BOYS: BIRTH TO 36 MONTHS
PHYSICAL GROWTH
NCHS PERCENTILES***

NAME_____ RECORD #_____

Provided as a
service of
Ross Laboratories

*Adapted from: National Center for Health Statistics: NCHS Growth Charts, 1976, Monthly Vital Statistics Report, Vol. 25, No. 3, Supp. (HRA) 76-1120. Health Resources Administration, Rockville, Maryland, June, 1976. Data from The Fels Research Institute, Yellow Springs, Ohio.

© 1976 ROSS LABORATORIES

Fig. A-1. Normal males, birth to 36 months. Length and weight. (Courtesy Ross Laboratories, Columbus, Ohio.)

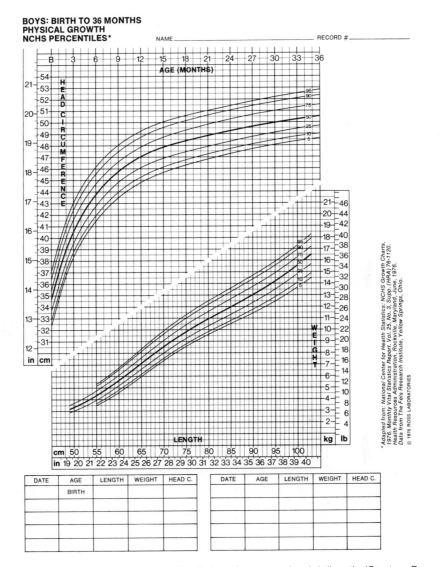

**BOYS: BIRTH TO 36 MONTHS
PHYSICAL GROWTH
NCHS PERCENTILES***

Fig. A-2. Normal males, birth to 36 months. Head circumference and weight/length. (Courtesy Ross Laboratories, Columbus, Ohio.)

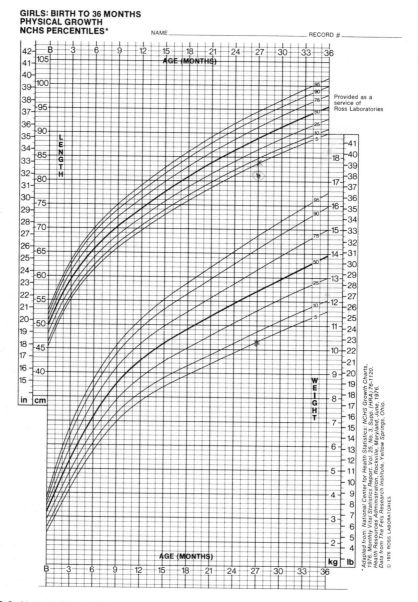

**GIRLS: BIRTH TO 36 MONTHS
PHYSICAL GROWTH
NCHS PERCENTILES***

NAME_____ RECORD #_____

Provided as a
service of
Ross Laboratories

*Adapted from: National Center for Health Statistics: NCHS Growth Charts, 1976, Monthly Vital Statistics Report, Vol. 25, No. 3, Supp. (HRA) 76-1120. Health Resources Administration, Rockville, Maryland, June, 1976. Data from The Fels Research Institute, Yellow Springs, Ohio.
© 1976 ROSS LABORATORIES

Fig. A-3. Normal females, birth to 36 months. Length and weight. (Courtesy Ross Laboratories, Columbus, Ohio.)

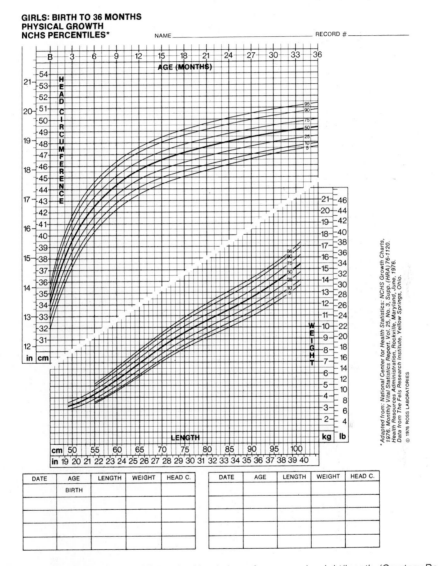

**GIRLS: BIRTH TO 36 MONTHS
PHYSICAL GROWTH
NCHS PERCENTILES***

Fig. A-4. Normal females, birth to 36 months. Head circumference and weight/length. (Courtesy Ross Laboratories, Columbus, Ohio.)

Table A-1. Changes in weight and length by low–birth weight and full-size infants during the first 3 years of life*

| Age interval (mo) | Size appropriate for gestational age (GA) | | | | | | | | | Size Small for GA | | |
| | GA 28–32 wk | | | GA 33–36 wk | | | GA 37–42 wk | | | GA 37–42 wk | | |
	N	Mean	SD	N	Mean	SD	N	Mean	SD	N	Mean	SD
Males—change in weight (kg)												
0–3	17	2.9	0.6	28	2.9	0.6	123	2.8	0.6	22	2.9	0.5
3–6	17	2.3	0.6	25	2.2	0.5	104	1.9	0.5	19	2.1	0.7
6–9	17	1.4	0.5	26	1.5	0.5	106	1.4	0.4	17	1.3	0.4
9–12	17	1.1	0.4	28	1.0	0.4	121	1.1	0.6	17	0.8	0.3
12–24	16	2.2	0.5	34	2.1	0.6	—	—	—	23	2.1	0.9
24–36	13	2.0	0.5	32	1.8	0.6	114	2.0	0.7	21	2.0	1.2
Males—change in length (cm)												
0–3	17	12.4	1.7	28	12.2	1.6	123	10.6	1.1	22	11.0	1.3
3–6	17	9.7	1.5	25	8.6	1.3	104	6.6	1.6	19	7.5	2.3
6–9	17	6.4	0.9	26	5.6	1.4	106	4.5	1.3	17	5.7	1.3
9–12	17	4.1	1.4	28	4.5	1.1	121	4.0	1.0	17	4.0	1.0
Females—change in weight (kg)												
0–3	22	2.4	0.5	34	2.7	0.5	136	2.4	0.5	32	2.5	0.6
3–6	18	2.1	0.4	34	2.1	0.6	78	1.9	0.5	28	1.8	0.4
6–9	16	1.4	0.3	32	1.4	0.3	78	1.4	0.5	26	1.2	0.4
9–12	18	1.2	0.4	28	0.9	0.4	86	1.0	0.4	27	1.0	0.4
12–24	21	2.6	0.6	34	2.4	0.7	—	—	—	35	2.1	0.6
24–36	21	2.2	0.9	29	2.0	0.7	79	2.2	0.7	35	1.9	0.9
Females—change in length (cm)												
0–3	22	11.7	1.8	34	11.0	1.1	136	10.0	1.1	32	10.9	1.4
3–6	18	9.1	1.5	34	7.9	1.4	78	6.5	1.4	28	6.9	1.3
6–9	16	5.9	1.5	32	4.9	1.0	78	4.8	1.2	26	4.9	0.5
9–12	18	4.6	1.0	28	4.8	1.4	86	4.1	1.0	27	3.8	1.0
12–24	21	12.8	2.1	34	12.3	1.7	—	—	—	35	11.8	1.7
24–36	21	8.8	1.9	29	8.5	1.6	79	8.5	1.2	35	7.9	1.5

*From Fomon, S. J.: Infant nutrition, ed. 2, Philadelphia, 1974, W. B. Saunders Co.

Table A-2. Skinfold measurements*

Age (mo)	Sex	Number	Biceps (mm) Mean	SD	Triceps (mm) Mean	SD	Subscapular (mm) Mean	SD	Subiliac (mm) Mean	SD
1	G	84	3.8	0.6	5.9	1.2	6.4	1.3	4.4	1.0
	B	114	3.6	0.7	5.5	1.3	5.7	1.3	4.1	1.1
3	G	84	5.6	1.2	8.4	1.7	7.9	1.6	7.3	1.9
	B	114	5.3	1.2	8.1	1.8	7.1	1.8	6.5	2.1
6	G	85	6.8	1.7	10.3	1.8	8.2	2.1	7.2	2.3
	B	113	6.4	1.6	9.9	1.8	7.4	1.8	6.6	2.3
9	G	83	6.3	1.1	10.1	1.7	7.9	1.6	5.7	1.5
	B	119	6.0	1.3	10.0	2.0	7.4	2.0	5.5	1.8
12	G	82	6.2	1.2	10.0	1.8	7.7	1.6	5.4	1.2
	B	120	6.0	1.3	10.0	1.9	7.4	1.8	5.2	1.5
18	G	74	6.1	1.2	10.2	1.7	7.2	1.5	5.1	1.2
	B	110	5.8	1.1	10.0	1.8	7.1	1.6	4.7	1.1
24	G	78	6.0	1.2	10.3	1.9	6.7	1.4	5.0	1.2
	B	112	5.9	1.2	10.0	2.1	6.6	1.8	4.8	1.7
36	G	80	6.3	1.6	10.4	2.0	6.6	2.0	5.0	1.2
	B	114	5.7	1.1	10.0	1.7	5.9	1.5	4.6	1.2

*From Karlberg, P., et al.: Acta Paediatr. Scand. **48**(suppl. 187):1, 1968.

Infant activity

Table B-1. Infant scheduling record*†

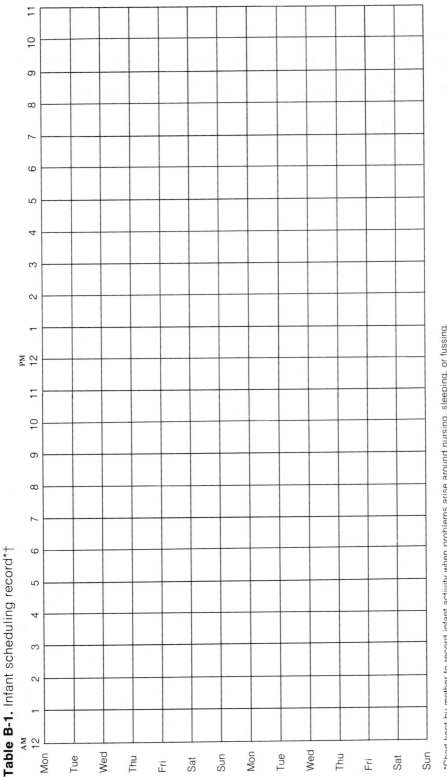

*Chart kept by mother to record infant activity when problems arise around nursing, sleeping, or fussing.
†Record with a line (—) time spent sleeping (—S—), feeding (—F—), and awake but not feeding (—A—), and crying or fussing (—cry—).

Dietary guidance during lactation

Table C-1. Tool A—Food record: diet history*

Name _____

Medical record no. _____

Date _____

Meals and snacks		Total food intake				Comments
		Description of food items				Any related factors?—associated activity, place, persons, money, feelings, hunger, etc.
Time	Place	Food	Amount	Type or preparation	With whom eaten?	

*From Williams, S.: Handbook of maternal and infant nutrition, Berkeley, Calif., 1976, SRW Productions, Inc.

Table C-2. Tool B—Nutrition interview: diet history*

Name _____ Date _____

Age _____ Height _____ Prepregnant weight _____

Gravida _____ EDC _____ Present weight _____

Activity-associated general day's food intake pattern

LIVING SITUATION

Housing _____

Members of household _____

Culture _____

Occupation: Husband _____

Self _____

Recreation, physical activity _____

PRESENT FOOD HABITS	**Place**	**Time**
Morning		
Noon		
Evening		
Snacks		
Comments		

Checklist

Protein foods	Breads, cereals, legumes	Vegetables
Milk	Breads (whole-grain	Dark Yellow
Cheese	enriched)	Deep green
Meat	Cereals	Potato
Fish	Pastas	Others
Poultry	Dried beans, peas,	Desserts, sweets
Eggs	lentils	Soft drinks, candy
Fruits	Fats and oils	Alcohol
Citrus	Butter	Vitamin, mineral
Others	Margarine	supplements
	Others	Medication, drugs

*From Williams, S.: Handbook of maternal and infant nutrition, Berkeley, Calif., 1976, SRW Productions, Inc.

Table C-3. Tool C—Nutritional analysis sheet*

Food groups	Major nutrient contributions	Recommended daily intake (number of servings)	Patient intake	Analysis of food needs
Protein-rich foods				
Milk and cheese	Protein (complete, high biological value); Ca, P, Mg; vitamin D; riboflavin	1 qt milk 2 oz cheese or ½ cup cottage cheese		
Eggs and meat	Protein (complete, high biological value); B complex vitamins; folic acid (liver); vitamin A (liver); iron (liver especially)	2 eggs 2 servings meat (3-4 oz each) Liver once a week at least		
Vitamin- and mineral-rich foods				
Grains, whole or enriched, breads or cereals, legumes	Protein (incomplete, supplementary); B complex vitamins; iron, Ca, P, Mg; energy (protein sparing)	4 or more servings		
Green and yellow vegetables	Vitamin A; folic acid	1-2 servings		
Citrus fruits and other vitamin C-rich fruits and vegetables	Vitamin C	2 servings		
Potatoes and other vegetables and fruits	Energy (protein sparing); added vitamins and minerals	1 serving or as needed for calories		
Fats—margarine, butter, and oils	Vitamin A (butter, fortified margarine); vitamin E (vegetable oils); energy (protein sparing)	1-2 tbsp as needed for calories		
Iodized salt	Iodine	Use with food to taste		

*From Williams, S.: Handbook of maternal and infant nutrition, Berkeley, Calif., 1976, SRW Productions, Inc.

Table C-4. Vegetarian food guide*

GENERAL GUIDELINES

1. Follow nutrition guide for regular food plan during pregnancy.
2. Eat a wide variety of foods, including milk and milk products and eggs.
3. If no milk is allowed, use a supplement of 4 μg of vitamin B_{12} daily. If goat and soymilk are used, partial supplementation may be needed.
4. If no milk is taken, also use supplements of 12 mg of calcium and 400 IU of vitamin D daily. Partial supplementation will be necessary if less than four servings of milk and milk products are consumed.
5. Select a variety of plant foods (especially grains, legumes, nuts, and seeds) to obtain "complete" proteins by complementary combinations, as indicated in the list below.
6. Use iodized salt.

	Complementary plant protein combinations	
Food	**Amino acids deficient**	**Complementary protein food combinations**
Grains	Isoleucine Lysine	Rice + legumes Corn + legumes Wheat + legumes Wheat + peanut + milk Wheat + sesame + soybean Rice + brewer's yeast
Legumes	Tryptophan Methionine	Legumes + rice Beans + wheat Beans + corn Soybeans + rice + wheat Soybeans + corn + milk Soybeans + wheat + sesame Soybeans + peanuts + sesame Soybeans + peanuts + wheat + rice Soybeans + sesame + wheat
Nuts and seeds	Isoleucine Lysine	Peanuts + sesame + soybeans Sesame + beans Sesame + soybeans + wheat Peanuts + sunflower seeds
Vegetables	Isoleucine Methionine	Lima beans Green beans Brussels sprouts } Sesame seeds or Cauliflower } + Brazil nuts or Broccoli } mushrooms Greens = millet or rice

*Modified from Lappé, F. M.: Diet for a small planet, New York, 1971, Friends of the Earth/Ballantine; from Worthington, B. S., Vermeersch, J., and Williams, S. R.: Nutrition in pregnancy and lactation, St. Louis, 1977, The C. V. Mosby Co.

Table C-5. Characteristic food choices of ethnic groups*

Black	Mexican-American	Japanese	Chinese	Filipino
Protein foods				
Meat	Meat	Meat	Meat	Meat
Beef	Beef	Beef	Pork	Pork
Pork, ham	Pork	Pork	Beef	Beef
Sausage	Lamb	Poultry	Organ meats	Goat
Pig's feet,	Tripe	Chicken	Poultry	Deer
ears, etc.	Sausage	Turkey	Chicken	Rabbit
Bacon	(chorizo)	Fish	Duck	Variety meats
Luncheon	Bologna	Tuna	Fish	Poultry
meats	Bologna	Tuna	Fish	Poultry
Organ meats	Bacon	Mackerel	White fish	Chicken
Poultry	Poultry	Sardines	Shrimp	Fish
Chicken	Chicken	(dried form:	Lobster	Sole
Turkey	Eggs	mezashi)	Oyster	Bonito
Fish	Legumes	Sea bass	Sardines	Herring
Catfish	Pinto beans	Shrimp	Eggs	Tuna
Perch	Pink beans	Abalone	Legumes	Mackerel
Red snapper	Garbanzo	Squid	Soybeans	Crab
	beans			
Tuna	Lentils	Octopus	Soybean	Mussels
Salmon	Nuts	Eggs	curd (tofu)	Shrimp
Sardines	Peanuts	Legumes	Black beans	Squid
Shrimp	Peanut butter	Soybean curd	Nuts	Eggs
		(tofu)		
Eggs		Soybean paste	Peanuts	Legumes
Legumes		(miso)	Almonds	Black beans
Kidney beans		Soybeans	Cashews	Chick peas
Red beans		Red beans		Black-eyed peas
Pinto beans		(azuki)		Lentils
Black-eyed		Lima beans		Mung beans
peas				
Nuts		Nuts		Lima beans
Peanuts		Chestnuts		White kidney
Peanut butter		(kuri)		beans
				Nuts
				Cashews
				Peanuts
				Pili nuts
Milk and milk products				
Milk	Milk	Milk	Milk	Milk
Fluid	Cheese	Fluid	Flavored	Flavored
Evaporated	Ice cream	Flavored	Whole milk	Evaporated
in coffee		Evaporated	(used in	Cheese
Buttermilk		Condensed	cooking)	Gouda
Cheese		Cheese	Ice cream	Cheddar
Cheddar		American		
Cottage		Monterey Jack		
Ice cream		Hoop		
		Ice cream		
Grain products				
Rice	Rice	Rice	Rice	Rice
Cornbread	Tortillas	Rice crackers	Noodles	Cooked cereals

*Modified from Nutrition during pregnancy and lactation, Sacramento, Calif., 1975, California Department of Health; from Worthington, B. S., Vermeersch, J., and Williams, S. R.: Nutrition in pregnancy and lactation, St. Louis, 1977, The C. V. Mosby Co.

Continued.

Table C-5. Characteristic food choices of ethnic groups—cont'd

Black	Mexican-American	Japanese	Chinese	Filipino
Grain products—cont'd				Cooked cereals—cont'd
Hominy grits	Corn	Noodles	White bread	Farina
Biscuits	Flour	(whole wheat:	Millet	Oatmeal
Muffins	Oatmeal	soba)		Dry cereals
White bread	Dry cereals	Spaghetti		Pastas
Dry cereal	Cornflakes	White bread		Rice noodles
Cooked cereal	Sugared	Oatmeal		Wheat noodles
Macaroni	Noodles	Dry cereal		Macaroni
Spaghetti	Spaghetti			Spaghetti
Crackers	White bread			
	Sweet bread			
	(pan dulce)			
Vegetables				
Broccoli	Avocado	Bamboo shoots	Bamboo shoots	Bamboo shoots
Cabbage	Cabbage	Bok choy	Beans	Beets
Carrots	Carrots	Broccoli	Green	Cabbage
Corn	Chilies	Burdock root	Yellow	Carrots
Green beans	Corn	Cabbage	Bean sprouts	Cauliflower
Greens	Green beans	Carrots	Bok choy	Celery
Mustard	Lettuce	Cauliflower	Broccoli	Chinese celery
Collard	Onion	Celery	Cabbage	Eggplant
Kale	Peas	Cucumbers	Carrots	Endive
Spinach	Potato	Eggplant	Celery	Green beans
Turnip	Prickly pear	Green beans	Chinese	Leeks
Lima beans	cactus leaf	Gourd	cabbage	Lettuce
Okra	(nopales)	(kampyo)	Corn	Mushrooms
Peas	Spinach	Mushrooms	Cucumbers	Okra
Potato	Sweet potato	Mustard	Eggplant	Onion
Pumpkin	Tomato	greens	Greens	Peppers
Sweet potato	Zucchini	Napa cabbage	Collard	Potato
Tomato		Peas	Chinese	Pumpkin
Yam		Peppers	broccoli	Radishes
		Radishes	Mustard	Snow peas
		(white radish:	Kale	Spinach
		daikon;	Spinach	Squash
		pickled white:	Leeks	Sweet potato
		takawan)	Lettuce	Tomato
		Snow peas	Mushrooms	Water chestnuts
		Spinach	Peppers	Watercress
		Squash	Potato	Yam
		Sweet potato	Scallions	
		Taro (Japanese	Snow peas	
		sweet potato)	Sweet potato	
		Tomato	Taro	
		Turnips	Tomato	
		Water	Water	
		chestnuts	chestnuts	
		Yam	White radish	
			White turnip	
			Winter melon	

Table C-5. Characteristic food choices of ethnic groups—cont'd

Black	Mexican-American	Japanese	Chinese	Filipino
Fruits				
Apple	Apple	Apple	Apple	Apple
Banana	Apricots	Apricots	Banana	Banana
Grapefruit	Banana	Banana	Figs	Grapes
Grapes	Guava	Cherries	Grapes	Guava
Nectarine	Lemon	Grapefruit	Kumquats	Lemon
Orange	Mango	Grapes	Loquats	Lime
Plums	Melons	Lemon	Mango	Mango
Tangerine	Orange	Lime	Melons	Melons
Watermelon	Peach	Melons	Orange	Orange
	Pear	Orange	Peach	Papaya
	Prickly pear	Peach	Pear	Pear
	cactus fruit	Pear	Persimmon	Pineapple
	(tuna)	Persimmon	Pineapple	Plums
	Zapote	Pineapple	Plums	Pomegranate
	(sapote)	Pomegranate	Tangerine	Rhubarb
		Plums		Strawberries
		(dried, pickled		Tangerine
		plums called		
		umeboshi)		
		Strawberries		
		Tangerine		
Other				
Salt pork	Salsa	Soy Sauce	Soy sauce	Soy sauce
(fat back)	(tomato-	Nori paste	Sweet and sour	Coffee
Carbonated	pepper-	(seasoned	sauce	Tea
beverages	onion relish)	rice)	Mustard sauce	
Fruit drinks	Chili sauce	Bean thread	Ginger	
Gravies	Guacamole	(konyaku)	Plum sauce	
Coffee	Lard	Ginger (shoga;	Red bean paste	
Iced tea	(manteca)	dried form	Black bean	
	Pork cracklings	called	sauce	
	Fruit drinks	denishoga)	Oyster sauce	
	Kool-aid	Tea	Tea	
	Carbonated	Coffee	Coffee	
	beverages			
	Beer			
	Coffee			

History form for evaluation of infant with failure to thrive*

No. _____

Date _____

Slow gaining special history

MOTHER

Name _____

A. Diet
1. Do you eat regular meals? _____ How do you rate the kind of food you eat? excellent ☐ good ☐ poor ☐
2. Do you take vitamins? _____ If so, what? _____
   _____
3. Do you take brewer's yeast? _____
4. Are you worried about your weight? _____

B. Health
1. Are you in good health _____ If not, describe problems _____
   _____
2. Are you taking any medications? _____ Birth control pills? _____
   Prescriptions? _____ Nonprescription medicines? _____
3. Have you had any thyroid problems at any time in your life? _____ Are thyroid medications being taken now? _____ What kind? _____
   _____
   Dosage _____ Last time you had your blood tested for thyroid
   _____
4. Do you have any blood pressure problems? _____

C. Habits
1. Do you smoke? _____ Which brand? _____
   How many per day? _____
2. Do you drink coffee? _____ How many cups per day? _____
   Do you drink caffeinated sodas? _____ How many caffeinated sodas per day? _____
3. Do you drink alcohol? _____ How much per day _____
   week _____ month _____ ?

D. Nursing
1. When the infant nurses, do you feel tingling ☐ burning ☐ filling feeling ☐
   leaking on other side ☐ nothing ☐
   other _____ ?
2. Do you have a quiet environment for nursing? _____ If not, why (describe)? (Example, loud music, freeway noise, dogs barking) _____
   _____
3. Do you own a rocking chair? _____

E. Social environment
1. Do you have a busy life-style? _____ If so, why (name activities)? _____
   _____
   _____
2. Marriage relationship is good ☐ average ☐ poor ☐.
3. Do you have other children? _____ Ages _____ Breast-fed?
   _____ How long? _____
4. Do you have any source of anxiety of tension? _____ If so, describe. _____
   _____

*Modified from form developed by Fleiss, P. M., and Frantz, K. B.

Continued.

Slow gaining special history—cont'd

INFANT

Name _____ Date of birth _____
1. How often is infant fed? _____
2. Breast milk only? _____ Other? _____
   Does he feed at each breast at each feeding? _____ How long on each breast? _____

3. How long does infant take to finish a feeding? _____ Does infant pause often during feeding? _____
4. Who initiates end of feeding? you ☐   infant ☐
5. How do you rate his sucking? poor ☐   weak ☐   average ☐   strong ☐
6. Is he burping easy? _____ What technique is used? _____ When burped? _____
7. Is a pacifier used? _____ What kind? _____ How much usage? _____
8. Number of wet diapers per day _____ Are paper diapers used? _____
9. Number of stools per day _____ consistency _____ color _____
10. Infant is active ☐   average ☐   placid ☐.
11. Night sleep pattern: time put to bed _____ Is this on a regular basis? _____
    List awake times _____
12. Is infant healthy? _____ Any problems since birth? _____ If so, what? _____
    _____
    Jaundice? _____ How high was the bilirubin level? _____
    Had any medications? _____ If so, what? _____
13. Ever had a urinalysis? _____ When? _____
    Any other test (especially those for slow weight gain)? _____
    If so, what? _____
    Where? _____

BIRTH HISTORY

1. Type of delivery: vaginal ☐   CS ☐   If CS, scheduled ☐   or emergency ☐ ?
2. Labor: yes ☐   no ☐   Length of time _____
3. Were medications given during labor or delivery? _____ If so, what? _____
   _____
4. Was it a difficult birth? _____ If so, describe problem _____
   _____
5. First time infant put to breast was _____ hr after birth. Did infant take to it easily? _____
6. Where was the birth? Home birth ☐   Hospital with rooming-in ☐   Hospital with infant only in the nursery ☐   Were you separated from infant for any length of time? _____
   If so, why? _____
7. Any medications taken during pregnancy? _____ If so, what? _____
   _____
8. Any medications taken after birth? _____ If so, what? _____
   _____

FAMILY HISTORY

1. Have previous infants or relatives with failure to thrive? yes ☐   no ☐
2. Have history of metabolic or malabsorption disease? yes ☐   no ☐
3. Infant has cystic fibrosis? yes ☐   no ☐
4. Infant has milk allergy? yes ☐   no ☐
5. Other? _____

Normal serum values for breast-fed infants

Table E-1. Serum chemical values of normal breast-fed infants*†

Concentration/100 ml of serum	Age 28 days			Age 56 days			Age 84 days			Age 112 days		
	N	Mean	SD	N	Mean	SD	N	Mean	SD	N	Mean	SD
Males												
Total protein (g)	22	5.87	0.50	36	5.96	0.42	29	6.16	0.57	51	6.29	0.51
Albumin (g)	22	4.02	0.35	36	4.14	0.34	29	4.27	0.39	51	4.38	0.40
Globulins (g)												
alpha$_1$	22	0.14	0.03	36	0.17	0.03	29	0.18	0.03	51	0.17	0.04
alpha$_2$	22	0.53	0.10	36	0.60	0.11	29	0.74	0.14	51	0.81	0.19
beta	22	0.61	0.11	36	0.67	0.13	29	0.69	0.20	51	0.67	0.11
gamma	22	0.57	0.14	36	0.38	0.09	29	0.28	0.08	51	0.26	0.10
Cholesterol (mg)	21	139	31	32	153	34	25	133	32	47	145	26
Triglycerides (mg)	18	122	36	32	106	57	25	170	76	46	148	57
Urea nitrogen (mg)	43	8.5	3.2	49	6.6	2.1	47	7.0	2.7	51	7.3	4.2
Calcium (mg)	41	10.2	0.8	47	10.3	1.0	42	10.4	0.8	48	10.3	0.8
Phosphorus (mg)	43	6.6	0.7	49	6.4	0.7	47	6.2	0.5	49	6.2	0.7
Alkaline phosphatase‡	31	**22**	6	40	**21**	7	35	21	8	44	18	7
Magnesium (mg)	40	2.0	0.2	47	2.1	0.2	45	2.1	0.2	50	2.2	0.2
Females												
Total protein (g)	18	6.04	0.40	27	5.86	0.44	21	6.21	0.57	42	6.31	0.62
Albumin (g)	18	4.07	0.27	27	4.03	0.35	21	4.29	0.37	42	4.36	0.42
Globulins (g)												
alpha$_1$	18	0.15	0.02	27	0.17	0.04	21	0.17	0.03	42	**0.19**	0.04
alpha$_2$	18	0.55	0.07	27	0.65	0.12	21	0.74	0.18	42	0.78	0.17
beta	18	0.70	0.18	27	0.63	0.11	21	0.71	0.13	42	0.67	0.16
gamma	18	0.57	0.10	27	0.38	0.10	21	0.30	0.06	42	**0.31**	0.10
Cholesterol (mg)	13	**180**	35	25	157	37	20	155	29	40	**165**	36
Triglycerides (mg)	9	**157**	43	24	112	53	18	195	56	38	**170**	52
Urea nitrogen (mg)	37	8.3	2.3	33	6.4	2.2	40	6.4	2.2	42	6.6	3.5
Calcium (mg)	37	10.3	0.8	33	10.3	0.8	40	10.3	0.8	42	10.7	0.7
Phosphorus (mg)	39	6.9	0.8	33	6.4	0.8	40	6.1	0.7	42	6.1	0.7
Alkaline phosphatase	31	19	5	28	17	5	32	17	5	36	17	5
Magnesium (mg)	39	2.0	0.4	32	2.0	0.2	40	2.1	0.2	41	2.1	0.3

*From Fomon, S. J. et al.: Acta Paediatr. Scand. suppl. 202:1, 1970.

†Bold figures indicate that value is greater than the corresponding value for infants of the opposite sex and that the difference is statistically significant at the 95% level of confidence.

‡King-Armstrong units.

Drugs in breast milk and the effect on the infant

The following list of drugs is provided to assist the clinician in making judgments about management for specific drugs in an individual mother and her infant. The clinician is referred to Chapter 10 for the discussion of interpretation of risks and benefits. It is also important to point out that the significance of a given blood level would vary with the pH and the binding capacity of the maternal plasma protein, which may differ for various ethnic and racial groups. Furthermore, it is not merely a matter of understanding the pharmacokinetics of a specific drug, but also of understanding the physiology of milk production and finally, most critically, understanding the absorption and excretion of the drug by the newborn, which changes with conceptual and chronological age.

The drugs have been grouped by their major use to provide an opportunity to compare therapeutic choices and select the medication that is best for both mother and infant. The classifications of the drugs listed are as follows:

Analgesics and anti-inflammatory drugs (nonnarcotic)
Antibiotics
Anticoagulants
Anticonvulsants and sedatives
Antihistaminics
Autonomic drugs
Cardiovascular drugs
Cathartics
Diagnostic materials and procedures
Diuretics
Environmental agents
Heavy metals
Hormones and contraceptives
Narcotics
Psychotropic and mood-changing drugs
Stimulants
Thyroid and antithyroid medications
Miscellaneous

Table F-1. Relationship of drugs to breast milk and effect on infant

Drug	Excreted in milk	Amount in milk after therapeutic dose	Effect on infant	Reference
Analgesics and anti-inflammatory drugs (nonnarcotic)				
Acetaminophen (Datril, Tylenol)	Yes		Detoxified in liver. Avoid in immediate postpartum period, otherwise no problems with therapeutic dose.	
Aspirin	Yes	1-3 mg/100 ml*	Long history of experience shows complications rare. Can cause interference with platelet aggregation and diminished factor XII (Hageman factor) at birth. When mother requires high, continuing level of medication for arthritis, apirin drug of choice. Observe infant for bruisability. Platelet aggregation can be evaluated. Salicylism only seen in maternal overdosing. Mother should increase vitamin C and vitamin K intake.	Bleyer and Breckenridge, 1970; Anderson, 1977
Donnatal (phenobarbital, hyoscyamine sulfate, atropine sulfate, hyoscine hydrobromide)	Yes		Consider for its component parts. Can be given to children but can accumulate in neonate.	PDR, 1979; personal observations
Flufenamic acid (Arlef)	Yes	0.50 μg/ml (mean)†	No apparent effect on infant when maternal dosage was 200 mg, three times a day. Infant able to excrete via urine.	Buchanan et al., 1969
Indomethacin (Indocin)	Yes		Convulsions in breast-fed neonate (case report). Used to close patent ductus arteriosus. Insufficient data as to effect on other vessels. May be nephrotoxic.	Eeg-Olofsson et al., 1978
Mefenamid acid (Ponstel)	Yes	Trace amounts‡	No apparent effect on infant at therapeutic doses; infant able to excrete via urine.	Buchanan et al., 1968
Naproxen (Naprosyn, synaxsyn, naprosine, naxen, proxen)	Yes	1% of maternal plasma; binds to plasma protein	Less toxic in adults than some other organic derivatives.	PDR, 1979; Roth, 1976
Oxyphenbutazone (Tandearil)	Yes	In milk of 2 of 55 mothers, 10% to 80% of maternal plasma level	No known effect.	O'Brien, 1974; Knowles, 1974

Pentazocine (Talwin)	No		Withdrawal in neonatal period from ingestion during pregnancy.	Kopelman, 1975; O'Brien, 1974
Percodan (oxycodone [derived from opiate thebaine] aspirin, phenacetin, caffeine)	Yes		Consider for its component parts. In neonatal period sleepiness and failure to feed, which increase maternal engorgement and neonatal weight loss, have been observed, probably due to oxycodone.	PDR, 1979; personal observations
Phenylbutazone (Butazolidin)	Yes	0.63 mg/ml 90 min after 750 mg given IM	Very potent drug; risk to infant not well defined but considerable. Not given directly to children; may accumulate in infant.	Gaginella, 1978; Shore, 1970
Propoxyphene (Darvon)	Yes	0.4% of maternal§ dose	Only symptoms detectable would be failure to feed and drowsiness. On daily, around-the-clock dosage infant could consume 1 mg/day.	O'Brien, 1974; Arena, 1970; Ananth, 1978
Antibiotics				
Amantadine (Symmetrel)	Yes	Not defined	Vomiting, urinary retention, rash. Contraindicated.	O'Brien, 1974
Ampicillin (Polycillin, Amcill, Omnipen, Penbritin)	Yes	0.07 μg/ml	Sensitivity due to repeated exposure; diarrhea or secondary candidiasis.	O'Brien, 1974; Savage, 1977; Gaginella, 1978
Carbenicillin (Pyopen, Geopen)	Yes	0.265 μg/ml 1 hr after 1 g given‖	Levels not significant. Drug is given to neonate.	O'Brien, 1974
Cefazolin (Ancef, Kefzol)	Yes	1.5 μg/ml or 0.075% dose given	Probably not significant.	Yoshioka et al., 1979
Cephalexin (Keflex)	No			
Cephalothin (Keflin)	No			
Chloramphenicol (Chloromycetin)	Yes	Half blood level; 2.5 mg/100 ml	Grey syndrome. Infant does not excrete drug well and small amounts may accumulate. Contraindicated. May be tolerated in older infant with mature glycuronide system.	Vorherr, 1974, 1976; Gaginella, 1978; Havelka et al., 1968
Chloroquine (Aralen)	Yes	2.7 mg in 2 days‖	Can be used to *treat* child under 6 mo of age who is wholly breast-fed.	Clyde and Shute, 1956
Colistin (Colymycin)	Yes	0.05-0.09 mg/100 ml	Not absorbed orally.	Vorherr, 1974

*Plasma level was 1-5 mg/100 ml.
†Shown when mean maternal plasma level was 6.41 μg/ml. Mean level in infant's plasma was 0.12 μg/ml; in infant's urine, 0.08 μg/ml. (Maternal plasma level was fifty times that of infant.)
‡0.91 μg/ml mean maternal plasma level showed 0.21 μg/ml mean milk level. Mean infant plasma level was 0.08 μg/ml and mean urine level. 9.8 μg/ml.
§Shown by animal experiments. Plasma/milk ratio (P/M) = ½.
‖Peaks in 6 hr.

Continued.

Table F-1. Relationship of drugs to breast milk and effect on infant—cont'd

Drug	Excreted in milk	Amount in milk after therapeutic dose	Effect on infant	Reference
Antibiotics—cont'd				
Demeclocycline (Declomycin)	Yes	0.2-0.3 mg/500 ml	Not significant in therapeutic doses. Can be given to infants.	O'Brien, 1974
Erythromycin (Ilosone, E-Mycin, Erythrocin)	Yes	0.05-0.1 mg/100 ml; 3.6-6.2 μg/ml	Higher concentrations have been reported in milk than in plasma. Should not be given under 1 mo of age because of risk of jaundice. Dose in milk higher when given IV to mother.	Gaginella, 1978; O'Brien, 1974
Gentamicin	Unknown		Not absorbed from gastrointestinal tract, may change gut flora. Drug is given to newborns directly.	Remington and Klein, 1976
Isoniazid (Nydrazid)	Yes	0.6-1.2 mg/100 ml*	Infant at risk for toxicity, but need for breast milk may outweigh risk.	Knowles, 1965; Jelliffe, 1978
Kanamycin (Kantrex)	Yes	18.4 μg/ml after 1 g given IM	Infant absorbs little from gastrointestinal tract. Infants can be given drug.	Anderson, 1977
Lincomycin (Lincocin)	Yes	0.5-2.4 mg/100 ml	Not significant in therapeutic doses to affect child.	O'Brien, 1974; *Toxicology Review*, 1978
Mandelic acid	Yes	0.3 g/24 hr after dose of 12 g/day	Not significant in therapeutic doses to affect child.	O'Brien, 1974; *Toxicology Review*, 1978
Methacycline (Rondomycin)	Yes	½ plasma level; 50-260 μg/100 ml	Same precautions as with tetracycline.	O'Brien, 1974; Vorherr
Methenamine (Hexamine)	Yes		Not significant in therapeutic doses to affect child.	O'Brien, 1974; *Toxicology Review*
Metronidazole (Flagyl)	Yes	Level comparable to serum†	Caution should be exercised due to its high milk concentrations. Contraindicated when infant under 6 mo, may cause neurologic disorders and blood dyscrasia.	Gray, 1961; Gaginella, 1978; Hervada, 1978
Nalidixic acid (Neggram)	Yes	0.4 mg/100 ml	Not significant in therapeutic doses beyond neonatal period. Hemolytic anemia in an infant attributed to nalidixic acid in G6PD deficiency or when mother has renal failure.	Catz and Giacoia, 1972; Vorherr, 1976
Nitrofurantoin (Furadantin)	Yes	Trace to 0.5 μg/ml	Not significant in therapeutic doses to affect child except in G6PD deficiency.	Varsano et al., 1973
Novobiocin (Albamycin, cathomycin)	Yes	0.36-0.54 mg/100 ml	Infant can be given drug directly.	Texeira and Scott, 1958

Drug		Amount in milk	Comment	Reference
Nystatin (Mycostatin)	No		Can be given to infant directly.	Knowles, 1974
Oxacillin (Prostaphlin)	No		Not absorbed orally	O'Brien, 1974
Para-aminosalicylic acid	No			O'Brien, 1974
Penethamate (Leocillin)	Yes	24-74 μg/100 ml	Animal study suggests it be avoided.	
Penicillin G, benzathine (Bicillin)	Yes	10-12 units/100 ml	Clinical need should supersede possible allergic responses.	Vorherr, 1976; Gaginella, 1978
Penicillin G, potassium	Yes	Up to 6 units/100 ml; 1.2-3.6 μg/100 ml	Infant can be given penicillin directly. Parents should be told to inform physician that infant has been exposed to penicillin because of potential sensitivity.	
Pyrimethamine (Daraprim)	Yes	0.3 mg/100 ml (3% of dose)	Significant in therapeutic doses when infant under 6 mo and entirely breast-fed.	Clyde and Shute, 1956
Quinine sulfate	Yes	0-0.1 mg/100 ml after maternal dose of 300-600 mg	In therapeutic doses, no affect to child except rare thrombocytopenia.	Terwilliger and Hatcher, 1939; *Medical Letter,* 1974
Sodium fusidate	Yes	0.02 μg/ml	Not significant in therapeutic doses to affect child.	O'Brien, 1974
Streptomycin	Yes	Present for long periods in slight amounts given as dihydrostreptomycin	Not to be given more than 2 wk. Ototoxic and nephrotoxic with long use. Is given to infants directly.	Knowles, 1965; Takyi, 1970
Sulfanilamide	Yes	9 mg/100 ml after dose of 2-4 g daily	Not significant in therapeutic doses; may cause a rash or hemolytic anemia. Should be avoided for first month postpartum.	Lein et al., 1974; Knowles, 1965; O'Brien, 1974
Sulfapyridine	Yes	3-13 mg/100 ml after dose of 3 g daily	To be avoided; has caused skin rash.	Lein et al., 1974; Knowles, 1965; O'Brien, 1974
Sulfathiazole	Yes	0.5 mg/100 ml after dose of 3 g/day	Not significant in therapeutic doses to affect child after 1 mo of age.	Lein et al., 1974; Knowles, 1965; O'Brien, 1974
Sulfisoxazole (Gantrisin)	Yes	Concentration similar to plasma level	To be avoided during first month postpartum; may cause kernicterus.	Lein et al., 1974; Knowles, 1965; O'Brien, 1974
Tetracycline HCl (Achromycin, Panmycin, Sumycin)	Yes	0.5-2.6 μg/ml after dose of 500 mg four times a day	Not enough to treat an infection in an infant. May cause discoloration of the teeth in the infant; the antibiotic, however, may be largely bound to the milk calcium. Do not give over 10 days or repeatedly.	Posner et al., 1955-1956; Shidlovsky et al., 1957-1958

*Same concentration in milk as in maternal serum.
†Gives serum levels in infants of 0.05 to 0.4 μg/ml.

Continued.

Table F-1. Relationship of drugs to breast milk and effect on infant—cont'd

Drug	Excreted in milk	Amount in milk after therapeutic dose	Effect on infant	Reference
Anticoagulants				
Coumarin derivatives Dicumarol (bishydroxycoumarin) Warfarin (Panwarfin)	Yes	Probably little but* may be cumulative	Monitor prothrombin time. Give vitamin K to infant. Discontinue if surgery or trauma occurs. Drug of choice if mother to continue nursing.	Brambel and Hunter, 1950; O'Brien, 1974; Savage, 1977; Baty et al., 1976; deSweet and Lewis, 1977
Ethyl biscoumacetate (Tromexan)	Yes	0-0.17 mg/100 ml†	Hemorrhage around umbilical stump and cephalhematoma reported. Prothrombin normal in infants with hemorrhage. Vitamin K has no effect. Contraindicated while nursing.	Illingworth, 1953; Knowles, 1974
Heparin	No		Heparin is not effective orally.	Goodman and Gilman, 1975
Phenindione (Hedulin) (Dindevan)	Yes		Breast milk a major route of excretion. Reports of serious hemorrhage in infant. Prothrombin times prolonged in infant. Contraindicated while nursing.	Eckstein and Jack, 1970; Knowles, 1974
Anticonvulsants and sedatives‡				
Barbital (Veronal)	Yes	8-10 mg/L after 500 mg dose	May produce sedation in infant. In general, barbiturates pass into milk but do not sedate infant. Watch for symptoms.	O'Brien, 1974
Carbamazepine (Tegretol)	Yes	60% of plasma levels§	Animal studies show lack of weight gain, unkempt appearance.	Pynnönen and Sillanpää, 1975
Chloral hydrate (Notec, Somnos)	Yes	Up to 1.5 mg/100 ml	No significant symptoms, can be given to infants directly.	Lacey, 1974
Diphenylhydantoin (Dilantin)	Yes	1.5 to 2.6 µg/ml after 300 mg/day dose	One case of hemolytic reaction reported. Other infants appear to tolerate the small doses. Therapeutic plasma level 10-20 µg/ml.	Mirkin, 1971
Mephenytoin (Mesantoin) (hydantoin homologue of mephobarbital)	Unknown		Detoxified in liver. No information.	
Pentobarbital (Nembutal)	Yes		Depends on liver for detoxification so may accumulate in first week of life until infant able to detoxify. No problem for older infant in usual doses.	
Phenobarbital (Luminal)	Yes	0.1-0.5 mg when plasma level 0.6 to 1.8 mg	Sleepiness and decreased sucking possible. On usual analeptic doses infants alert and feed well. On hypnotic doses infant depressed and hard to rouse.	Tyson et al., II, 1938

Drug	In milk	Amount in milk	Comments	References
Phensuximide (Milontin)			No specific data.	
Primidone (Mysoline)	Yes		Causes drowsiness and decreased feeds. May cause bleeding due to hypoprothrombinemia. Need vitamin K. Avoid drug during lactation.	O'Brien, 1974
Sodium bromide (Bromo-Seltzer and across-the-counter sleeping aids)	Yes	Up to 6.6 mg/100 ml	Drowsy, decreased crying, rash, decreased feeding	Tyson et al., III, 1938
Trimethadione (Tridione)			No specific data.	
Antihistaminics				
Brompheniramine (Dimetane) Diphenhydramine (Benadryl) Methdilazine (Tacaryl) Tripelennamine (Pyribenzamine)	Yes	No specific data available. All pass into milk.	Drug is used in neonates. May cause sedation, decreased feeding, or may produce stimulation and tachycardia. Should avoid long-acting preparations, which may accumulate in infant. When combined with decongestants, may cause decrease in milk.	Arena, 1970; Rivera-Calimlim, 1977; Oseid, 1975
Autonomic drugs				
Atropine sulfate‖	Yes	0.1 mg/100 ml	Hyperthermia, atropine toxicity, infants especially sensitive; also inhibits lactation. Infant dose 0.01 mg/kg	O'Brien, 1974; Rivera-Calimlim, 1977
Carisprodol (Soma, Rela)	Yes	Two to four times maternal plasma	Blocks interneuronal activity in descending reticular formation and spinal cord; drowsiness, hypotonia, poor feed.	O'Brien, 1974; *PDR*, 1979
Ergot (Cafergot)	Yes	Unknown	90% of infants had symptoms of ergotism. Vomiting and diarrhea to weak pulse and unstable blood pressure. Short-term therapy for migraine should not exceed 6 mg. Cafergot also contains caffeine, 100 mg.	Riviera-Calimlim, 1977; O'Brien, 1974; Knowles, 1965
Mepenzolate bromide (Cantil)	No		Postganglionic parasympathetic inhibitor used to diminish gastric acidity and decrease spasm of colon. Oral absorption low.	O'Brien, 1974; *PDR*, 1979
Methocarbamol (Robaxin)	Yes	Minimal	Too little in milk to produce effect.	O'Brien, 1974

*Reports conflict.
†No correlation with dosage, continues in milk after plasma clear.
‡All barbitals appear in breast milk.
§When plasma 13.0 µmol/L, 7.5 µmol/L in milk.
‖Ingredient in many prescription and nonprescription drugs.

Continued.

Table F-1. Relationship of drugs to breast milk and effect on infant—cont'd

Drug	Excreted in milk	Amount in milk following therapeutic dose	Effect on infant	Reference
Autonomic drugs—cont'd				
Neostigmine	No		No known harm to infant.	McNall and Jafarnia, 1965
Propantheline bromide (Pro-Banthine)	No	Uncontrolled data indicate no measurable levels	Drug rapidly metabolized in maternal system to inactive metabolite. Mother should avoid long-acting preparations, however.	O'Brien, 1974; Takyi, 1970
Scopolamine (hyoscine)	Yes		Usually given as single dose and of no problem to neonate. No data on repeated doses.	Arena, 1970
Cardiovascular drugs				
Diazoxide (Hyperstat)			Arteriolar dilators and antihypertensive, only given IV, not active orally.	PDR, 1979
Dibenzyline†			No data available	
Digoxin	Yes	0.96-0.61 ng/ml*	Digoxin 20% bound to protein; infant receives < 1/100 of dose. If mother at toxic level of 5 ng/ml, milk would have 4.4 ng/ml and infant would receive only $^1/_{20}$ daily dose.	Loughnan, 1978; Levy et al., 1977
Guanethidine (Ismelin)‡	Yes		Not significant in therapeutic doses to affect child.	O'Brien, 1974; Takyi, 1976
Hydralazine (Apresoline)‡	Yes		Jaundice, thrombocytopenia, electrolyte disturbances possible.	
Methyldopa (Aldomet)‡	Yes		Galactorrhea. No specific data except as affects mother's milk production.	Takyi, 1970; Redmond, 1976
Propranolol (Inderal)§	Yes	40 ng/ml of maternal plasma‖	Insignificant amount. Infants reported had no symptoms noted. Should watch for hypoglycemia and/or "β-blocking effects."	Anderson and Salter, 1976
Quinidine	Yes		Arrhythmia may occur.	Oseid, 1975
Reserpine (Serpasil)‡	Yes		May produce galactorrhea, lethargy, diarrhea, or nasal stuffiness.	O'Brien, 1974; Medical Letter, 1974
Cathartics				
Aloin	Yes	Low	Occasionally gave symptoms, caused colic and diarrhea in infant.	Tyson, I, 1937
Anthraquinone laxatives such as dihydroxyanthraquinone (Dorbane and Dorbantyl)	Yes	High	Caused colic and diarrhea in infant.	Hervada et al., 1978

Calomel	No	None	None	Tyson, I, 1937
Cascara	Yes	Low	Caused colic and diarrhea in infant.	Hervada et al., 1978
Milk of magnesia	No	None	No effect.	Hervada et al., 1978
Mineral oil	No	None	No effect.	Tyson, I, 1937
Phenolphthalein	Unknown	Unknown¶	Reported to cause symptoms in some.	Tyson, I, 1937
Rhubarb	Unknown	None	None in syrup form. Fresh rhubarb may give symptoms of colic and diarrhea.	Tyson, I, 1937
Saline cathartics	No	None	No effect.	Hervada et al., 1978
Senna	No	None	None.	Tyson, I, 1937
Stool softeners and bulk-forming laxatives	No	None	No effect.	Hervada et al., 1978
Suppositories (for constipation)	No	None	Not absorbed.	Shore, 1970
Diagnostic materials and procedures				
Barium	No		Not absorbed.	
Iopanoic acid (Telepaque)	Yes		Not sufficient to produce problem in infant on single dose. Does contain iodine radical.	O'Brien, 1974
Radioactive compounds				
Radioactive sodium	Yes	0.5-1.3% of dose/L**	Diminished after 24 hr; discontinue nursing 24 hr.	Knowles, 1974
[^{67}Ga] citrate	Yes		Discontinue nursing until ^{67}Ga has cleared, usually 24 hr.	O'Brien, 1974
^{125}I, ^{131}I	Yes	M/P = 0.13 μCi/0.002 μCi††	^{131}I content in milk proportional to amount of milk. Most excreted in 24 hr. Discontinue nursing for 48 hr or check milk prior to resuming feeding if under 48 hr.	Weaver et al., 1960
^{90}Sr	Yes	M/P = $^{1}/_{10}$	Less than in cow's milk. Bottle infant doubles stores in 1 mo.	Widdowson et al., 1960

*Peak level occurs 4 to 6 hr after dose given. Maternal plasma level was higher, M/P = 0.9 and 0.8; infant's plasma level was 0.
†α blocking agent.
‡Adrenergic blocking agent.
§β blocking agent.
‖Total daily dose to infant via milk is 15-20 μg.
¶Reports differ.
**Peak in 2 hr; detectable for 96 hr.
††27% of dose in 48 hr.

Continued.

Table F-1. Relationship of drugs to breast milk and effect on infant—cont'd

Drug	Excreted in milk	Amount in milk after therapeutic dose	Effect on infant	Reference
Diagnostic materials and procedures—cont'd				
^{99m}Tc	Yes		Reported to clear in 6 to 22 hr. Discontinue breast-feeding 24 hr. ^{99m}Tc preferentially picked up by breast tissue.	O'Connell and Sutton, 1976
Tuberculin test	No		Tuberculin-sensitive mothers can adoptively immunize their infants through breast milk and that immunity may last several years.	Mohr, 1973
X rays	No		No effect.	
Diuretics				
Acetazolamine (Diamox)	Probable	No specific data available but probably similar to sulfonamide	Acts as enzyme inhibitor on carbonic anhydrase non-bacteriostatic sulfonamide. Observe only for dehydration and electrolyte loss by monitoring urine and turgor.	Rothermel and Faber, 1975
Furosemide (sulfamoylanthranilic acid) (Lasix)	No		Drug is given to children under medical management	Takyi, 1970; O'Brien, 1974
Mercurial diuretics (Dicurin, Thiomerin)	Yes		In addition to diuretic effect, there is risk of mercury deposition. However, drug not absorbed orally.	O'Brien, 1974
Spironolactone (Aldactone)	Yes	Canrenone, a metabolite, appears	Acts as antagonist of aldosterone; causes sodium excretion and potassium retention. The metabolite apparently has some activity.	
Thiazides (Diuril, Enduron, Esidrix, Hydrodiuril, Oretic, Thiuretic tablets)	Yes	> 0.1 mg/100 ml*	Risk of dehydration and electrolyte imbalance, especially sodium loss, which would require monitoring. Watching weight and wet diapers and taking an occasional specific gravity reading of the urine and serum sodium would assure status of infant. Risk, however, is extremely low. May suppress lactation due to dehydration in mother.	Werthmann and Krees, 1972; Catz and Giacoia, 1972
Environmental agents				
Aldrin	Yes	Varies by location	Not a reason to wean from breast. No need to test milk unless inordinate exposure.	Bakken and Seip, 1976

Benzene hexachloride (BHC)	Yes	Varies by location	Not a reason to wean from breast. No need to test milk unless inordinate exposure.	Bakken and Seip, 1976
Dichlorodiphenyltrichloroethane (DDT or DDE)	Yes	Varies by location	Not a reason to wean from breast. No need to test milk unless inordinate exposure.	Wurster, 1970
Dieldrin	Yes	Varies by location	Also found in permanently mothproofed garments. Avoid these. Not a reason to wean.	Bakken and Seip, 1976
Hexachlorobenzene (HCB)	Yes	Varies by location	Not a reason to wean from breast. No need to test milk unless inordinate exposure.	Bakken and Seip, 1976
Heptachlorepoxide	Yes	Varies by location	Not a reason to wean from breast. No need to test milk unless inordinate exposure.	Bakken and Seip, 1976
Methyl mercury	Yes	500-1000 ng/ml†	Infant blood level 600 ng/ml in heavy exposure. Only in excessive exposure is testing and/or weaning necessary.	Amin-Zaki et al., 1976
Polybrominated biphenyl (PBB)	Yes	Varies by location	If mother at high risk from the environment or the diet, milk sample should be measured. If level in milk is high, then breast-feeding should be discontinued. Those at risk are (1) workers who handle PBB/PCB, (2) individuals who eat game fish from contaminated waters. Crash diets mobilize fats and should be avoided especially if PBB or PCB present.	AAP Committee on Environmental Hazards, 1978
Polychlorinated biphenyl (PCB)	Yes	Varies by location		
^{90}Sr, ^{89}Sr (strontium)	Yes	$^{1}/_{10}$ of that in maternal diet	Cow's milk has six times as much as human milk. Cow's milk-fed infant doubles amount in body in 1 mo.	Staub and Murthy, 1965; Widdowson et al., 1960
Heavy metals				
Arsenic	Yes	Can be measured for given patient	Can accumulate. Check infant's blood level if there is reason to suspect exposure.	Arena, 1970
Copper	Yes			
Fluorine	Yes		Monitor for excessive dose.	Arena, 1970
Gold thiomalate (Myocrisin)	Yes	0.022 µg/ml when mother given 50 mg/wk	No proteinuria or aminoaciduria observed.	Bell and Dale, 1976
Halothane	Yes	2 ppm	Nursing mothers who work in environment with halothane should be checked.	

*Linear relationship between plasma and milk. In 1 L of milk at 0.1 mg/100 ml there would be 1 mg/day. Infant dose is 20 mg/kg/day.

†M/P = 8.6% in heavy exposure.

Continued.

Table F-1. Relationship of drugs to breast milk and effect on infant—cont'd

Drug	Excreted in milk	Amount in milk after therapeutic dose	Effect on infant	Reference
Heavy metals—cont'd				
Iron	Yes			
Lead	Unknown		Nursing contraindicated if maternal serum 40 μg; conflicting reports, breast milk not always cause of lead poisoning in breast-fed infant.	Perkins and Oski, 1976
Magnesium	Yes		Not sufficient to be toxic.	Arena, 1970
Mercury	Yes		Hazardous to infant.	O'Brien, 1974
Hormones and contraceptives				
Carbimazole (neo-mercazole)	Yes		Antithyroid effect may cause goiter.	O'Brien, 1974
Chlorotrianisene (Tace)	Yes		Has estrogenic effect although does not change consistency of milk. May have feminizing effect on infant.	
Contraceptives (oral) Ethinyl estradiol Mestranol 19-Nortestosterone Norethindrone (Norlutin) Norethynodrel (Enovid)	Yes		May diminish milk supply. May decrease vitamins, protein, and fat in milk. Velázquez showed no difference when mothers took norethindrone. Most significant concern is long-range impact of hormone on young infant, which is not certain. Reports of feminization of infant.	Briggs and Briggs, 1974; Barsivala and Virkar, 1973; Ibrahim and El-Tawil, 1968; Kora, 1969; Miller and Hughes, 1970; Velázquez et al., 1976; Ramadan et al., 1972; Nilsson et al., 1977
Corticotropin	Yes		Destroyed in gastrointestinal tract of infant. No effect.	Catz and Giacoia, 1972
Cortisone	Yes		Animal studies show 50% lower weight than controls and retarded sexual development and exophthalmos.	Catz and Giacoia, 1972
Dihydrotachysterol (Hytakerol)	Yes		May cause hypercalcemia; need monitoring of infant serum and urine calcium.	Catz and Giacoia, 1972
Epinephrine (Adrenalin)	Yes		Destroyed in GI tract of infant.	Catz and Giacoia, 1972
Estrogen	Yes	0.17 μg/100 ml after 1 g	Risks as with oral contraceptives.	Knowles, 1974
Fluoxymesterone (Halotestin, Ora-Testryl, Ultandren)	Yes		Suppresses lactation; masculinizing.	O'Brien, 1974

Drug	Secreted	Amount in milk	Comments	References
Insulin	Unknown		Destroyed in gastrointestinal tract.	Catz and Giacoia, 1972
Liothyronine (Cytomel)	No		Synthetic form of natural thyroid.	O'Brien, 1974
Medroxyprogesterone acetate (Provera)	No			O'Brien, 1974
Phenformin HCl	Yes	Minimal	Not sufficient to cause symptoms in infant. Does not cause hypoglycemia in normal infants. No case reports available.	O'Brien, 1974
Prednisone	Yes	0.07–0.23% dose/L after 5 mg dose*	Minimal amount not likely to cause effect on infant in short course.	Katz and Duncan, 1975; McKenzie et al., 1975
Pregnanediol	Yes		Unknown risk as with other female hormones over a long period of time.	
Tolbutamide (Orinase)	Yes		Not recommended in the childbearing years.	
Narcotics				
Codeine		0 to trace after 32 mg every 4 hr (6 doses)	No effect in therapeutic level and transient usage. Can accumulate. Individual variation. Watch for neonatal depression.	Knowles, 1965; Oseid, 1975; Kwit and Hatcher, 1935
Heroin	Yes		13 of 22 infants had withdrawal; historically breast-feeding had been used to wean addict's infant. This is no longer recommended.	Savage, 1977; Catz and Giacoia, 1972
Marihuana (*Cannabis*)	Yes		Shown in laboratory animals to produce structural changes in nursling's brain cell; impairs DNA and RNA formation. Infant at risk of inhaling smoke during feeding or when held while smoking.	Nahas, 1974, 1975, 1976; Crumpton and Brill, 1971; Clark et al., 1970; Campbell et al., 1971; Talbott, 1969
Meperidine (Demerol)	Yes	> 0.1 mg/100 ml‡	Trace amounts may accumulate if drug taken around the clock when infant is neonate. Watch for drowsiness and poor feeding.	O'Brien, 1974; Oseid, 1975
Methadone	Yes	0.03 µg/ml or 0.023–0.028 mg/day†	When dosage not excessive, infant can be breast-fed if monitored for evidence of depression and failure to thrive.	Blinick et al., 1975 and 1976; Kreek et al., 1974
Morphine	Yes	Trace amount	Single doses have minimal effect. Potential for accumulation. May be addicting to neonate. No longer considered appropriate means of weaning infant of an addict.	Arena, 1970; O'Brien, 1974; Vorherr, 1974, 1976

*0.16 µg/ml after 10 mg dose; 2.67 µg/ml after 2 hr.
†Mother received 50 mg/day; M/P = 0.83. Peak level 4 hr after oral dose. Results obscured if addict also taking the herbal root golden seal.
‡Plasma 0.07–0.1 mg/100 ml.

Continued.

Table F-1. Relationship of drugs to breast milk and effect on infant—cont'd

Drug	Excreted in milk	Amount in milk after therapeutic dose	Effect on infant	Reference
Psychotropic and mood-changing drugs				
Alcohol	Yes	Similar to plasma level	Ordinarily no problem and can be therapeutic in moderation. Infants are more susceptible to effects. Chronic drinking reported to cause obesity in one infant. Ethanol in doses of 1 to 2 g/kg to the mother causes depression of milk-ejection reflex (dose dependent). No acetaldehyde found in infants.	Ananth, 1978; *Medical Letter*, 1974
Amphetamine	Yes		Has caused stimulation in infants with jitteriness, irritability, sleeplessness. Long-acting preparations cumulative.	Arena, 1970; Knowles, 1965, 1974; Vorherr, 1974
Benzodiazepines*				
Chlordiazepoxide HCl (Librium)	Yes		Not sufficient to affect infant first week when glucuronyl system needed for detoxification. May accumulate. Older infant, no apparent problem.	Catz and Giacoia, 1972; Takyi, 1970; O'Brien, 1974
Diazepam (Valium)	Yes	90 μg/L†	Detoxified in glucuronyl system. In first weeks of life may contribute to jaundice. Metabolite active. Effect on infant: hypoventilation, drowsiness, lethargy, and weight loss. Single doses over 10 mg contraindicated during nursing. Accumulation in infant possible.	Erkkola and Kanto, 1972; Brandt, 1976; Patrick et al., 1972; Cole and Hailey, 1970; Catz, 1973
Pineazepam	Yes	5-11.2 ng of metabolite/ml; > 1.0 ng of pineazepam/ml‡	No data, probably similar to diazepam.	Pacifici and Placidi, 1977
Haloperidol (Haldol)	Yes	Unknown	A butyrophenone antidepressant; animal studies in nurslings show behavior abnormalities.	Lundberg, 1972
Lithium carbonate (Eskalith, Lithane, Lithonate)	Yes	⅓-½ maternal plasma level§	Measurable lithium in infant's serum. Infant kidney can clear lithium; however, lithium inhibits adenosine 3':5'-cyclic monophosphate, significant to brain growth. Also affects amine metabolism. Real effects not measurable immediately. Report of cyanosis and poor muscle tone and ECG changes in nursing infant.	Schou and Amdisen, 1973; Sykes et al., 1976; Tupin and Hopkin, 1978; O'Brien, 1974; Tunnessen and Hertz, 1972
Monoamine oxidase (MAO) inhibitors (Eutonyl, Nardil)			Inhibits lactation.	Dickey and Stone, 1975

Drug	Excreted in milk	Amount in milk	Comments	References
Meprobamate (Miltown, Equanil)‖	Yes	2 to 4 times maternal plasma level	If therapy continued, infant should be followed closely.	O'Brien, 1974; Ananth, 1978
Penfluridol‖	Yes	Unknown	Animal studies show learning abnormalities in sucklings. This is a potent long-acting oral neuroleptic drug.	Janssen et al., 1970; Athlenius et al., 1973
Phenothiazines				
Chlorpromazine (Thorazine)	Yes	1/3 plasma level¶	Can be safely nursed; minimum in milk. Increases maternal prolactin. No symptoms in infants reported; 5 yr follow-up showed infants normal.	Ananth, 1978; Blacker et al., 1962; Milkovich and Van den Berg, 1976; Vorherr, 1974
Mesoridazine (Serentil)	Yes	Minimal	Probably no effect.	O'Brien, 1974
Piperacetazine (Quide)	Yes	Minimal		O'Brien, 1974
Thioridozine (Mellaril)	Yes	No information	Thioridoxine is less potent in general than other phenothiazines. Probably quite safe.	O'Brien, 1974
Trifluoperazine (Stelazine)	Yes	Minimal		O'Brien, 1974
Tricyclic antidepressants			Apparently no accumulation. No infants that have been followed showed symptoms. Watch for depression or failure to feed. Increases maternal prolactin secretion.	Ananth, 1978; Ayd, 1973; Vorherr, 1974
Amitriptyline HCl (Elavil)	Yes	Minimal amounts		
Desipramine HCl (Norpramin, Pertofrane)	Yes	Minimal amounts		
Imipramine HCl (Tofranil)	Yes	0.1 mg/100 ml**		
Stimulants				
Caffeine	Yes	1% of dose	Accumulates when intake moderate and continual. Causes jitteriness, wakefulness, and irritability. Caffeine present in many hot and cold drinks. Consider if infant very wakeful.	Horning, 1975; Rivera-Calimlim, 1977
Theobromine	Yes	3.7-8.2 mg/L after 240 mg dose††	No adverse symptoms observed in the infants. Chocolate most common cause of exposure.	Resman et al., 1977
Theophylline	Yes	10% of maternal dose§§	Irritability, fretfulness	Yurchak et al., 1976; Knowles, 1974

*Alcohol enhances effect of this group.

†10 mg or less yields 45 ng of diazepam/ml and 85 ng of metabolite/ml. P/M ratio is variable. Mean P/M ratio of diazepam is 6.14; of metabolite is 3.64. Effect lasts about 4 days.

‡Both drug and active metabolite appear for about 4 days after dose, 5-11.2 ng/ml metabolite, less than 1.0 ng/ml pineazepam.

§0.030 mmol/L in infant's serum, 0.57 mmol/L in infant's urine. Milk level was half of maternal serum level in case report by Sykes et al.

‖Neuroleptic drug.

¶If dose < 200 mg, milk contains bare trace. Dose of 1200 mg showed trace.

**Plasma level 0.2-1.3 mg/100 ml.

††113 g chocolate bar.

§§M/P = 0.7.

Continued.

Table F-1. Relationship of drugs to breast milk and effect on infant—cont'd

Drug	Excreted in milk	Amount in milk after therapeutic dose	Effect on infant	Reference
Thyroid and antithyroid medications				
Carbimazole (neo-mercazole)	Yes		May cause goiter.	O'Brien, 1974
Methimazole (Tapazole)	Yes	M/P > 1	Inhibits synthesis of thyroid hormone but does not inactivate existing thyroid. Can inhibit infant thyroid. ⅛ grain/day of thyroid can be given to infant simultaneously.	Vorherr, 1976; Gaginella, 1978; Kwit and Hatcher, 1935
Potassium iodide	Yes	3 mg/100 ml*	May alter thyroid function of infant; may cause goiter in infant.	Gaginella, 1978; Knowles, 1965, 1974
Propylthiouracil	Yes	M/P > 1; 4.5-6% of dose	Risk of goiter and agranulocytosis. With present microtechniques for T₃, T₄ and TSH, close monitoring of infant is possible, as with methimazole.	Vorherr, 1976
Radioactive iodine ¹²⁵I, ¹³¹I (as a treatment)	Yes	M/P > 1	*Treatment* doses are excreted via the breast for 1 to 3 wk. Milk can be checked by Geiger counter if there is a question. Breast-feeding should be discontinued until milk is clear.	Knowles, 1965, 1974; Weaver et al., 1960
Thiouracil	Yes	9-12 mg/100 ml†	Same as for propylthiouracil.	Williams et al., 1944
Thyroid and thyroxine	Yes		Does not produce adverse symptoms on long-range follow-up. Noted to improve milk supply of hypothyroid mothers. No contraindication.	Vorherr, 1976; O'Brien, 1974

Miscellaneous

	Secreted in Milk	Amount	Significance	Reference
Cyclophosphamide	Yes	Present‡	Antineoplastic agent. Any amounts contraindicated.	Wienik and Duncan, 1971
DPT	Yes	Minimal	Does not interfere with immunization schedule.	ACOG, 1971
Methotrexate	Yes	Minor route of excretion: M/P = 0.08/1.0	Antimetabolite. Infant would receive 0.26 μg/100 ml, which researchers consider nontoxic for infant.	Johns et al., 1972
Nicotine	Yes	Mean 91 ppb (20-512 ppb)§	Decreases milk production. No apparent effect on infant—perhaps a tolerance is developed in utero. Smoking may interfere with let-down if smoking started prior to onset of a feeding.	Ferguson et al., 1976; Perlman et al., 1942; AAP Committee on Environmental Hazards, 1976; Lancet, editorial, 1974
Poliovirus vaccine	No		Live vaccine taken orally. Not necessary to withhold nursing 30 min before and after dose. Provide booster after infant no longer nursing.	DeForest et al., 1973
Rh antibodies	Yes		Destroyed in gastrointestinal tract; not effective orally.	Knowles, 1965, 1974
Rubella virus vaccine	Yes	Minimal	Will not confer passive immunity. Mother should not be given vaccine when at risk for pregnancy.	ACOG, 1971
Smallpox vaccine	No		Exposure is by direct contact. Live virus. Contraindicated when mother has infant under 1 yr. No longer given to children routinely.	ACOG, 1971

*Dose was 325-650 mg three times a day.
†Maternal plasma level was 3.4 mg/100 ml after a 1.0 g dose; M/P = 3.
‡Single 500 mg IV dose in milk at 1, 3, 5, and 6 hr. after injection.
§At ½ to 1½ packs/day. Large variation from single donor.

BIBLIOGRAPHY

Alexander, L., and Moloney, L.: Marijuana, depression and drug dependency, Med. Counterpoint **4:**12, Sept. 1972.

Ahlenius, S., Brown, R., and Engel, J.: Learning deficits in a 4 week old offspring of nursing mothers treated with neuroleptic drug, penfluridol, Naunyn Schmeidebergs Arch. Pharmacol. **279:**31, 1973.

American Academy of Pediatrics Committee on Environmental Hazards: Effects of cigarette-smoking on the fetus and child, Pediatrics **57:**411, 1976.

American Academy of Pediatrics Committee on Environmental Hazards: PCBs in breast milk, Pediatrics **62:**407, 1978.

American College of Obstetrics and Gynecology: Recommendations regarding rubella vaccination for women, ACOG Newslett., Jan., 1971.

American Medical Association: Queries and minor notes. Magnesium sulfate and breast milk, J.A.M.A. **146:**298, 1951.

Amin-Zaki, L., et al.: Perinatal methylmercury poisoning in Iraq, Am. J. Dis. Child. **130:**1070, 1976.

Ananth, J.: Side effects in the neonate from psychotropic agents excreted through breast feeding, Am. J. Psychiatry **135:**801, 1978.

Anderson, P.: Drugs and breast feeding—a review, Drug Intell. Clin. Pharm. **11:**208, 1977.

Anderson, P., and Salter, F.: Propranolol therapy during pregnancy and lactation, Am. J. Cardiol. **37:**325, 1976.

Arena, J.: Contamination of the ideal food, Nutr. Today, **5:**2, 1970.

Ayd, F.: Excretion of psychotropic drugs in human breast milk, Int. Drug Ther. Newslett. **8:**33, 1973.

Bakken, A., and Seip, M.: Insecticides in human breast milk, Acta Paediatr. Scand. **65:**535, 1976.

Baldwin, W.: Clinical study of senna administration to nursing mothers: assessment of effects on infant bowel habits, Can. Med. Assoc. J. **89:**566, 1963.

Barsivala, V., and Virkar, K.: The effects of oral contraceptives on concentrations of various components of human milk, Contraception **7:**307, 1973.

Bartig, D., and Cohen, M.: Excretion of drugs in human milk, Hosp. Formul. Manag. **4:**26, 1969.

Baty, J. D., et al.: May mothers taking warfarin breast feed their infants? Br. J. Clin. Pharmacol. **3:**969, 1976.

Bell, R. A. F., and Dale, I. M.: Gold secretion in maternal milk, Arthritis Rheum. **19**(2)1374, 1976.

Bergman, A., and Wiesner, L.: Relation of passive cigarette smoking to sudden infant death syndrome, Pediatrics **58:**665, 1976.

Berke, R.: Radiation dose to breast-feeding child, J. Nucl. Med. **14:**51, 1973.

Blacker, K. H., Weinstein, B. J., and Ellman, G. L.: Mother's milk and chlorpromazine, Am. J. Psychiatry **119:**178, 1962.

Bland, E., et al.: Radioactive iodine uptake by thyroid of breast-fed infants after maternal blood-volume measurements, Lancet **2:**1039, 1969.

Bleyer, W. A., and Breckenridge, R. T.: Studies on the detection of adverse drug reactions in the newborn, II. The effect of prenatal aspirin on newborn hemostasis, J.A.M.A. **213:**2049, 1970.

Blinick, G., Jerez, E., and Wallach, R. C.: Drug addiction in pregnancy and the neonate, Am. J. Obstet. Gynecol. **125:**135, 1976.

Blinick, G., et al.: Methadone assays in pregnant women and progeny, Am. J. Obstet. Gynecol. **121:**617, 1975.

Borglin, N. E., and Sandholm, L. E.: Effect of oral contraceptives on lactation, Fertil. Steril. **22:**39, 1971.

Bounameaux, Y., and Durenne, J.: Un cas de leucèmie chez une Femme allaitante: effects du traitment par le busulfan sur la nourrisson, J. Ann. Soc. Belg. Med. Trop. **44:**381, 1964.

Brambel, C., and Hunter, R.: Effect of dicumarol on the nursing infant, Am. J. Obstet. Gynecol. **59:**1153, 1950.

Brandt, R.: Passage of diazepam and desmethyldiazepam into breast milk, Arzneim Forsch **26:**454, 1976.

Breast feeding and drugs in human milk, Rev. Vet. Hum. Toxicol. **20:**346, 1978.

Briggs, M., and Briggs, M.: Oral contraceptives and vitamin nutrition, Lancet **1:**1436, 1974.

Buchanan, R., et al.: The breast milk excretion of mefenamic acid, Curr. Ther. Res. **10:**592, 1968.

Buchanan, R. A., et al.: The breast milk excretion of flufenamic acid, Curr. Ther. Res. **11:**533, 1969.

Campbell, A. M. G., et al.: Cerebral atrophy in young *Cannabis* smokers, Lancet **2:**1219, 1971.

Catz, C. S.: Diazepam in breast milk, Drug Ther. Jan., 1973.

Catz, C. S., and Giacoia, G.: Drugs and breast milk, Pediatr. Clin. North Am. **19:**151, 1972.

Clark, L., Hughes, R., and Nakashima, E.: Behavioral effects of marijuana: experimental studies, Arch. Gen. Psychiatry **23:**193, 1970.

Clyde, D., and Shute, G.: Transfer of pyrimethamine in human milk, J. Trop. Med. Hyg. **59:**277, 1956.

Cobrink, R. W., Hood, T., and Chusid, E.: The effect of maternal narcotic addiction on the newborn infant, Pediatrics **24**:288, 1956.

Cole, A. P., and Hailey, D. M.: Diazepam and active metabolite in breast milk and their transfer to the neonate, Arch. Dis. Child. **50**:741, 1975.

Colley, J., Holland, W. W., and Corkhill, R. T.: Influence of passive smoking and parental phlegm on pneumonia and bronchitis in early childhood, Lancet **2**:1031, 1974.

Crumpton, E., and Brill, N.: Personality factors associated with frequency of marijuana use, Calif. Med. **115**:11, 1971.

Curtis, E.: Oral-contraceptive feminization of a normal male infant, Obstet. Gynecol. **23**:295, 1964.

Davis, S., and Wedgwood, R.: Antibiotic prophylaxis in acute viral respiratory diseases, Am. J. Dis. Child. **109**:544, 1965.

Deforest, A., et al.: The effect of breast-feeding on the antibody response of infants to trivalent oral poliovirus vaccine, J. Pediatr. **83**:93, 1973.

deSweet, M., and Lewis, P. J.: Excretion of anticoagulants in human milk, N. Engl. J. Med. **297**:1471, 1977.

Dickey, R. P., and Stone, S. C.: Drugs that affect the breast and lactation, Clin. Obstet. Gynecol. **18**:95, 1975.

Dillon, H., Wilson, D., and Schaffner, W.: Lead concentrations in human milk, Am. J. Dis. Child. **4**:91, 1974.

Drugs in breast milk, Med. Lett. Drugs Ther. **16**(6):25, March 15, 1974.

Eckstein, H. B., and Jack, B.: Breast-feeding and anticoagulant therapy, Lancet **1**:672, 1970.

Editorial, tobacco smoke and the non-smoker, Lancet **1**:1201, 1974.

Eeg-Olofsson, O., et al.: Convulsions in a breast-fed infant after maternal indomethacin, Lancet **2**:215, 1978.

Erkkola, R., and Kanto, J.: Diazepam and breast-feeding, Lancet **1**:1235, 1972.

Fahim, M., and King, T.: Effect of phenobarbital on lactation and the nursing neonate, Am. J. Obstet. Gynecol. **101**:1103, 1968.

Ferguson, B., Wilson, D. J., and Schaffner, W.: Determination of nicotine concentrations in human milk, Am. J. Dis. Child. **130**:837, 1976.

Gaginella, T. S.: Drugs and the nursing mother—infant, U.S. Pharm. **3**:39, 1978.

Galloway, C.: Follow-up on a patient with myasthenia gravis, Am. J. Obstet. Gynecol. **79**:1031, 1960.

Goodman, L., and Gilman, A., editors: The pharmacological basis of therapeutics, ed. 5, New York, 1975, The Macmillan Co.

Gray, M. S., Kane, P. O., and Squires, S.: Further observations on metronidazole (Flagyl), Br. J. Vener. Dis. **37**:278, 1961.

Halikas, J., Goodwin, D., and Guse, S.: Marijuana use and psychiatric illness, Arch. Gen. Psychiatry **27**:162, 1972.

Harlap, S., and Davies, A.: Infant admissions to hospital and maternal smoking, Lancet **1**:529, 1974.

Havelka, J., et al.: Excretion of chloramphenicol in human milk, Chemotherapy **13**:204, 1968.

Hervada, A. R., Feit, E., and Sagraves, R.: Drugs in breast milk, Perinatal Care **2**:19, 1978.

Hirsh, J.: Fetal effects of Coumadin administered during pregnancy, Blood **36**:623, 1970.

Horning, M., et al.: Identification and quantification of drugs and drug metabolites in human breast milk using GC-MS-COM methods, Clin. Chem. **21**:1282, 1975.

Hosbach, R., and Foster, R.: Absence of nitrofurantoin from human milk, J.A.M.A. **202**:1057, 1967.

Ibrahim, A., and El-Tawil, N.: The effect of a new low-dosage oral contraceptive pill on lactation, Int. Surg. **49**:561, 1968.

Illingworth, R. S.: Abnormal substances excreted in human milk, Practitioner **171**:533, 1953.

Illingworth, R. S., and Finch, E.: Ethyl biscoumacetate (Tromexan) in human milk, J. Obstet. Gynecol. Br. Empire **66**:487, 1959.

Ingall, D., and Zuckerstatter, M.: Diagnosis and treatment of the passively addicted newborn, Hosp. Pract. **5**:101, 1970.

Jakubovič, A., Hattori, T., and McGeer, P.: Radioactivity in suckled rats after giving ^{14}C-tetrahydrocannibinol to the mother, Eur. J. Pharmacol. **22**:221, 1973.

Jakubovič, A., Tait, R., and McGeer, P.: Excretion of THC and its metabolites in ewe's milk, Toxicol. Appl. Pharm. **28**:38, 1974.

Janssen, P. A. J., Niemegeers, C. J. E., and Schellekens, K. H. L.: The pharmacology of penfluridol (R1634), a new potent and orally long-acting neuroleptic drug, Eur. J. Pharmacol. **11**:139, 1970.

Jelliffe, D., and Jelliffe, E. F. P.: Human milk in the modern world, Oxford, 1978, Oxford University Press.

John, T. J., et al.: Effect of breast-feeding on seroresponse of infants to oral poliovirus vaccination, Pediatrics **57**:47, 1976.

Johns, D. G., et al.: Secretion of methotrexate into human milk, Am. J. Obstet. Gynecol. **112**:978, 1972.

Jukes, T.: When friends or patients ask about . . . DDT, J.A.M.A. **229:**571, 1974.

Kaern, T.: Effect of oral contraceptives immediately postpartum on initiation of lactation, Br. Med. J. **3:**644, 1967.

Kan, M., Hopkins, G.: Unilateral breast uptake of ^{67}Ga from breast feeding, Radiology **121:**668, 1976.

Katz, F. H., and Duncan B. R.: Entry of prednisone into human milk, N. Engl. J. Med. **293:** 1154, 1975.

Kesäniemi, Y.: Ethanol and acetaldehyde in the milk and peripheral blood of lactating women after ethanol administration, J. Obstet. Gynaecol. Br. Comm. **81:**84, 1974.

Kitto, W.: Breast feeding and tolbutamide, J.A.M.A. **199:**680, 1967.

Knowles, J. A.: Excretion of drugs in milk—a review, J. Pediatr. **66:**1068, 1965.

Knowles, J. A.: What is treatment? J. Pediatr. **69:**508, 1966.

Knowles, J. A.: Breast milk: a source of more than nutrition for the neonate, Clin. Toxicol. **7:**69, 1974.

Kolansky, H., and Moore, W.: Effects of marijuana on adolescents and young adults, J.A.M.A. **216:**486, 1971.

Kopelman, A. E.: Fetal addiction to pentazocine, Pediatrics **55:**888, 1975.

Kora, S.: Effect of oral contraceptives on lactation, Fertil. Steril. **20:**419, 1969.

Krajnovič, P., and Ferič, V.: Untersuchungen zur Frage der Arzheimittelsicherheit in der Frauenheilkunde, Arzneim Forsch **24:**1061, 1974.

Kreek, M. J., et al.: Analysis of methadone and other drugs in maternal and neonatal body fluids, Am. J. Drug Alcohol Abuse, **1:**409, 1974.

Kreuz, D., and Axelrod, J.: Delta-9-tetrahydrocannabinol localization in body fat, Science **179:**391, 1973.

Kris, E. B., and Carmichael, D. M.: Chlorpromazine maintenance therapy during pregnancy and confinement, Psychiatry Quart. **31:**690, 1957.

Kwit, N. T., and Hatcher, R. A.: Excretion of drugs in milk, Am. J. Dis. Child. **49:**900, 1935.

Lacey, J.: Dichloralphenazone and breast milk, Br. Med. J. **4:**684, 1971.

Laumas, R. K., et al.: Radioactivity in the breast milk of lactating women after oral administration of ^{3}H-norethynodrel, Am. J. Obstet. Gynecol. **98:**411, 1967.

Lebowitz, M., and Burrows, B.: Respiratory symptoms related to smoking habits of family adults, Chest **69:**48, 1976.

Le Orme, M., et al.: May mothers given warfarin breast-feed their infants? Br. Med. J. **1:**1564, 1977.

Levitan, A., and Manion, J.: Propranolol therapy during pregnancy and lactation, Am. J. Cardiol. **32:**247, 1973.

Levy, M., Granit, L., and Laufer, N.: Excretion of drugs in human milk, N. Engl. J. Med. **297:**798, 1977.

Lien, E. J., Kuwahara, J., and Koda, R. T.: Diffusion of drugs into prostatic fluid and milk, Drug. Intell. Clin. Pharm. **8:**470, 1974.

Lipman, A.: Antimicrobial agents in breast milk, Mod. Med. **45:**89, 1977.

Livingston, S.: Treatment of epilepsy with diphenylhydantoin sodium, Postgrad. Med. **20:**584, 1956.

Llewellyn-Jones, D.: Inhibition of lactation by oestrogens, Br. Med. J. **4:**387, 1968.

Loughman, P. M.: Digoxin excretion in human breast milk, J. Pediatr. **92:**1019, 1978.

Lundberg, P.: Abnormal otogeny in young rabbits after chronic administration of haloperidol to the nursing mothers, Brain Res. **40:**395, 1972.

McCracken, G., Nelson, J.: The current status of gentamicin for the neonate and young infant, Am. J. Dis. Child. **124:**13, 1972.

McKenzie, S. A., Selley, J. A., and Agnew, J. E.: Secretion of prednisolone into breast milk, Arch. Dis. Child. **50:**894, 1975.

McNall, P., and Jafarnia, M.: Management of myasthenia gravis in the obstetrical patient, Am. J. Obstet. Gynecol. **92:**518, 1965.

Milkovich, L., and Van Den Berg, B.: An evaluation of the teratogenicity of certain antinauseant drugs, Am. J. Obststet. Gynecol. **125:** 244, 1976.

Miller, G. H., and Hughes, L. R.: Lactation and genital involution effects of a new low-dose oral contraceptive on breast feeding mothers and their infants, Obstet. Gynecol. **35:**44, 1970.

Mirkin, B.: Diphenylhydantoin: placental transport, fetal localization, neonatal metabolism, and possible teratogenic effects, J. Pediatr. **78:** 329, 1971.

Mohr, J. A.: The possible induction and/or acquisition of cellular hypersensitivity associated with ingestion of colostrum, J. Pediatr. **82:**1062, 1973.

Nahas, G.: Inhibition of cellular mediated immunity in marihuana smokers, Science **183:** 419, 1974.

Nahas, G.: Marihuana: toxicity, tolerance, and therapeutic efficacy, Drug Ther. Jan. 1974, p. 33.

Nahas, G.: Marihuana, J.A.M.A. **233:**79, 1975.

Nahas, G., and Paton, W., editors: Marihuana: chemistry, biochemistry and cellular effects, New York, 1976, Springer-Verlag New York, Inc.

Nilsson, S., Nygren, K. G., and Johanson,

E. D. B.: d-Norgestrel concentrations in maternal plasma, milk, and child plasma during administration of oral counterceptives to nursing women, Am. J. Obstet. Gynecol. **129**:179, 1977.

Nurnberger, C., and Lipscomb, A.: Transmission of radio-iodine (I^{131}) to infants through human maternal milk, J.A.M.A. **150**:1398, 1952.

O'Brien, T.: Excretion of drugs in human milk, Am. J. Hosp. Pharm. **31**:844, 1974.

O'Brien, T.: Excretion of diphenylhydantoin in human milk, Am. J. Hosp. Pharm. **32**:14, 1975.

O'Connell, M. E. A., and Sutton, H.: Excretion of radioactivity in breast milk following $^mTc^{99}$-Sn polyphosphate, Br. J. Radiol. **49**:377, 1976.

Oseid, B. J.: Breast feeding and infant health, Clin. Obstet. Gynecol. **18**:149, 1975.

Overbach, A.: Drugs used with neonates and during pregnancy: part 3. Drugs that may cause fetal damage or cross into breast milk, R.N. **37**:39, 1974.

Pacifici, G. M., and Placidi, G. F.: Rapid and sensitive electron-capture gas chromatographic method for determination of pineazepam and its metabolites in human plasma, urine and milk, J. Chromatography **135**:133, 1977.

Patrick, M. J., Tilstone, W. J., and Reavey, P.: Diazepam and breast feeding, Lancet **I**(7740):542, 1972.

Perkins, K., and Oski, F.: Elevated blood lead in a 6-month old breast-fed infant: the role of newsprint logs, Pediatrics **57**:426, 1976.

Perlman, H. H., Dannenberg, A. M., and Sokoloff, N.: The excretion of nicotine in breast milk and urine from cigaret smoking, J.A.M.A. **120**:1003, 1942.

Perry, J., and LeBlanc, A.: Transfer of nitrofurantoin across the human placenta, Tex. Rep. Biol. Med. **25**:265, 1967.

Physicians' desk reference, Oradell, N.Y., 1978, Medical Economics Co.

Posner, C., and Konicoff, N.: Tetracycline in obstetric infections. In Welch, H., and Marti-Ibañez, F., editors: Antibiotic Annual, 1955-56, New York, Medical Encyclopedia, Inc., p. 345.

Pynnönen, S., and Sillanpää, M.: Carbamazepine and mother's milk, Lancet **2**:563, 1975.

Ramadan, M. A., et al.: The effect of the oral contraceptive ovosiston on the composition of human milk, J. Reprod. Med. **9**:81, 1972.

Redman, C.: Fetal outcome in trial of antihypertensive treatment in pregnancy, Lancet **2**:753, 1976.

Remmington, J. S., and Klein, J. O.: Infectious diseases of the fetus and newborn infant, Philadelphia, 1976, W. B. Saunders Co.

Resman, B., Blumenthal, H. P., and Jusko, W. J.: Breast milk distribution of theobromine from chocolate, J. Pediatr. **91**:477, 1977.

Rivera-Calimlim, L.: Drugs in breast milk, Drug Ther. **2**(12):20, 1977.

Rose, D. P., et al.: Effect of oral contraceptives and vitamin B_6 deficiency on carbohydrate metabolism, Am. J. Clin. Nutr. **28**:872, 1975.

Roth, S.: Anti-inflammatories: exploring new options, Curr. Prescrib. May, 1976, p. 46.

Rothermel, P., and Faber, M.: Drugs in breast-milk—a consumer's guide, Birth Fam. J. **2**:76, 1975.

Savage, R.: Drugs and breast milk, J. Hum. Nutr. **31**:459, 1977.

Schlesinger, E.: Dietary fluorides and caries prevention, Am. J. Public Health **55**:1123, 1965.

Schou, M., and Amdisen, A.: Lithium and pregnancy: III. Lithium ingestion by children breast-fed by women on lithium treatment, Br. Med. J. **2**:138, 1973.

Shambaugh, G., Jr.: Prophylactic antibiotics? Arch. Otolaryngol. **77**:459, 1963.

Shore, M.: Drugs can be dangerous during pregnancy and lactation, Can. Pharm. J. **103**:8, 1970.

Shidlovsky, B. A., Prigot, A., and Maynard, A.: Absorbtion, diffusion, and excretion studies on the phosphate complex salt of tetracycline. In Welch, H., and Marti-Ibañez, F., editors: Antibiotic Annual, 1957-1958, New York, Medical Encyclopedia, Inc., p. 459.

Smith, D.: Marijuana: Some notes, queries, and answers, Med. Counterpoint 1971, p. 29.

Smith, D., and Mehl, C.: The new social drug: cultural, legal and medical perspectives on marijuana, vol. 3, Englewood Cliffs, N.J., 1970, Prentice-Hall, Inc.

Stone, O., and Willis, C.: The effect of stannous fluoride and stannous chloride on inflammation, Toxicol. Appl. Pharmacol. **13**:332, 1968.

Straub, C., and Murthy, G.: A comparison of Sr^{90} component and cow's milk, Pediatrics **36**:732, 1965.

Sykes, P., Quarrie, J., and Alexander, F.: Lithium carbonate and breast-feeding, Br. Med. J. **2**:1299, 1976.

Takyi, B. E.: Excretion of drugs in human milk, J. Hosp. Pharm. **28**:317, 1970.

Talbott, J.: Marihuana psychosis, J.A.M.A. **210**:299, 1969.

Tank, G., and Storvick, C.: Caries experience of children one to six years old in two Oregon communities (Corvallis and Albany): III. Relation of diet to variation of dental caries, J. Am. Dent. Assoc. **70**:394, 1965.

Terwilliger, W. G., and Hatcher, R. A.: Morphine and quinine in human milk, Surg. Gynecol. Obstet. **58:**823, 1939.

Texeira, G. C., and Scott, R. B.: Further clinical and laboratory studies with novobiocin, II. Novobiocin concentration in the blood of new-born infants and in the breast milk of lactating mothers, Antibiot. Med. **5:**577, 1958.

Toddywalla, V. S., Joshi, L., and Virkar, K.: Effect of contraceptive steroids on human lactation, Am. J. Obstet. Gynecol. **127:**245, 1977.

Toxicology review. Breast feeding and drugs in human milk, Rev. Vet. Hum. Toxicol. **20:**346, 1978.

Tunnessen, W., and Hertz, C.: Toxic effects of lithium in newborn infants: a commentary, J. Pediatr. **81:**804, 1972.

Tupin, J. P., and Hopkin, J. T.: Lithium for mood disturbances, Rational Drug Ther. **12**(9):1, 1978.

Tyson, R. M., Shrader, E. A., and Perlman, H. H.: Drugs transmitted through breast milk: I. Laxatives, J. Pediatr. **12:**824, 1937.

Tyson, R. M., Shrader, E. A., and Perlman, H. H.: Durgs transmitted through breast milk: II. Barbiturates, J. Pediatr. **13:**86, 1938.

Tyson, R. M., Shrader, E. A., and Perlman, H. H.: Drugs transmitted through breast milk: III. Bromides, J. Pediatr. **13:**91, 1938.

Vagenakis, A., Abreau, C., and Braverman, L.: Duration of radioactivity in the milk of a nursing mother following ^{99m}Tc administration, J. Nucl. Med. **12:**188, 1971.

Varsano, I., Fischl, J., and Tikvah, P.: Letters, the excretion of orally ingested nitrofurantoin in human milk, J. Pediatr. **82:**886, 1973.

Veláquez, J. G., et al.: Effecto de al administracion oral diaria de 0.350 mg. de noretindrona en la lactancia y en la composicion de la leche, Ginecol. Obstet. Mex. **40:**31, 1976.

Vorherr, H.: Drug excretion in breast milk, Postgrad. Med. **56:**97, 1974.

Vorherr, H.: Drug excretion in breast milk, Senologia **1:**27, 1976.

Wagner, J.: Drug bioavailability studies, Hosp. Pract., Jan., 1977, p. 119.

Weaver, J. C., Kamm, M. L., and Dobson, R. L.: Excretion of radioiodine in human milk, J.A.M.A. **173:**872, 1960.

Werthmann, M., and Krees, S.: Excretion of chlorothiazide in breast milk, J. Pediatr. **81:**781, 1972.

Widdowson, E. M., et al.: Absorption, excretion, and retention of strontium by breast-fed and bottle-fed babies, Lancet **2:**941, 1960.

Wiernik, P. H., and Duncan, J. H.: Cyclophosphamide in human milk, Lancet **1:**912, 1971.

Williams, R. H., Kay, G. H., and Jandorf, B. J.: Thiouracil: its absorption, distribution and excretion, J. Clin. Invest. **23:**613, 1944.

Wurster, C. F.: DDT in mother's milk, ICEA News, Nov.-Dec., 1970, vol. 9.

Yoshioka, H., et al.: Transfer of cefazolin into human milk, J. Pediatr. **94:**151, 1979.

Yurchak, A. M., and Jusko, W. J.: Theophylline secretion into breast milk, Pediatics **57:**518, 1976.

The Whittlestone physiological breast milker*

The Whittlestone physiological breast milker has been designed especially for home or hospital, on sound physiological principles to simulate the action of a sucking baby. It is effective and comfortable!

The breast cups have a soft foam rubber pad and liner which contracts rhythmically behind the nipple area (areola)—gently stimulating the breasts, compressing the milk ducts and encouraging the ejection of milk into the breast cups. The vacuum can be controlled by the mother to suit her own level of comfort and effectiveness. The vacuum also helps to keep the breast cups in place, and removes the milk to the collecting bottles. (Obsolete breast pumps relied on suction alone, which could be damaging to the breast tissue and was often painful and ineffective).

This New Zealand designed milker is the only one which provides two breast cups. Both breasts are milked simultaneously thus taking advantage of the natural let-down reflex and reducing the time involved in expressing breast milk.

---

*Available from Y Procuta, P. O. Box 17, Cambridge, New Zealand.

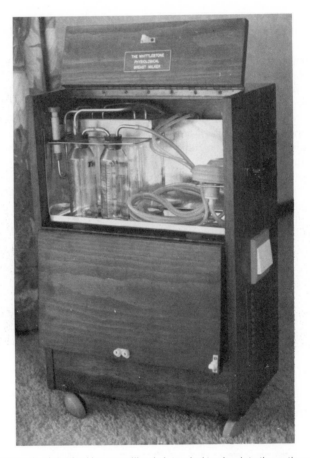

Fig. G-1. Whittlestone physiological breast milker is intended to simulate the action of suckling infant. This is the only breast milker which applies enough stimulation to increase milk secretion and induce fully effective emptying of breasts. (Courtesy Y Procuta, P.O. Box 17, Cambridge, New Zealand.)

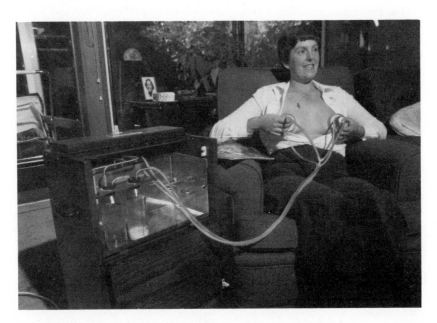

Fig. G-2. Whittlestone physiological breast milker in use. The breast cups have a foam rubber pad and liner, which contract rhythmically behind the areola, gently stimulating the breast, compressing the milk ducts, and encouraging the ejection of milk into the breast cup. Both breasts are milked simultaneously. Milk is kept sterile and immediately refrigerated in water bath. (Courtesy Y Procuta, P.O. Box 17, Cambridge, New Zealand.)

The Lact-Aid nursing supplementer

Lact-Aid is made up of four parts: (1) the body with permanently attached nursing tube, (2) the clamp ring, (3) the extension tube, and (4) the presterilized Lact-Aid bag with 4 oz capacity.

For convenience in filling and assembling Lact-Aid, a bag hanger and funnel have been specially designed. Six T-shaped end tabs provide easy attachment to the nursing bra.

The filled Lact-Aid is attached to the nursing bra or neck cord between the breasts and is positioned so that the supplement cannot siphon out. The presterilized bag is attached to the body by the clamp ring. The infant suckles the tip of the nursing tube and the nipple of the breast at the same time. As the infant nurses, supplement is drawn from the bottom of the presterilized bag by the extension tube attached to the bottom of the body. This keeps the infant from swallowing any air that might be trapped in the top of the bag. The body has an orifice designed to provide the best rate of flow, slower than milk flows from the breast, but fast enough to keep from overtiring the infant. The nursing tube carries the supplement to the infant's mouth. It is clear, very soft, and flexible and will not cause the infant's mouth or the nipple any discomfort.

When the infant is put to breast, the flow of supplement rewards his nursing efforts. This provides a pleasant incentive for the infant to continue nursing, which in turn provides the breasts with suckling stimulation to build up the milk supply. The Lact-Aid is small enough, even when it contains the full 4 oz capacity of supplement, to enable one to nurse discreetly without it showing.

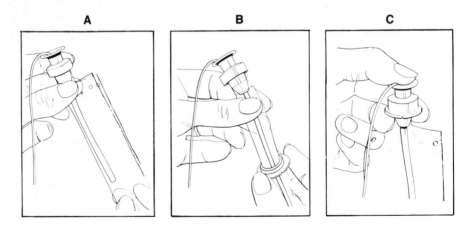

Fig. H-1. A, Gently press trapped air out of bag. Fold bag in half vertically, along extension tube, and continue to wrap folded sides of bag around tube. **B,** Insert end of rolled bag into clamp ring. Narrow vertical rim of ring should be toward body. As ring is pushed up, it hugs neck of bag and wedges tightly under skirt of body. **C,** Press upward on notched rim of clamp ring with fingers, and press down on top of body with thumb to assure a tight fit. (From Avery, J. J.: Lact-Aid nursing supplementer instruction book, Denver, 1977, Resources in Human Nurturing, International.)

LACT-AID PARTS

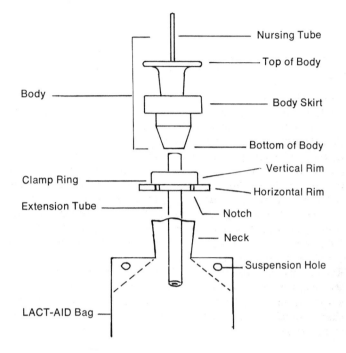

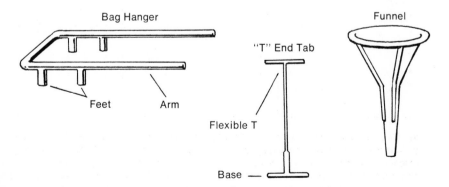

Fig. H-2. Lact-Aid parts. (From Avery, J. J.: Lact-Aid nursing supplementer instruction book, Denver, 1977, Resources in Human Nurturing, International.)

BIBLIOGRAPHY

Avery, J. L.: A brief discussion of adoptive-nursing: an introduction to the topic, Denver, Resources in Human Nurturing, International.*

Avery, J. L.: Induced lactation: a guide for counseling and management, Denver, Resources in Human Nurturing, International.*

---

*Available from Resources in Human Nurturing, International, Lact-Aid division, Box 6861, Denver, Colo. 80206.

Organizations interested in supporting breast-feeding

Ammehjelpen
Postboks 15
Holmen, Oslo 3, Norway

Arbeitsgruppe and Dritte Welt
Postbach 1007
Bern 300, Switzerland

Association for Improvement of Maternity
   Services
61 Dartmouth Park Road
London NW 5, United Kingdom

Baby Foods Action Group
103 Gower Street
London WC1E 6AW, United Kingdom

Center for Science in the Public Interest
1779 Church Street, NW
Washington, D.C. 20036

International Childbirth Education Association
2763 NW 70th Street
Seattle, Wash. 98167

La Leche League International, Inc.
9616 Minneapolis Avenue
Franklin Park, Ill. 60131

National Childbirth Trust
Breast-feeding Promotion Group
9 Queensborough Terrace
London W2 3TB, United Kingdom

Nursing Mothers' Association of Australia
99 Burwood Road
Hawthorn, Victoria, Australia 3122

Parents Centres of Australia
148 Hereford Street
Forest Lodge, NSW, Australia 2229

Resources in Human Nurturing, International
P.O. Box 6861
3885 Forest Street
Denver, Colo. 80206

War on Want
467 Caledonian Road
London N.7, United Kingdom

Publications for the patient and family

Applebaum, R. M.: Abreast of the times, breast feeding for the modern mother, Miami, 1969, R. M. Applebaum.

Avery, J. L.: Induced lactation: a guide for counseling and management, Denver, 1973, Resources in Human Nurturing, International.

Eiger, M., and Olds, S.: The complete book of breast-feeding, New York, 1972, Workman Publishing Co., Inc.

Gerard, A.: Please breast-feed your baby, New York, 1972, New American Library, Inc.

Hormann, E.: A study of induced lactation, information sheet no. 85, Franklin Park, Ill., 1971, La Leche League International, Inc.

Hormann, E.: Relactation: a guide for breast feeding the adopted baby, Franklin Park, Ill., 1958, La Leche League International, Inc.

Kippley, S., and Kippley, K.: Breast-feeding and natural child spacing, New York, 1974, Harper & Row, Publishers.

La Leche League International, Inc.: The womanly art of breast-feeding, Franklin Park, Ill., 1958, Interstate Publishers (English, French, Spanish, and Japanese).

Matsumura, T.: Breast-feed your children, Tokyo, 1972, Horiuchi Bunjiro (Japanese).

Phillips, V.: Successful breast-feeding, Melbourne, 1976, Nursing Mothers' Association of Australia.

Pryor, K.: Nursing your baby, New York, 1973, Harper & Row, Publishers.

Raphael, D.: The tender gift: breast-feeding, Englewood Cliffs, N.J., 1973, Prentice-Hall, Inc.

Prenatal dietary prophylaxis of atopic disease*

In addition to heredity, the prophylaxis of allergic disease in the potentially allergic child involves four major considerations:

1. The possibility of intrauterine sensitization
2. The nutrition of the newborn infant with particular respect to the fact that human breast milk is the best and only natural food
3. The role of secretory immunoglobulin A (SIgA)
4. The fact that food ingested by the nursing mother may pass through with the breast milk and be immunologically capable of sensitizing a potentially allergic infant or of causing a reaction in a previously sensitized infant

Because specific food allergies occasionally appear to be inherited, the pregnant mother of a potentially allergic child should exclude from her diet not only those foods to which she is allergic but also those foods to which other members of the immediate family are sensitive. Overindulgence in any particular food (pica) is to be avoided, particularly the peanut, which is a rather common offender.

An absolute indication for a strict dietary regimen is the presence in the immediate family of significant asthma or atopic dermatitis. If the prospective mother is sensitive to milk, she should be on a milk-free diet. All of the protein required by the mother may be obtained from beef and other meats and soybean. Adequate vitamins should be supplied, bearing in mind that some of the synthetic coloring, of which tartrazine (FD&C yellow no. 5) is the most common offender, as well as some artificial flavoring materials may cause problems. It is hoped that vitamin products completely free of these materials will eventually be available. Adequate calcium should be supplied and is least expensive when obtained as calcium carbonate powder, reagent quality, one-half teaspoon (0.4 g calcium) per day during pregnancy and two-thirds teaspoon (0.5 g calcium) per day during lactation.

If there is no milk allergy in the immediate family a pint of milk (500 ml) daily, boiled 10 minutes, or the same amount of half evaporated milk and half water may be given. In these preparations, bovine γ-globulin, the most heat labile of the milk allergens, followed closely by bovine serum albumin, is rendered immunologically inactive. As a result, milk-allergic individuals sensitive only to these proteins are the only milk-allergic individuals who can tolerate boiled or evaporated milk.

---

*From Glaser, J., Dreyfuss, E. M., and Logan, J.: Prenatal dietary prophylaxis of atopic disease. In Kelley, V. C., editor: Practice of pediatrics, vol. 2, Hagerstown, Md., 1976, Harper & Row, Publishers, Inc.

One of the least allergenic substitutes for cow's milk is soybean milk. The preparations designed primarily for infants are rather tasty to adults and may be used as desired. Detailed instructions for their use may be obtained from the manufacturers.

The superheated proprietary milks have been shown to be only somewhat more allergenic than soybean milk. If soybean milk is objectionable, it is reasonable to substitute these milks, not to exceed 1½ pints a day. Bremil, Enfamil, Similac, and SMA are some of the preparations readily obtained at drug stores and supermarkets.

Glossary

acinus The tube leading to the smallest lobule of a compound gland; it is characterized by a narrow lumen.

adipose tissue *See* panniculus adiposus.

afferent Conducting inwards to, or toward, the center of an organ, gland, or other structure or area. Applies to sensory nerves, arteries, and lymph vessels.

alveolus A glandular acinus or terminal portion of the alveolar gland where milk is secreted and stored, 0.12 mm in diameter. From 10 to 100 alveoli, or tubulosaccular secretory units, make up a lobulus.

apocrine A term descriptive of a gland cell that loses part of its protoplasmic substance when secreting.

arborization Developing a branched appearance.

areola mammae Areola. The pigmented area surrounding the papilla mammae, or nipple.

autophagic vacuole Autophagosome. A membrane-bound body within a cell containing degenerating cell organelles.

basal lamina The layer of material, 50 to 80 nm thick, that lies adjacent to the plasma membrane of the basal surfaces of epithelial cells. It contains collagen and certain carbohydrates. It is often called the basement membrane.

casein A derivative of caseinogen. The fraction of milk protein that forms the tough curd.

colostrum The first milk. It is a yellow sticky fluid secreted during the first few days postpartum, which provides nutrition and protection against infectious disease. It contains more protein, less sugar, and much less fat than mature breast milk.

columnar secretory cells A type of secretory cell in the shape of a hexagonal prism, which appears rectangular when sectioned across the long axis, the length being considerably greater than the width.

Cooper's ligaments Triangularly shaped ligaments stretching between the mammary gland, the skin, the retinacula cutis, the pectineal ligament, and the chorda obliqua. These underlie the breasts.

corpus mammae The mammary gland; breast mass after freeing breast from deep attachments and removal of skin, subcutaneous connective tissue, and fat.

cuboidal secretory cells A secretory cell whose height and breadth are of similar size.

cytosol Cell fluid.

doula An individual who surrounds, interacts with, and aids the mother at any time within the period that includes pregnancy, birth, and lactation. She may be a relative, friend, or neighbor and is usually but not necessarily female. One who gives psychological encouragement and physical assistance to a new mother.

efferent Carrying impulses away from a nerve center.

ejection reflex A reflex initiated by the suckling of the infant at the breast, which triggers the pituitary gland to release oxytocin into the bloodstream. The oxytocin causes the myoepithelial cells to contract and eject the milk from the collecting ductules. (Also called let-down reflex or draught.)

347

engorgement The swelling and distention of the breasts, usually in the early days of initiation of lactation, due to vascular dilation as well as the arrival of the early milk.

eosinophil A granular leukocyte possessing large conspicuous granules in the cytoplasm and containing a bilobed nucleus.

foremilk The first milk obtained at the onset of suckling or expression. Contains less fat than later milk of that feeding (i.e., the hind milk).

galactocele A cystic tumor in the ducts of the breast, which contains a milky fluid.

galactogogue A material or action that stimulates the production of milk.

galactopoiesis The development of milk in the mammary gland. The maintenance of established lactation.

galactorrhea Abnormal or inappropriate lactation.

galactose ($C_6H_{12}O_6$) A simple sugar that is a component of the disaccharide lactose, or milk sugar.

galactosemia A congenital metabolic disorder in which there is an inability to metabolize galactose due to a deficiency of the enzyme galactose-1-phosphate uridyl transferase. It causes failure to thrive, hepatomegaly, and splenomegaly.

Golgi apparatus A specialized region of the cytoplasm, often close to the nucleus, which is composed of flattened cisternae, numerous vesicles, and some larger vacuoles. In secretory cells it is concerned with packaging the secretory product. It is also probably concerned with the secretion of polysaccharides in some cells, but its full range of functions has not yet been elucidated.

heterophagic vacuole Heterophagosome. A membrane-bound body within a cell, containing ingested material.

hind milk Milk obtained later during nursing period, that is, the end of the feeding. This milk is usually high in fat and probably controls appetite.

homocystinuria A rare inborn error of amino acid metabolism characterized by mental deficiency, epilepsy, dislocation of the lens, growth disturbance, thromboses, and defective hair growth.

hyperadenia The existence of mammary tissue without nipples.

hypermastia The existence of accessory mammary glands.

hyperthelia The existence of abundant, more or less developed, nipples without accompanying mammary tissue.

immunoglobulin Protein fraction of globulin, which has been demonstrated to have immunological properties. These include IgA, IgG, and IgM—factors in breast milk, which protect against infection.

induced lactation Process by which a nonpuerperal female (or male) is stimulated to lactate.

lactiferous ducts The main ducts of the mammary gland, which number from 15 to 30 and open onto the nipple. They carry milk to the nipple.

lactiferous sinuses Dilations on the lactiferous ducts at the base of the nipple.

Lactobacillus bifidus Organism of the intestinal tract of breast-fed infants.

lactocele Cystic tumor of the breast due to the dilation and obstruction of a milk duct usually filled with milk.

lactoferrin An iron-binding protein of external secretions, including human milk. It inhibits the growth of iron-dependent microorganisms in the gut.

lactogenesis Initiation of milk secretion.

let-down reflex *See* ejection reflex.

lobulus A subunit of the parenchymal structure of the breast made up of 10 to 100 alveoli, or tubulosaccular secretory units. From 20 to 40 lobuli make up a lobus.

lobus A subunit of the parenchymal structure of the breast made up of 20 to 40 lobuli. From 15 to 25 lobi are arranged like the spokes of a wheel with the nipple as the central point.

lymphocyte A mature leucocyte derived through the intermediate stage of lymphoblast from the reticuloendothelium found in lymphatic tissue.

mamilla The nipple; any teatlike structure.

mammogenesis Growth of the mammary gland.

mastitis Inflammation of the breast, including cellulitis, and occasionally abscess formation.

matrescence The state of becoming a mother or motherhood as a new event in an individual's life.

megaloblastic anemia Defective red blood cell formation due to megaloblastic hyperplasia of the marrow; there are often megaloblasts, or primitive nucleated red cells in the peripheral blood.

merocrine Pertaining to the type of secretion in which the active cell remains intact while forming and discharging the secretory product.

mesencephalon The midbrain.

methylmalonic aciduria The condition of the urine being acidic from an accumulation of methylmalonic acid due to an inborn error of metabolism.

milk fever A syndrome of fever and general malaise associated with early engorgement of the breasts or with sudden weaning from the breast.

mitogen A substance capable of stimulating cells to enter mitosis.

Montgomery glands Small prominences, sebaceous glands in the areola of the breast, which become more marked in pregnancy. They number 20 to 24 and secrete a fluid that lubricates the nipple area.

Morgagni's tubercle Small sinuses into which the miniature ducts of the Montgomery glands open in the epidermis of the areola.

myoepithelial cell An epithelial cell, usually lying around a glandular acinus, in which part of the cytoplasm has contractile properties, serving to empty the sinus of its secretion.

nonnutritive sucking The act of suckling the breast with little or no secretion of milk. Infant may suckle when distressed or to be calmed or quieted.

nonpuerperal lactation The production of milk in a woman who has not given birth.

nucleotides Compounds derived from nucleic acid by hydrolysis and consisting of phosphoric acid combined with a sugar and a purine or pyrimidine derivative. The milk nucleotides are secreted from glandular epithelial cells.

opsonic Belonging to or characterized by opsonin, a substance in mammalian blood having the power to render microorganisms and blood cells more easily absorbed by phagocytes.

oxytocin An octapeptide synthesized in the cell bodies of neurons located mainly in the paraventricular nucleus and in smaller amounts in the supraoptic nucleus of the hypothalamus. Oxytocin stimulates the ejection reflex by stimulation of the myoepithelial cells in the mammary gland.

panniculus adiposus Adipose tissue. The superficial fascia, which contains fatty pellicles.

papilla mammae Mamilla. The nipple of the breast.

perinatal Around birth. The time from conception though birth, delivery, lactation, and at least 28 days postpartum.

plasma cell Cell derived from the B cell series, which manufactures and secretes antibodies.

prolactin A hormone present in both male and female and at all ages. During pregnancy it stimulates and prepares the mammary alveolar epithelium for secretory activity. During lactation it stimulates synthesis and secretion of milk. At other ages and in the male it interacts with other steroids.

rachitic Relating to, characterized by, or affected with rickets.

relactation Process by which a woman who has given birth but did not initially breast-feed is stimulated to lactate (also applies to reinstituting lactation after it has been discontinued).

squamous epithelium A sheet of flattened, scalelike epithelium adhering edge to edge.

stroma The connective tissue basis or framework of an organ.

subependymal matrix The layer beneath the ependyma, the layer of ciliated epithelium that lines the central canal of the spinal cord and the ventricles of the brain.

tail of Spence The axillary tail of the breast.

transitional milk The milk produced early in the postpartum period as the colostrum diminishes and the mature milk develops.

tubuloalveolar Having both tubular and alveolar qualities.

tubulosaccular Having both tubular and saccular character.

turgescence The swelling up of a part. The unusual turgid feeling resulting from swelling with fluid.

whey protein Protein remaining when the curds of casein have been removed. The mixture of proteins present is complex and includes β-lactoglobulin and α-lactalbumin and enzymes.

witch's milk Product of neonatal galactorrhea due to absorption of placental prolactin.

Index

A

A and D ointment, use with cracked nipples, 124
Abscesses, breast, in staphylococcal epidemics, 224-225
Absorption of drugs from gastrointestinal tract, 162
Accessory mammary glands, 16-17
Accumulation of various nutritional components during last trimester of pregnancy, 197
Acid; *see* specific acids
Acrodermatitis enteropathica, 65, 204-205
ACTH; *see* Adrenocorticotropic hormone
Active transport of drugs into milk, 160, 161
Activity of infant, 300-301
Admission of mother to hospital, 245-247
Adrenocorticotropic hormone, 28
Age, chronological and gestational, affecting infant's ability to detoxify and excrete drug agent, 162
Alcohol
  let-down reflex and, 35, 126, 182
  moderate use of, in colic, 133
Aldomet; *see* Methyldopa
Aldrin, 169
Allergic disease(s)
  development of, heredity and, 249
  increase in, abandonment of breast-feeding and, 249
Allergic protective properties of human milk, 88-89
Allergy
  to cow's milk, allergic syndromes associated with, 89
  development of, in offspring of allergic parents, 250
  diet and, 149
  human milk as prophylaxis in, 249-253
Aluminum, 65-66
Alum-precipitated toxoid test, 125, 217
Alveoli, 17
  growth of, and progesterone, 28
Amenorrhea as a result of lactation, 96, 266
American Academy of Pediatrics
  recommendation about formulas, 51
  statement by, in support of human milk, 292
Amino acid
  components of, in human milk, 54

Amino acid—cont'd
  essential, in management of premature infants, 192-196
Amitriptyline, 169
Ammehjelpen, 290
Amphetamines, 167
Ampicillin in listerosis, 227
Analgesics, appearance of, in milk, 165
Anatomy of human breast, 16-27
Anesthesia in cesarean section, 221
Antibacterial factors
  in breast milk, 286
  in colostrum and mature milk, 84
Antibiotics, appearance of, in milk, 165
Antibody(ies)
  colostrum and, 46
  maternal, transmitted to fetus, 73
  type of, relationship with transplacental transfer, 79
Antibody-facilitated digestion, 250
Anticholinergics, appearance of, in milk, 165
Anticoagulants
  in milk, 166
  therapy with, in venous thrombosis and pulmonary embolism, 223
Antidepressants, tricyclic, 168
"Antistaphylococcal factor," 85
Antithyroid drugs in milk, 166
Antiviral factors in breast milk, 286
Anxiety, interfering with milk let-down, 127
Apocrine secretion, 158, 160
  mechanism of, 36
Appetite, weight changes related to, 141
Appliance, orthopedic, in cleft palate, 213-214
Apresoline; *see* Hydralazine in toxemia
APT test; *see* Alum-precipitated toxoid test
Arbovirus, substances in human milk active against, 88
Areola, 18-19, 21
  compressing, to assure infant grasp of, 122
  examination of, 113
  pigmentation of, 19
Areola mammae; *see* Areola
Areolar engorgement, 120